AF616286

PERGAMON MATERIALS SERIES
VOLUME 4

Structural Biological Materials: Design and Structure-Property Relationships

PERGAMON MATERIALS SERIES

Series Editor: Robert W. Cahn FRS
Department of Materials Science and Metallurgy, University of Cambridge, UK

Vol. 1 **CALPHAD (Calculation of Phase Diagrams): A Comprehensive Guide** by N. Saunders and A. P. Miodownik
Vol. 2 **Non-equilibrium Processing of Materials** edited by C. Suryanarayana
Vol. 3 **Wettability at High Temperatures** by N. Eustathopoulos, M. G. Nicholas and B. Drevet
Vol. 4 **Structural Biological Materials: Design and Structure - Property Relationships** edited by M. Elices

A selection of forthcoming titles in this series:

Ostwald Ripening by S. Marsh
Underneath the Bragg Peaks: Structural Analysis of Complex Materials by T. Egami and S. J. L. Billinge
Phase Transformations in Titanium- and Zirconium-based Alloys by S. Banerjee and P. Mukhopadhyay
The Coming of Materials Science by R. W. Cahn
Nucleation by A. L. Greer and K. F. Kelton
Multinuclear Solid State NMR of Inorganic Materials by K. J. D. MacKenzie and M. E. Smith
Thermally Activated Mechanisms in Crystal Plasticity by D. Caillard and J. L. Martin

PERGAMON MATERIALS SERIES

Structural Biological Materials

Design and Structure-Property Relationships

edited by

Manuel Elices

Departamento de Ciencia de Materiales
Escuela Técnica Superior de Ingenieros de Caminos
Universidad Politécnica de Madrid
Madrid – España

2000

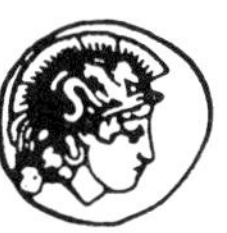

PERGAMON
An Imprint of Elsevier Science
Amsterdam – Lausanne – New York – Oxford – Singapore - Tokyo

ELSEVIER SCIENCE Ltd
The Boulevard, Langford Lane
Kidlington, Oxford OX5 1GB, UK

First edition 2000

Library of Congress Cataloging in Publication Data

Structural biological materials : design and structure--property relationships / edited by Manuel Elices.
p. cm. -- (Pergamon materials series)
Includes bibliographical references and index.
ISBN 0-08-043416-9 (hc)
1. Biomedical materials. I. Elices, Manuel. II. Series.

R857.M3 S77 2000
610'.28--dc21

ISBN: 0 08 043416 9

⊗ The paper used in this publication meets the requirements of ANSI/NISO Z39.48-1992 (Permanence of Paper).
Printed in The Netherlands.

Series Preface

My editorial objective in this Series is to present to the scientific public a collection of texts that satisfies one of two criteria: the systematic presentation of a specialised but important topic within materials science or engineering that has not previously (or recently) been the subject of full-length treatment and is in rapid development; or the systematic account of a broad theme in materials science or engineering. The books are not, in general, designed as undergraduate texts, but rather are intended for use at graduate level and by established research workers. However, teaching methods are in such rapid evolution that some of the books may well find use at an earlier stage in university education.

I have long editorial experience both in covering the whole of a huge field – physical metallurgy or materials science and technology – and in arranging for specialised subsidiary topics to be presented in monographs. My intention is to apply the lessons learned in 40 years of editing to the objectives stated above. Authors (and in some instances, as here, editors) have been invited for their up-to-date expertise and also for their ability to see their subject in a wider perspective.

I am grateful to Elsevier Science Ltd., who own the Pergamon imprint, and equally to my authors and editors, for their confidence, and to Dr. Rumen Duhlev of Elsevier Science Ltd. for his efforts on behalf of the Series.

Herewith, I am pleased to present to the public the fourth title in this Series, on a topic of great current concern.

ROBERT W. CAHN, FRS
(Cambridge University, UK)

Acknowledgements

This book would not have been possible without the contribution of all the authors, experts of international prestige, who have made every effort to synthesize the enormous amount of literature available on the subject, collaborating to the best of their ability in the preparation of the various chapters.

Neither would the work have been possible without the support of the Menéndez Pelayo International University in the organization of a Workshop on Biological Materials in ideal conditions, or without the financial aid of the Alfonso Martín Escudero Foundation whose objectives are developed in teaching activities and natural science research. Both these institutions were extremely helpful and beneficent.

The book owes a great deal to the encouragement, the juvenile energy and continued support of Professor Robert Cahn, and to the unfailing understanding of the Senior Publishing Editor, Dr. Duhlev.

The collaboration of the professors and research students of the Department of Materials Science of the Polytechnic University of Madrid has been of great value, and my special thanks are due to Rosa Morera for her rewriting of all the manuscripts and to José Miguel Martínez for his help with the Figures. Finally I would like to thank my family, particularly my wife Marga, for all their support during the preparation of this volume.

MANUEL ELICES
(Universidad Politécnica de Madrid, Spain)

List of Contributors

C. APARICIO
Departamento de Ciencia de Materiales e Ingeniería, E.T.S. Ingenieros Industriales, Universidad Politécnica de Cataluña, Avenida Diagonal 647, 08028 Barcelona, Spain.

D. BADER
Department of Engineering and IRC in Biomedical Materials, Queen Mary and Westfield College, Mile End Road, London E1 4NS, U.K.

R. BROWN
Department of Plastic & Reconstructive Surgery, University College London, 67, Riding House St., London W1P 7LD, U.K.

R.W. CAHN
Department of Materials Science and Metallurgy, University of Cambridge, Pembroke Street, Cambridge CB2 3QZ, U.K.

M. ELICES
Departamento de Ciencia de Materiales, E.T.S. Ingenieros de Caminos, Canales y Puertos, Universidad Politécnica de Madrid, Ciudad Universitaria, 28040 Madrid, Spain.

T. FERNANDEZ OTERO
Laboratorio de Electroquímica, Facultad de Químicas, UPV/EHU, Apartado 1072, 20080 San Sebastián, Spain.

M.P. GINEBRA
Departamento de Ciencia de Materiales e Ingeniería, E.T.S. Ingenieros Industriales, Universidad Politécnica de Cataluña, Avenida Diagonal 647, 08028 Barcelona, Spain.

G. JERONIMIDIS
Centre for Biomimetics, Department of Engineering, The University of Reading, Whiteknights, Reading RG6 2AY, U.K.

D. LEE
Department of Engineering and IRC in Biomedical Materials, Queen Mary and Westfield College, Mile End Road, London E1 4NS, U.K.

M. ONTAÑON
Departamento de Ciencia de Materiales e Ingeniería, E.T.S. Ingenieros Industriales, Universidad Politécnica de Cataluña, Avenida Diagonal 647, 08028 Barcelona, Spain.

J.A. PLANELL
Departamento de Ciencia de Materiales e Ingeniería, E.T.S. Ingenieros Industriales, Universidad Politécnica de Cataluña, Avenida Diagonal 647, 08028 Barcelona, Spain.

E. RENUART
Department of Materials Science & Engineering, Stanford University, Palo Alto, CA 94305-2205, U.S.A.

H. SCHECHTMAN
PROCC – Programa de Computaçao Cientifica, FIOCRUZ – Fundaçao Oswaldo Cruz, Avenida Brasil 4365, Residência Oficial, 21045-900 Rio de Janeiro, RJ, Brazil.

Y. TERMONIA
Central Research and Development, E.I. du Pont de Nemours, Inc., Experimental Station, Wilmington, DE 19880-0356, U.S.A.

C. VINEY
Department of Chemistry, Heriot-Watt University, Edinburgh EH14 4AS, Scotland.

INTRODUCTION

1. THE RELEVANCE OF BIOLOGICAL MATERIALS

Biological materials have evolved to fit their purpose and represent the success stories of four billion years of research and development by Nature. Nature has achieved materials with properties, durability, mechanisms of programmed supramolecular self-assembly and biodegradability that go far beyond the current know-how of materials industries. The ability to appreciate Nature's lessons on biological materials —as in the book you have in your hands— is the output of multidisciplinary research teams and has advanced greatly as a result of parallel advances in Physics, Chemistry and Molecular Biology.

Biological materials not only enjoy optimised properties —as strength, toughness or compliance— they exhibit several optimised properties simultaneously. Such materials are said to be *multifunctional*, like insect antennae; they are mechanically robust, self repairing, they can detect chemical and thermal information and convey this information for processing, and can undergo controlled and rapid changes in shape and orientation. In fact, survival in Nature depends on the ability to sense what is happening externally, to integrate the inputs, to predict events and to adapt to new conditions (Vincent 1992). Some biological materials are able to perform these tasks and are also said to be *smart*. All of them are a source of inspiration and a challenge to materials scientists (Janocha 1999).

Yet Nature's lessons do not stop here; *processing* and *recycling* are two subjects of major concern. Biological materials offer the attractions of *biosynthesis* —they are produced from renewable resources—, *benign processing* conditions —they are assembled and shaped in an aqueous environment and at mild temperatures— and *biodegradability* —they break down into harmless components when exposed to specific environments—. One of the great values of biological materials is their potential to serve as models for the advanced materials of the future. They provide endless inspiration, and the perfection with which they fulfil their roles displays boundless ingenuity (Ball 1997).

The field of biological materials is a *multidisciplinary* arena; those interested in mechanical properties have much to learn from studies in biology and vice versa, those whose interest is in biomimetics will profit from chemistry and physics and so on. Certainly this interdisciplinary field is gratifying, with challenges that are often very different and rewarding from those in traditional disciplines. The last four chapters of this book are devoted to fibres and in particular to silks. Silks are an intriguing class of fibrous proteins that attract scientific inquiry from a variety of disciplines (Kaplan et al. 1999). For example; *biologists* explore the functional attributes of orb webs, *textile engineers* are intrigued by the lustre and mechanical properties of silkworm fibres, *molecular biologists* find opportunities to study multigene families, and polymer chemists are interested in structure-function relationships with respect to protein folding and assembly. Clearly, this is a *multidisciplinary* approach and *interdisciplinary* research strategies are required if one is to understand and then apply the technological lessons afforded by studying biological materials.

Multidisciplinary teams of investigators are not often found. It is not easy to bring together scientists of such varying backgrounds, and more difficult to get them to work side by side. Aware of these difficulties, but convinced of the benefits of a meeting of this kind, the Menéndez Pelayo Intenational University organised a Workshop of biological materials, sponsored by the Alfonso Martín Escudero Foundation. It was held in the early summer of 1998 in Santander, in the magnificent setting of the Palacio de la Magdalena, focusing on the study of the relationships between the structure and the properties of some biological materials, considering their multifunctional and "smart" characteristics and the techniques of their processing and recycling. All these aspects provide the backdrop for the diverse chapters of this book.

2. CONTENTS OUTLOOK

The variety of biological materials is so wide that even if we restricted it to structural materials, a mere introduction would run into several volumes. So a selection had to be made, for subjective and circumstantial reasons, of a few materials. The contributions are grouped loosely into three main blocks: that of hard materials, considering only bone; soft materials, with special emphasis on tissues; and finally fibrous materials, particularly silk fibres. Priority is given in all the chapters to the relationship between structure and properties and to some aspects of design and engineering with these particular materials.

In two introductory chapters, G. Jeronimidis presents the main concepts of structure-property relationships in biological materials; the composite nature of these materials is underlined and the importance of hierarchies is illustrated. The design and function of structural biological materials are also considered; design in nature offers many examples of effective integration between the efficiency attributes of the materials themselves and of the structures.

Chapter 3 on *structure and mechanical properties of cortical bone*, by J.A. Planell and collaborators, provides the basis for the relationship between bone structure and the measured mechanical properties. The hierarchical structural organisation of bone is rationalised in terms of specific local structural features. Some models of the Young's modulus seem to work well, but it is not so for other mechanical properties. Further research is needed if general constitutive equations for bone are sought.

Chapter 4, by D. Bader and D. Lee, concentrates on *articular cartilage*, which has traditionally attracted much research interest in the fields of biomechanics and biomaterials. This chapter attempts to provide an insight in the biomechanical performance of articular cartilage over a range of hierarchical levels. However, despite the large amount of research activity invested in tissue mechanics it is still very difficult to characterise the mechanical behaviour of normal and damaged articular cartilage in terms of discrete values for established material parameters.

Tissue engineering, a new and evolving field, is the subject of chapter 5 by R.A. Brown. Its interdependence on a range of other highly developed disciplines —such as cell biology, biomaterials, bioengineering and surgery— has allowed its rapid growth. The attempt here was to rationalise these approaches within concepts of design imperatives operating within the process of biological repair and the control requirements of mammalian cells. Examples are shown, ranging from nerve repair to major blood vessels.

Chapter 6, by D. Bader and H. Schenchtman, highlights the problems associated with *biomechanical testing of tendons*. Specific test conditions were established to examine the *in vitro* behaviour of selected tendons, such as those found in the human foot. Several parameters, for both static and dynamic conditions, were obtained and used in a design template. Here, again the hierarchical structure of tendon poses problems in selecting the appropriate parameters and the need was felt to develop models to account for the predicted healing behaviour *in vivo*.

The part of the book devoted to soft tissues closes with Chapter 7, by T. Fernández-Otero on *Biomimicking with smart polymers*. Conducting polymers are envisaged as soft, wet, multifunctional materials. Large and reverse composition changes are related to large and reverse changes in properties which mimic most of the biological functions characteristic of mammalian organs.

The last part of the book is devoted to fibres because of the fibrous composite nature of most biological materials. In chapter 8, C. Viney and E. Renuart, focus on general properties of *fibres* and on *fibrous materials*. A great variety of Nature's structural materials are deposited in fibrous form. All are characterised by hierarchical molecular order. Studies of natural fibres promise a number of potentially useful lessons and several examples are discussed in this chapter.

Computer modelling of mechanical properties of fibres is the subject of chapter 9, by Y. Termonia. In essence, it is a Monte-Carlo model for the study of the mechanical behaviour of synthetic and biological polymer fibres. The model is built on molecular parameters —such as molecular weight, density of entanglements, crystalline fraction, etc.— which can be easily determined from experimental data. The model is applied to polyethylene, the simplest and most widely studied synthetic polymer.

Chapter 10, by C. Viney, concentrates on *Natural silks*, highlighting specific characteristics of silks that provide insight into how the synthesis, processing, hierarchical microstructure and mechanical property control of industrial fibres might be advanced or refined. Throughout, the specific ideas stimulated by studies of silk from the golden orb weaver spiders are regarded here as generalisable in the context of lyotropic polymer fiber production.

Last chapter, by Y. Termonia, is devoted to model the *stress-strain behaviour of spider dragline*. Spider dragline represents one of the strongest materials available to date. Spider dragline is a strongly hydrogen-bonded polymer in which the crystalline size and molecular weight distribution plays a crucial role. The model developed in chapter 9 is quite successful in reproducing the complex stress-strain curves found experimentally for the dragline in both the wet and the dry states.

A glossary is included of the terms that appear often in the book. The disparity of the themes under discussion, of the techniques adopted, and of the fields of investigation in which the authors are involved —in their various languages— might confuse some of the issues. The glossary is intended to remove some of these obstacles.

Several excellent books have been published in recent years on the subject of Biological Materials (Vincent 1990, Byrom 1991, Viney et al. 1993, among others). This book covers new ground, as some topics are updated and deals with themes not mentioned in earlier publications. The scope of structural biological materials is so vast and so impressive, with so much still to be discovered, that every contribution is welcomed.

3. MODELLING AND HIERARCHICAL STRUCTURE OF BIOLOGICAL MATERIALS

Two topics appear in most of the chapters of the book: the *hierarchical structure* of the biological materials, and the *lack of models* that would be general enough to predict their mechanical behaviour. These two features are interwoven.

Hierarchical structures are assemblages of molecular units, or higher aggregates, embedded with other phases, which in turn are similarly organised at increasing size levels. The hierarchical order of a material may be defined as the number of levels of scale with recognised structure. Such multilevel architectures are capable of conferring unique properties to the structure (Lakes 1993).

Hierarchical structures arise in both natural and in man-made materials. In practically all complex systems, and particularly in biological materials, the unifying theme is the pervasiveness of hierarchical structures. As G. Jeronimidis points out, the most immediate reaction when studying the mechanical properties of biological materials is that the traditional distinction between *material* and *structure* is far more elusive then in man-made objects. In artificial structures, the idea of macroscopic hierarchical frameworks can be traced back at least to Eiffel's design for his tower, and the above comments are exemplified in Fig. 1.1.

Hierarchical structures in biological materials span many orders of magnitude; from the macromolecular level (tropocollagen units, 10^{-9} m in diameter) up to whole organisms such as trees (giant redwood, 10 m, trunk diameter at the base). Several examples appear along the book; wood (Fig. 1.3), tendon (Figs. 1.4 and 6.1), bone (Figs. 1.6 and 3.6), osteon (Fig. 3.1), viral spikes (Fig. 8.10) and spider silk (Fig. 10.5) among others. Integrated sub-structuring is the common theme of biological materials, far more subtle and extensive than in any man-made material or structure.

Stiffness, strength, fracture toughness and other mechanical properties are modulated, tailored and optimised by controlled interactions between the hierarchies. How can we *predict* those properties, keeping in mind the hierarchical structure? The *sky-scraper analogy* (developed during the workshop) may help in clarifying this topic. We might consider a skyscraper as a hierarchical structure, similar to a femur or a tree, and try to predict its mechanical behaviour under applied "loads"; an earthquake, a differential settlement or an accidental high load.

The simplest and clumsiest approach would be to test a full-size copy of the skyscraper submitted to the stresses we wish to study. This would obviously entail an enormous cost and possible destruction, and the information would apply only to that particular case. Paradoxically, full-scale testing of structures and structural components is used in engineering only when no other options are found. And the same situation arises in the sphere of biomaterials when testing, for example, a femur or a tendon.

The next approach would be to test one or more storeys of the skyscraper, or a reduced-scale model (even though it is very difficult to scale *all* the magnitudes). Here again, the test would have a very *limited* validity —only for that structure and the type of solicitation— and the cost would still be high. In the case of biomaterils, this is the method adopted to test a piece of bone or tendon, and the findings are purely local and not susceptible to generalisation, as indicated by Planell et al. in Chapter 3 and by Dan Bader et al. in Chapters 4 and 6.

The ideal approach would be one capable of detecting the type of material that is relevant to the properties to be predicted, or in other words the hierarchical level relevant to the problem under study. In the case of the skyscraper, most of the mechanical properties can be predicted only from a few parameters related to the steel and concrete used in the construction; usually the Young's modulus and yield stress or strength are enough. The characteristics of the insulating materials, or others that are not structural —windows, partitions, bathroom fittings or the grand piano on the third floor— are almost irrelevant for computing natural frequencies or displacements of the skyscraper.

The hierarchical order of a biological material is much higher than that of a complex structure such as the Eiffel Tower. Unfortunately, in most biological materials we still do not know the relevant order when a specific property is sought. Once the "steel" and "concrete" of that particular material are known, efforts should be concentrated on measuring their properties relevant for the model under consideration.

When problems arise on another scale they cannot be solved with previous parameters. To continue with the example of concrete and steel, consider two well known pathologies; the *alkali-silica reaction* in concrete or the *hydrogen embrittlement* in prestressed steel tendons. To understand these phenomena it is necessary to go down to other hierarchical levels; to capture the subleties of hydrated cement gels or the behaviour of steel interfaces and dislocations. Only by working at these levels is it possible to solve the problems: to manufacture materials that are immune to these infirmities and to predict the behaviour of the structure.

Many biological materials exhibit hierarchical structure and the hierarchical aspects of structure are useful in the design of both novel materials and structures, provided the relevant scale for the property sought is identified. Among the useful properties that may be conferred by hierarchical structure, that of simultaneously achieving values of strength and fracture toughness is of paramount importance. However, in modern structural engineering the tendency seems to be away from hierarchical structures; even though these contain less material to achieve the desired strength, the costs associated with fabrication and maintenance currently exceed any saving in material cost (Lakes 1993). Nevertheless a thrust of recent work is being done in this area (Tadmor et al. 2000).

In conclusion, the aim of this book is to show some examples of the relationships between structure and properties of biological materials, features that represent desirable objectives in the design and manufacture of synthetic structural materials. Biological materials are characterised by hierarchical architectural design with length scales ranging from molecular to macroscopic. They are multifunctional and smart, self-healing and remarkably durable. Yet Nature's lessons do not stop even here, self-organisation and self-assembly are used by Nature to produce all its structures and devices, although at slow rates. Nature is parsimonious in its use of constituent materials and works at room temperature and under benign conditions. A formidable example to follow!

REFERENCES

Ball, P. (1997) *Made to Measure*, Princeton University Press, Princeton, NJ.

Byrom, D. (Ed.) (1991) *Biomaterials*, MacMillan Publishers Ltd., U.K.

Janocha, H. (Ed.) (1999) *Adaptronics and Smart Structures*, Springer.

Kaplan, D., Viney, C., Former, B. and Adams, W. (1999) *Silk Symposium*, Special issue of Int. J. of Biological Macromolecules, **24**, 2 and 3.

Lakes, R. (1993) Nature **361**, 511.

Tadmor, E.B., Phillips, R., Ortiz, M. (2000) *Int. J. of Solids and Structures* **37**, 379.

Vincent, J.F.V. (1990) *Structural Biomaterials*, Princeton University Press, Princeton, NJ.

Vincent, J.P. (1992) *Metals and Materials*, January 13.

Viney, C., Case, S.T., Waite, J.H. (Eds.) (1993) *Biomolecular Materials*, MRS, Vol. 292, Pittsburgh, Pennsylvania.

Vogel, S. (1992) *Biomimetics*, **1**(1), 63.

Contents

Chapter 1

Structure-Property Relationships in Biological Materials

Chapter 1

Structure-Property Relationships in Biological Materials

GEORGE JERONIMIDIS

1.1. INTRODUCTION

The study of the mechanical properties of biological materials offers a unique opportunity to understand how materials science and engineering principles are applied in Nature. It should also provide inspiration and stimulation to scientists and engineers for new materials concepts, efficient design strategies and structural optimisation. In many respects the book is aimed at the materials and engineering communities which, we believe, will benefit from ideas, concepts and solutions tuned by biological evolution.

Since the early pioneering work of D'Arcy Thompson (Thompson 1952), who studied the relationship between growth and shape of living things, the subject has been developed considerably, especially in the past twenty years. The impetus has come from a variety of disciplines and reasons: medicine and veterinary science (mechanical properties of soft and hard tissues such as skin, tendons, bone, etc., prosthetic devices, replacement materials); biology (mechanical aspects of adaptation, evolution, physiology, behaviour); agriculture and forestry (plant biomechanics in relation to crops, wood production, etc.); food industries (food quality, textural attributes related to mechanical properties, food processing and manufacture). In parallel, materials science and engineering principles, theories and techniques have also evolved and been refined providing the means to measure, interpret, analyse, quantify and model the relationships between materials, structures, design and function. The most recent addition to the list of disciplines interested in biological systems is biomimetics, the purpose of which can be summarised simply as "the abstraction of good design from Nature" (Vincent 1995).

There are several books covering various aspects of the subject (Wainwright et al. 1975, Vincent and Currey 1980 and Vincent 1990) and an increasing number of scientific papers and review articles are being published in the literature. The contribution made by James E. Gordon in the late 70' and 80's (Gordon 1976 and 1978) has provided perhaps the most effective catalyst for the current and growing level of interest in biological materials and structures. His books have stimulated biology, engineering, materials science and medicine to approach the subject in a truly interdisciplinary manner and to look more closely at the design aspects of biological systems for, in his words, "...nothing attracts less attention that total success".

The most striking feature of biological systems is perhaps the way in which their mechanical properties are related to highly organised and integrated hierarchical assemblies of load-bearing units. These span many orders of magnitude, from the macromolecular level (tropocollagen units, 10^{-9} m in diameter) up to whole organisms such as large animals and trees (giant redwood, 10 m. trunk diameter at the base). Stiffness, strength, toughness, etc. are modulated, tailored and optimized by controlled interactions between the hierarchies. Integrated sub-structuring is the common theme of biology, far more subtle and extensive than in any man-made material or structure.

This creates difficulties in writing on the subject because the traditional division between "materials" and "structures' in the engineering sense is far less clear-cut than in man-made artifacts and somewhat arbitrary. However, in the first two chapters of this book greater emphasis has been given on the materials aspects in the first and on the structural ones in the second. They provide a general background and examples against which the specific topics dealt with in greater detail by the various authors can be set.

The subjects covered in this publication are by no means exhaustive; they have been selected to give the reader an informed insight into new developments, state of the art scientific and technological achievements and areas of application. The common thread being the study of biological materials and structures as paradigms for the education and stimulation of material scientists and engineers (Jeronimidis and Atkins 1995 and French 1988).

1.2. BIOLOGICAL MATERIALS: SCALE, HETEROGENEITY, REPRESENTATIVE VOLUME ELEMENTS (RVE)

The most immediate reaction when studying the mechanical properties of tissues from plants and animals is, as remarked above, that the traditional distinction between "material" and "structure" is far more elusive than in man-made objects.

The nature of this dilemma is illustrated in Fig. 1.1. In practice it is convenient to be flexible and to wear the appropriate hat, material or structural, according to need, i.e. depending on the type of information sought. In fact one must be prepared to zoom in and out of the picture, as it were, analysing details or integrating data. It is true that all engineering materials, metals, plastics or ceramics, have also

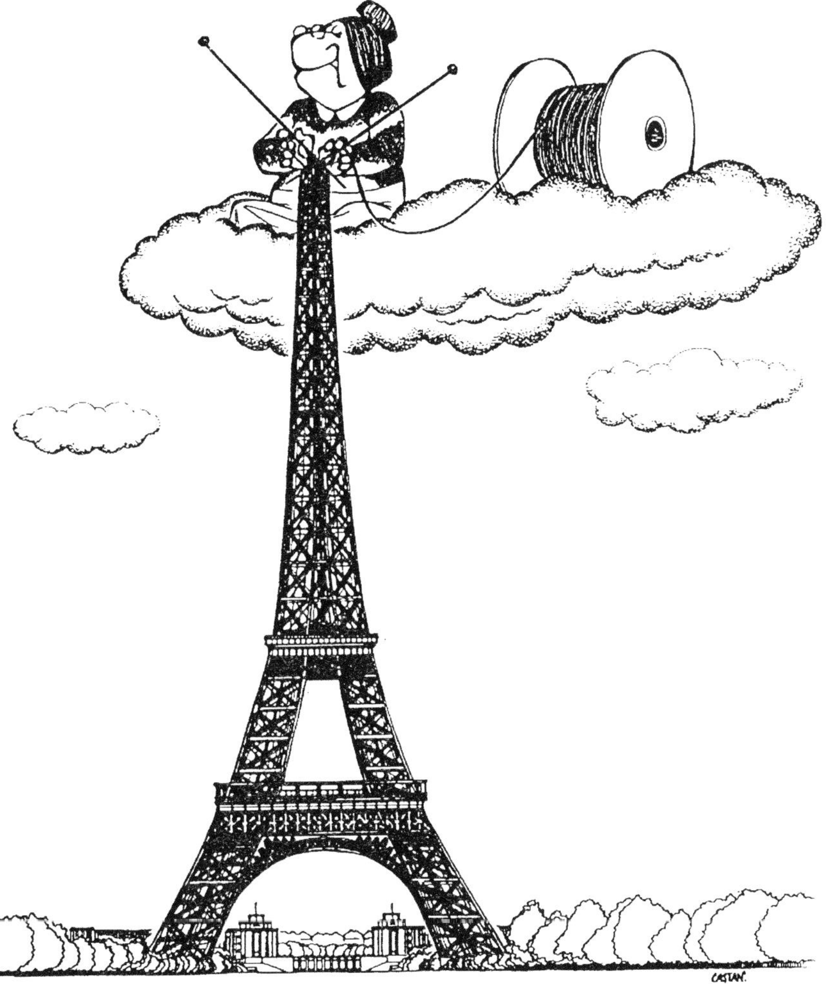

Fig. 1.1. Material or structure?

microstructure but, in general, their Representative Volume Element (RVE) is very small compared to the linear dimensions of the structures or structural components they are used for. The RVE of a material is the smallest volume over which the average of mechanical or physical properties, such as Young's modulus or coefficient of thermal expansion, for example, are representative of the whole. In a metal, the grain size may be of the order of 10 μm; hence, a volume of 0.1 mm^3 will contain 10^5 grains. Even if the grains have different orientations, with different properties in different directions, owing to anisotropy of their crystalline structure, the average

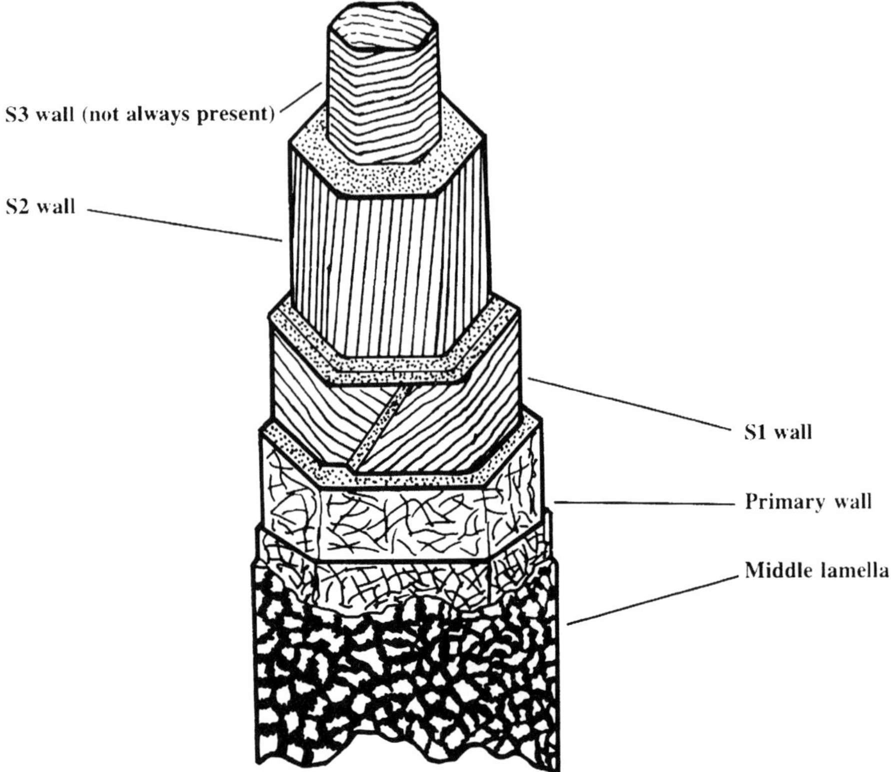

Fig. 1.2. Typical wood cell and cell wall laminated structure

value of the property over the RVE can be considered constant throughout the material. In more heterogeneous materials such as glass or carbon fibre-reinforced composites, typical fibre diameters of 5-10 μm generally mean RVEs of the order of a few mm^3.

On the other hand, even a very familiar biological material such as wood offers an amazing array of hierarchies spanning in typical dimensions from nanometres (cellulose microfibrils) to the centimetre level (wood tissue). The RVEs of the various substructures cover therefore a range from 10^3 mm^3 down to 10^{-12} mm^3 i.e. fifteen orders of magnitude with perhaps seven hierarchical levels: tissue, cell, laminated cell walls, individual walls, cellulose fibres, microfibrils and protofibrils. A typical wood cell (approx. 30 μm in diameter) is illustrated in Fig. 1.2 showing the fibre orientation in the various walls. The transition from wood cell to wood tissue is shown in Fig. 1.3.

This situation is common to virtually all biological materials and Figs. 1.4 to 1.6 show the hierarchical structures of tendon, muscle and bone.

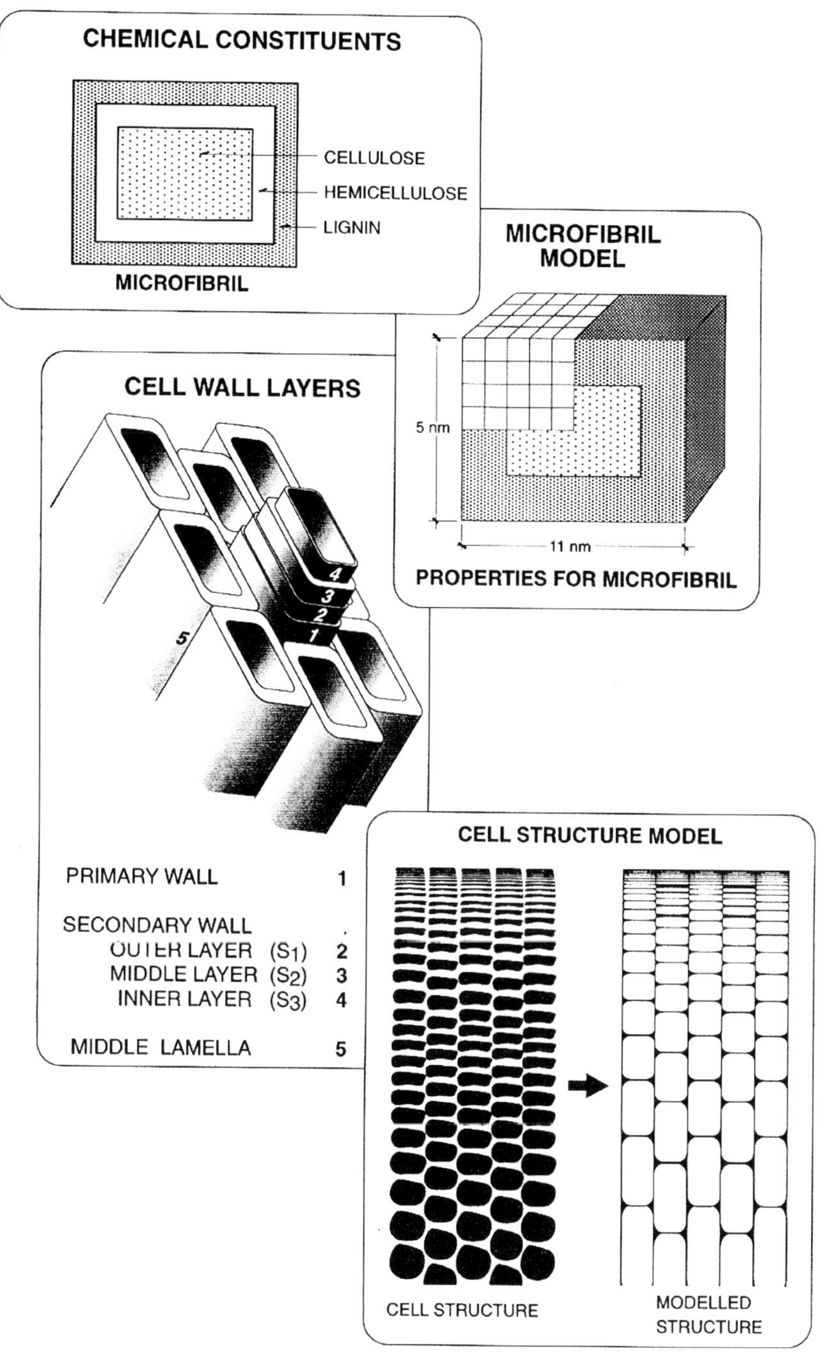

Fig. 1.3. Transition from cells to tissue in wood

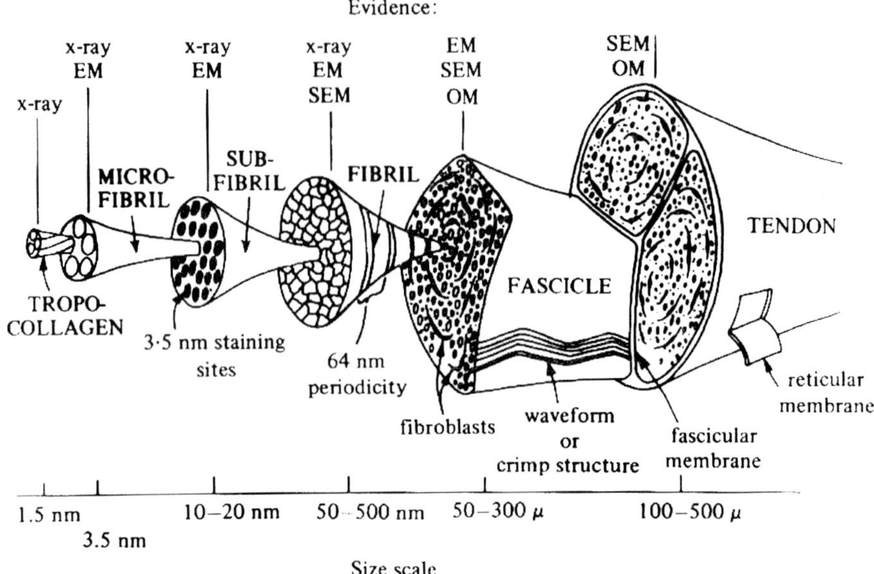

Fig. 1.4. Hierarchical structure of tendon

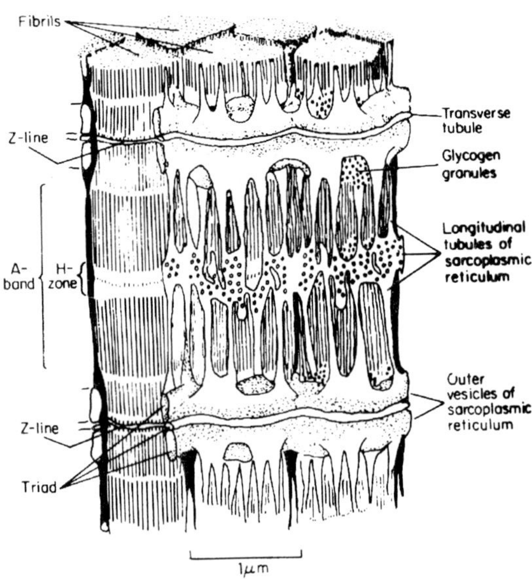

Fig. 1.5. Architecture of striated muscle

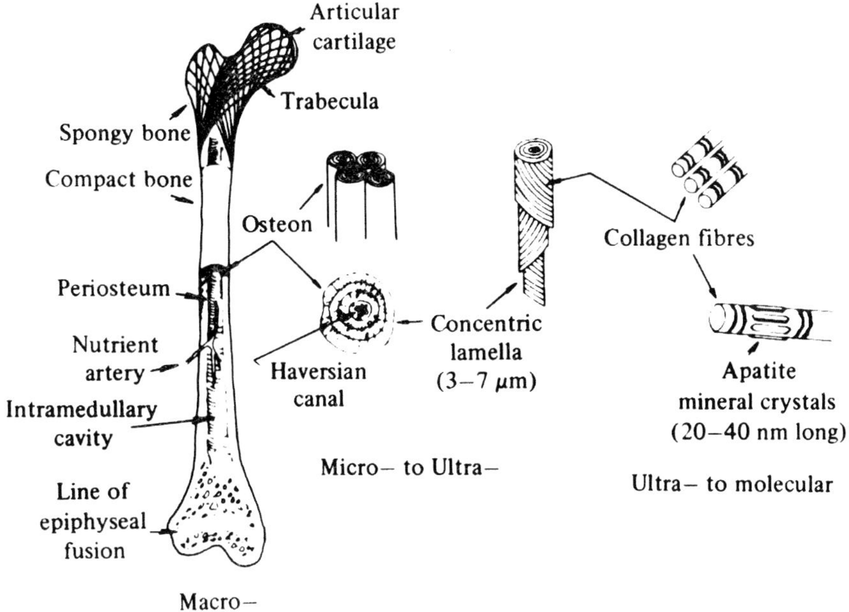

Fig.1.6. Hierarchical structures in bone

For the purpose of this contribution it is convenient and more appropriate perhaps to identify the various hierarchies of biological systems using definitions such as organism, organ, tissue, cell, cell wall, etc. borrowed from by biology. The engineering equivalents, structure, component, element, material are not as effective. In the case of trees and wood, for example, the tree is the organism, trunk, branches, leaves and fruits are organs; organs are made of one or more tissues (wood, for example) and the tissues themselves are organised structures (assembly of cells and extracellular substances) made of several materials (cellulose and lignin) which, themselves are often hierarchical and heterogeneous. In bone too, one can identify the organ itself (femur, for example), the tissue (osteate, lamellar or cancellous bone), tissue components such as osteons, made of concentric lamellae, each of which contains collagen fibres and hydroxyapatite crystals. Figs. 1.7 and 1.8 show a number of hierarchies in antler, for example. In the limit one may argue that the only substances recognisable as "materials" in biology are the basic chemicals which are at the start of the assembly process of the load-bearing structures (fibres, tissues, organs, etc.). These are comparatively few. Polypeptides (collagen, elastin, keratin, muscle), polysaccarrides (cellulose, hemicelluloses,), polyphenols (lignin, tannins), hybrids such as chitin (polyacetylglucosamine) and minerals, mostly calcium salts (hydroxyapatite in bone, calcium carbonate in mollusc shells).

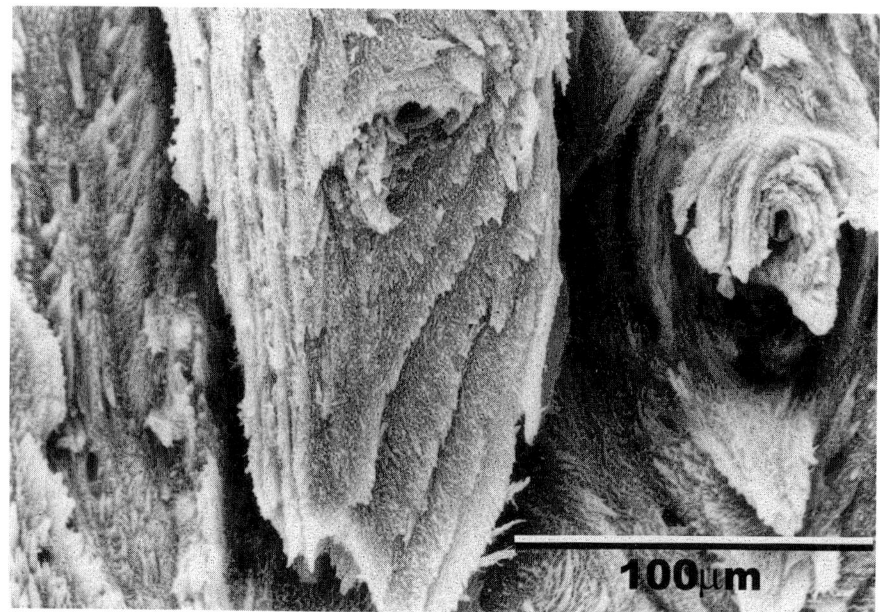

Fig. 1.7. Hierarchies in antler: osteons, lamellae and calcified fibres

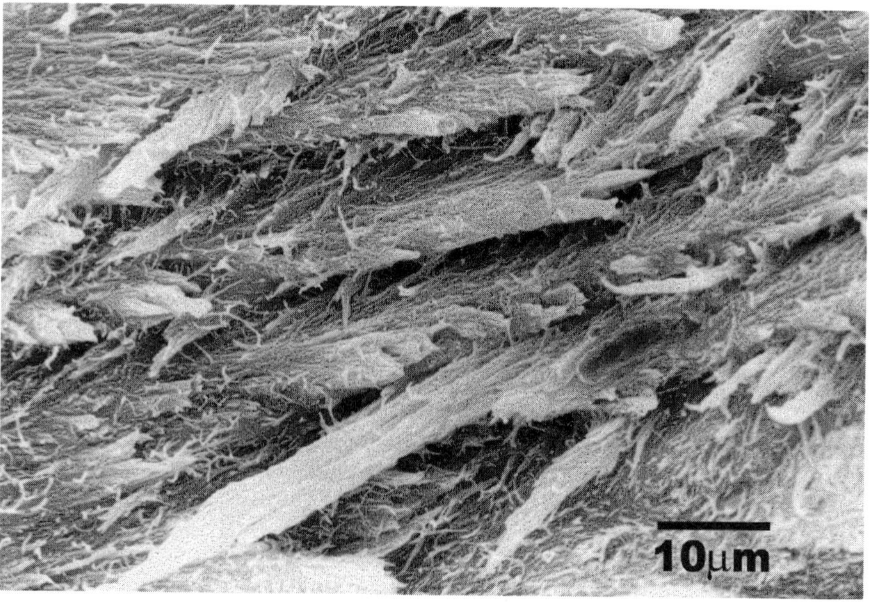

Fig. 1.8. Detail of concentric lamellar structure in antler.

These material ingredients are used in a wide range of tissues such as skin and tendons (collagen, elastin, mucopolysaccharides), bone (collagen, hyrdroxyapatite), horns, feathers, nails, hooves (keratin), wood and turgid plant tissues (cellulose, hemicelluloses and lignin), soft and hard cuticles (chitin, tannins, ceramic), mollusc shells, etc. (Turner et al. 1994).

To a large extent, the study of the mechanical properties of biological materials consists in developing the connections within and between the various RVEs, using averaging techniques from solid mechanics theories (rule of mixtures for composites, for example). However, it is important to remember that in averaging properties within a RVE and between RVEs, some information on the subsystem is lost in the process. This is particularly relevant in relation to mechanical events occurring at local levels, such as damage initiation and growth, for example, as opposed to global events such as elastic behaviour or structural instabilities of the kind associated with buckling and fracture.

1.3. FIBRES: THE KEY BUILDING BLOCKS FOR PERFORMANCE AND VERSATILITY

It may be argued that without structural fibres a great deal of evolutionary development in biology, from unicellular organisms in water to higher forms of life, marine, terrestrial and aerial would have impossible, or at the very least extremely difficult. It is a fact that almost all biological load-bearing materials, tissues and organs are fibrous composites. As a result, the mechanical behaviour of biological systems is optimised by extracting every drop of performance from the fibres themselves and from the virtually unlimited range of fibrous structures, architectures and patterns which are topologically possible (Neville 1993). Fibres are metabollically expensive to produce and it makes a great deal of sense to use them as efficiently as possible.

A measure of the compromise between metabolic and information economies on the one hand and versatility on the other is perhaps the fact that there are only three main fibre-forming polymers in nature: polypeptides (collagen, elastin, silks, keratins), polysaccharides (cellulose, hemicelluloses) and the hybrid polypeptide-polysaccharide, chitin (insect cuticles and crustacean shells). The specific tailored composite designs which incorporate these fibres are countless.

By their very nature, long and thin, the use of fibres for structural purposes has a number of consequences: a) anisotropy due to the directionality of properties imparted by the fibres to the composites, b) hierarchies due to the assembly of microfibrils into fibres, etc., c) heterogeneity and d) strong non-linearity in stress-strain behaviour due to fibre architectures, low bending stiffness of fibres and use of relatively compliant matrices in many "soft" tissues (Jeronimidis and Vincent 1984).

Since in most of the fibres being discussed the preferential molecular orientation is in the fibre direction, it follows also that the tensile mechanical properties in the fibre direction are much, much better than the compressive ones. In this respect, all polymeric fibres with enhanced molecular orientation in the fibre direction are very similar, biological (cellulose, silk, collagen, etc.) or man-made high performance ones (aramid, high molecular weight polyethylene). Unfortunately, direct measurements of tensile properties of the true natural fibres (often microfibrils) are impossible, except for silks, because they cannot be isolated and tested. Generally, the properties of the fibres are inferred from measurements on tissues or fibre aggregates, taking into account volume fractions and fibre orientation and deriving the fibre properties from micromechanics models.

The measured tensile Young's modulus of biological fibre aggregates or bundles varies a great deal (Vincent and Currey 1980), from about 100 GPa in cellulose down to 1 GPa in non-mineralised collagen. Similarly, the tensile strength in the fibre direction can be as high as 300-400 MPa in some plant fibres such as flax (structures rather than single fibres) and close to 5000 MPa for some silks [see Chapters 10 and 11]. In practice, so long as the primary carbon-carbon bonds of the main chain can be used effectively, the expected tensile properties are similar to those which can be predicted for highly aligned macromolecular systems. The range of observed properties in natural fibrous elements is a reflection of the composite hierarchical structure of most natural fibres and of the interactions between units.

From an engineering point of view it is obvious that fibres are ideal tension elements where their relative efficiency is directly proportional to the specific Young's modulus (for stiffness controlled structures) or to the specific tensile strength (for strength controlled structures). It can also be shown (Gordon 1976 and Cox 1965) that the efficiency of tensile structures increases by subdividing the load bearing area into as many sub-elements as possible. This has an obvious advantage in terms of multiple load paths, redundancy and hence resistance to crack propagation. There is a more subtle advantage arising from the fact that in order to get loads in and out of tension structures it is more efficient, in terms of weight of "terminations", to attach many small elements individually rather than a single one of the same cross-sectional area. This principle is clearly applied in many biological tensile structures such as tendons and their attachment to bones, anchor points in spiders' webs and connections between cartilage and bone [Chapters 4, 5 and 6]. Similar considerations govern the design of suspension cables in bridges, mooring lines in oil extraction platforms, tents, sails and all manner of fabric-based civil engineering structures.

Of course, the problem of designing efficient terminations for bundles of fibres in tension disappears if no terminations are needed. This solution is very popular in nature and can be found in the multicellular tissues of turgid plants parenchyma, illustrated in Fig. 1.9, as well as in many invertebrates such as worms, tunicates, sea anemonae and even sharks (Wainwright et al. 1975). Fig. 1.10 shows the structure of squid. In all these examples and in many others, the load bearing fibres have no detectable beginning or end, i.e. they form a two-dimensional fibrous architecture without terminations, enclosing a fluid which can be pressurised by chemical (osmotic pressure) or physiological (muscles) means. The fibrous structure is put into tension, balancing the internal pressure. This is extremely efficient in terms of optimum usage of expensive high strength fibres.

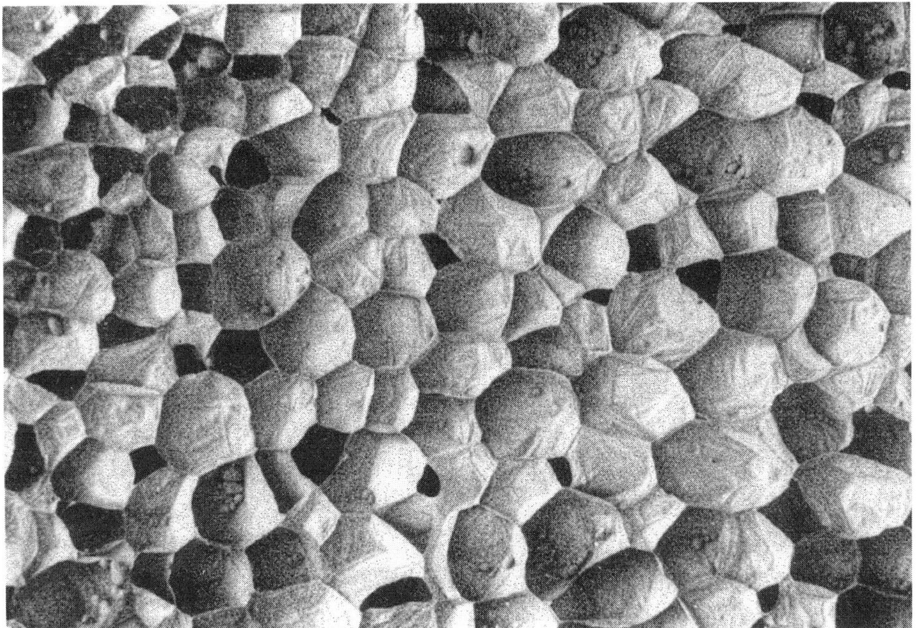

Fig. 1.9. Parenchyma cells in potato

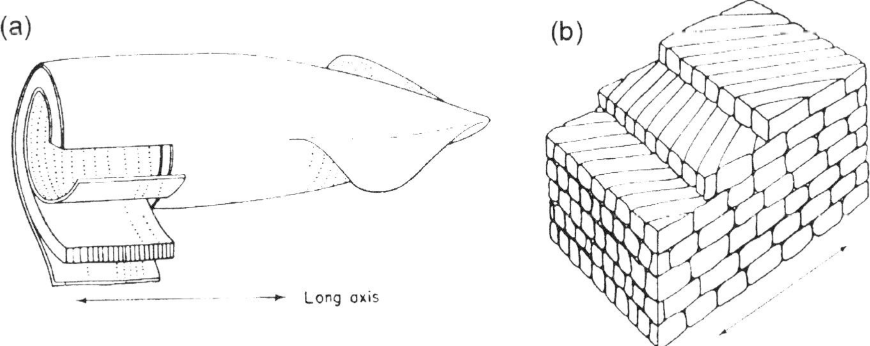

Fig. 1.10. The structure of tunicates (a) and the arrangement of fibres in the tunicae (b).

As mentioned earlier, a major drawback of high modulus - high tensile strength polymeric fibres, natural or artificial, is that the high molecular orientation in the fibre direction and the weak, secondary bond lateral interactions between polymer chains result in very poor compressive properties. If the fibres have to be used in applications where stiffness and strength are needed in bending and direct compression, then they become very inefficient owing to fibre buckling (slender columns in compression) or to compression kinks within the fibres. In a liquid environment many biological structures can be designed as flexible fibrous composite pressure vessels where the tensile strain in the fibres arising from the stretching of the fluid container under pressure pre-stresses the fibres in tension, minimising the risk of buckling or kinking in compression. The same mechanism of fibre pre-stressing is found also in mammalian skin, blood vessels, tendons, non-lignified plant cells and many other pliant biological tissues.

However, in order to survive end evolve on land and to fly , resistance to bending and compression is also beneficial. Mammals, insects and higher plants need load-bearing structures capable of carrying bending and compressive stresses but the available structural fibres have the same weakness in compression as those used efficiently in the pure tensile structures. The same dilemma exists in the utilisation of man-made composites in structures other than ropes or sails but there are artificial fibres, such as boron, with exceptional compressive strength, albeit extremely expensive. Nature has a much more limited choice of fibres and, indeed, has never developed a totally ceramic fibre. It has solved the problem of lack of compressive strength in four main ways:

1.- by incorporating a ceramic phase which can support the fibres laterally in compression, preventing buckling and kinking (bone, mineralised tendons);
2.- by making fibrous composite structures with very high degree of cross-linking in the matrix and also between fibres and matrix (tanned insect cuticle, lignified plant cell walls);
3.- by pre-stressing fibres in tension via pressure or growth (turgid plant cell walls, skin and blood vessels);
4.- by pre-stressing in tension parts of structures vulnerable to compression at the expense of higher compressive stresses in less vulnerable parts - in practice by mechanisms similar to those used in pre-stressed concrete - (in trees the periphery of the trunk is in tension and the centre in compression).

These solutions can be very efficient in terms of structural weight penalty, especially 3 and 4. Solutions 1 and 2 are really compromises because nothing else is available but quite effective too, in particular when the supporting function of the ceramic phase or the highly crosslinked matrix is implemented at the appropriate hierarchical level, generally the microfibrillar one.

1.4. CONCLUSIONS

In this chapter the main concepts of structure-property relationships in biological materials have been introduced and discussed at a general level. The composite nature of most biological materials has been underlined, together with its mechanical and design consequences. The importance and benefit of hierarchies for efficient utilization of fibre properties and for widening the range of available structural solutions beyond the narrow spectrum of available polymeric fibres has been illustrated. More detailed information on selected examples will be found in the other chapters of this book.

ACKNOWLEDGEMENTS

The author gratefully acknowledge the following sources of illustrations reproduced in this chapter and thank the authors and publishers who have granted their permission: Fig. 1.1.- Castan and A. Regie, France. Fig.1.3.- From K. Persson, H. Petersson and F. Stefansson – Cell structure modelling for determination of mechanical properties of wood. In *Plant Biomechanics*, G. Jeronimidis and J.F.V. Vincent Eds., 1977, Volume I, pp. 171-177, The University of Reading, Reading. Fig. 1.4.- From J. Kestelic and E. Baer – Deformation in tendon collagen. In The Mechanical Properties of Biological Materials. J.F.V. Vincent and J.D. Currey Eds., 1980, pp. 397-435, Cambridge University Press (ISBN 0 521 23478 6, Copyright: Society for Experimental Biology). Fig. 1.5.- From L.D. Peachy – The sarcoplasmic reticulum and transverse tubules of frog's sartorius, 1965, *J. Cell Biol.*, **25**, pp. 209.232. Fig. 1.6.- From J.B. Park – *Biomaterials: An Introduction.* 1979, Plenum Press, New York. Figs. 1.7 and 1.8.- From M. Watkins – PhD Thesis, Reading University, 1986. Fig. 1.10.- From D.V. Ward and S.A. Wainwright – Locomotory aspects of squid mantle structure. 1972, *J. Zoology, London*, **167**, pp. 437-449 (Printed in Great Britain by Henry Ling Ltd., the Dorchester Press, Dorchester).

REFERENCES

Cox, H.L. (1965) *The Design of Structures of Least Weight.* (Pergamon. Oxford).

French, M. (1988) *Invention and Evolution: Design in Nature and Engineering.* (Cambridge University Press).

Gordon, J.E. (1976) *The New Science of Strong Materials. 2nd Ed.* (Penguin Books, London).

Gordon, J.E. (1978) *Structures.* (Penguin Books, London).

Jeronimidis, G. and Atkins, A.G. (1995) *Proc. Instn. Mech. Engnrs.*, **209**, 221.

Jeronimidis, G. and Vincent, J.F.V. (1984) In *Connective Tissue Matrix.* ed. D.W.L. Hukins, (Macmillan. London), p. 188.

Neville, A.C. (1993) *Biology of Fibrous Composites.* (Cambridge University Press).

Thompson, D' A., W. (1952) *On Growth and Form. 2nd Ed.* (Cambridge University Press).

Turner, R.M., Vincent, J.F.V. and Jeronimidis, G. (1994) In *Encyclopedia of Advanced Materials.* ed. D. Bloor, R.J. Brook, M.C. Fleming, S. Mahajan and R.W. Cahan, (Pergamon. Oxford), .p. 244.

Vincent, J.F.V. (1990) *Structural Biomaterials.* (Princeton University Press).

Vincent, J.F.V. (1995) in *Encyclopaedia Britannica Yearbook*, (Bettman Archive), p.169.

Vincent, J.F.V. and Currey, J.D. (1980) *The Mechanical Properties of Biological Materials.* (Cambridge Universiry Press).

Wainwright, S.A., Biggs, W.D., Currey, J.D. and Gosline, J.M. (1975) *Mechanical Design of Organisms.* (Arnold).

Chapter 2

Design and Function of Structural Biological Materials

Chapter 2

Design and Function of Structural Biological Materials

GEORGE JERONIMIDIS

2.1. INTRODUCTION

The importance of structural materials, man-made or grown by nature, lies not so much in their intrinsic properties, discussed in Chapter I, but rather in the way in which these properties are used for specific functions. Design is the expression of function and design consists very often in achieving compromises between conflicting requirements as well as extracting maximum benefit from the materials used. In biology there is also a strong pressure to be energetically and metabolically efficient. It is often this last requirement which, in nature, drives the successful integration of material properties, architecture and shape, providing a wide range of optimised designs, tailored to specific functions.

The fundamental mechanical and engineering rules, which govern the design of biological structures, are obviously the same as those used in the design of man-made structures. There are no surprises there; but biology appears very often to have been able to achieve a great deal more efficiency and functionality by clever ways of putting things together rather than by developing fanciful high performance materials. This does not mean that the solutions found in nature are "optimum" in an absolute sense, but rather that the point reached under evolutionary and selection pressures at any particular time represent a "local" optimum in relation to the existing conditions.

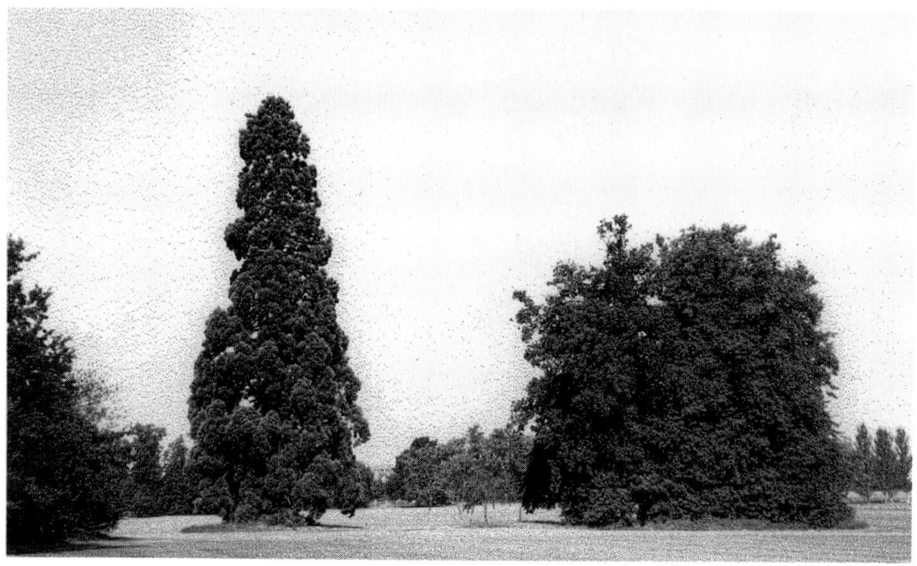

Fig. 2.1. Trees

In designing structures to resist mechanical loads nature has a number of advantages over the more traditional approaches used by engineers: the extensive use of fibrous composite materials, the hierarchical nature of the load-bearing elements and, more importantly perhaps, the fact that biological structures are grown rather than "made". Growth, i.e. the possibility of adding (and sometimes removing material as in bone), means that mechanical inputs from the environment (forces, temperatures, etc.) are already present, detected and processed by the organism and used as a blueprint for the design. This information is used to best effect, together with the genetic memory, to redirect the deposition of new material, modify interactions between hierarchies, reorient structural fibres and modify shape to optimise performance. In practice biological structures are designed "under stress and strain", interacting all the time with the short and long term loads that they have to resist. This is the essence of adaptive mechanical design.

As yet, we cannot replicate these processes. The nearest that we can get to this design approach is to rely on analytical, simulation and modelling techniques, such as solid mechanics, structural engineering, finite elements, etc., to quantify the relationships between external loads, geometry, material properties, design and function. However good and sophisticated these tools may be, they still are comparatively crude compared to the biological ones. Some recent approaches which "mimic" growth processes, i.e. the addition and removal of material according to some engineering rule (maximum von Mises stress, for example), have been quite successful

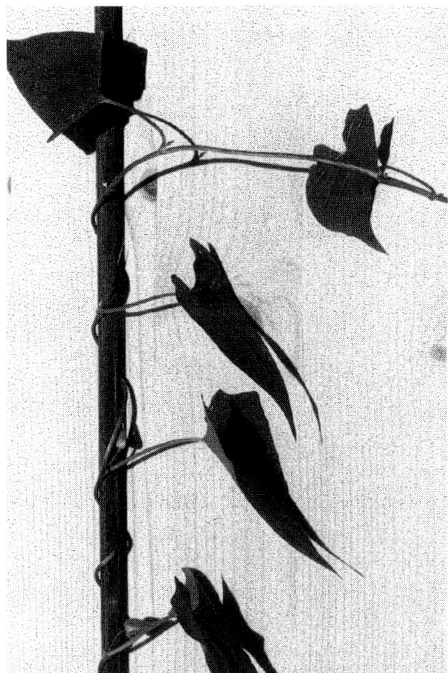

Fig. 2.2. Bindweed supported by cane

in "designing" optimal shapes based on a number of criteria (minimum mass, fatigue life, etc.). These techniques fall into the general group of "genetic algorithms" (Matteck and Vorberg 1989, Worden and Tomlinson 1995 and Steven et al. 1999).

Rather than attempt a general description of the points mentioned above, this chapter will illustrate the concepts through the presentation and discussion of examples, from which some general principles can be derived. The subdivision into sections is somewhat arbitrary, dealing first with biological structures where no locomotion and nervous system are involved (mainly plants) and moving on to more complicated organisms.

2.2. DESIGN FOR STIFFNESS AND DESIGN FOR STRENGTH

Most plants, and trees in particular - especially large ones -, are excellent examples of stiffness controlled engineering design. Their main requirement is to stand up, gather sunlight for photosynthesis and compete if necessary with neighbours by growing taller or faster (Fig. 2.1). The main external loads on plants are self-weight and wind loads. There are exceptions such as lianas, vines and climbing plants (Fig. 2.2), which

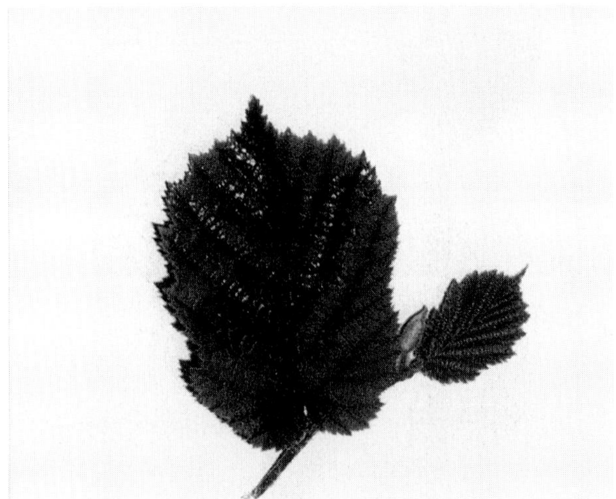

Fig. 2.3. Open and budding leaves in beech

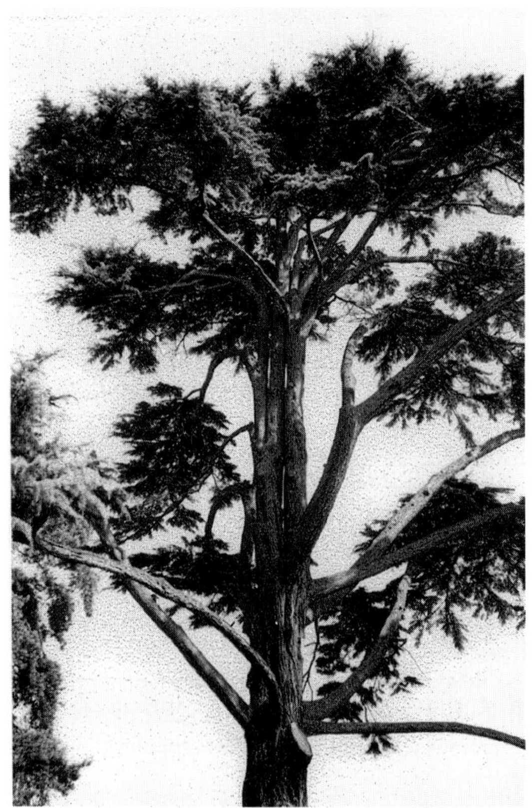

Fig. 2.4. Branching in Lebanon Cedar

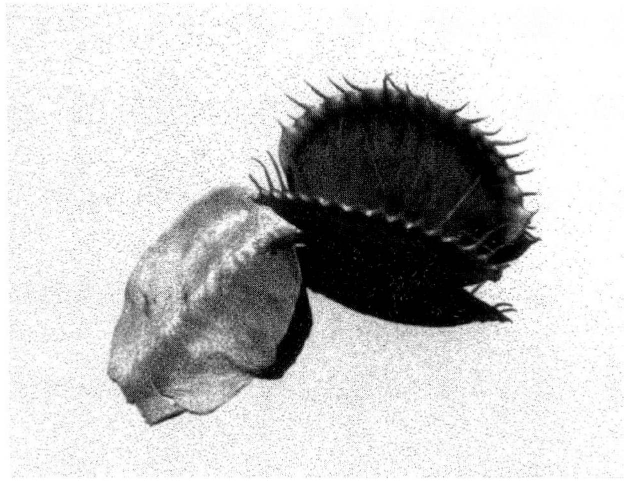

Fig. 2.5. Open leaves of Venus Flytrap

rely on the support provided by other plants or by other rigid structures to reach for sunlight (Rowe and Speck 1996). But even lianas (common ivy does this too) can switch the mechanical properties of their main stem from flexible to rigid in bending when the need arises.

In many respects plants are intuitively simple to analyse, being similar, as it were, to many "static" engineering structures. In spite of this apparent simplicity, it must be remembered that a tree, for example, integrates in its tissues, form and function the wisdom of many engineering disciplines. With reference to Fig. 2.3 and 2.4, one can think of structural mechanics (stressed trunk and branches), composite materials and cellular structures (tissues), joining technology with fibrous matcrials (branch junctions), fluid mechanics and heat transfer (water transport, transpiration), soil mechanics (roots), solar energy collection (leaves and their deployment from buds) and aerodynamics (wind loads on leaves and limbs). In addition, a great deal of optimisation is carried out all the time by other mechanisms associated with growth, such as pre-stressing, and formation of reaction wood (Jeronimidis and Vincent 1997). It should not be surprising to realise that it would be possible to cover a great deal of a traditional engineering university curriculum just by studying trees.

Different considerations apply to plants, which rely on turgor pressure, rather than lignification and they will be discussed later in this chapter. However, it is worth mentioning at this stage that in such systems the pressure inside parenchyma cells provides not only structural benefits but also the main mechanisms for "rapid" movements in plants. The best example of this is the well known closing of the Venus Flytrap (Fig. 2.5).

In *stiffness-controlled design* the principles, which govern optimisation, are well known. What is not so well developed is the integration of materials properties, on the one hand, and intrinsic attributes of the structure such as loads, geometry, etc. These concepts have been worked out in great detail by Cox (Cox 1965) and can be found also in other publications (Gordon 1978 and Ashby and Jones 1980). The idea behind them is to derive expressions for the efficiency of a structure, defined as the ratio between the load carried and the weight of the structure itself, separating the contribution which is due to the material (material efficiency index) from that of the loads and geometry of the structure (structural loading coefficients). In this way, comparisons between different materials can be made in relation to the function that they have to perform in the structure which may be purely tensile (rope, cable, spider drag-line, tendons), purely compressive (brick, stone, intervertebral disc) or a bit of both as in bending of beams and plates (branches of trees, limb bones, engineering beams, etc.)

For stiffness-controlled structures, where excessive deflections constitute failure even though the materials may not brake, there are major differences between purely tensile and purely compressive loading, especially when the latter is likely to lead to buckling as the most likely failure mode.

The equations which give the efficiency under various situations are given below, where P is the load carried (= P_{crit} for buckling in compression), W the weight of the structure itself, ℓ is the distance over which the load is carried and n is the number of elements acting in parallel to carry the load:

Stiffness Controlled Tensile Structure

$$Efficiency = \frac{P}{W} \propto \frac{E}{\rho} \cdot \frac{n^{1/2}}{\ell n^{1/2} + kP^{1/2}\sigma^{-1/2}} \tag{2.1}$$

where E is the Young's modulus, ρ the density, σ the tensile strength and k a coefficient connected with the cunning of the designer.

Stiffness Controlled Compressive Structure

$$Efficiency = \frac{P_{crit}}{W} \propto \frac{E^{1/2}}{\rho} \cdot \frac{P_{crit}^{1/2}}{\ell^2 n^{1/2}} \quad \text{Column} \tag{2.2}$$

$$Efficiency = \frac{P_{crit}}{W} \propto \frac{E^{1/3}}{\rho} \cdot \frac{P_{crit}^{2/3}}{\ell^{5/3} n^{2/3}} \quad \text{Panel} \tag{2.3}$$

In each of the three equations, the first term represents the "material efficiency criterion" and the second the "structural loading coefficient".

In tension (Eq. (2.1)) the structural efficiency increases with the specific modulus of the material, E/ρ, as expected, but also with the *number* of tensile elements acting in parallel n. This is because end-fittings are needed to transmit the tensile forces in and out of the tension element (their efficiency being a function of the material strength σ). One can show that their additional weight (one end-fitting per element) decreases with n. Also, all other things being equal, a tensile structure becomes more efficient as the length over which the forces have to be carried increases (the penalty of the end fittings decreases) and when the loads are not very high ($P^{1/2}$). These principles are very well illustrated by biological structures such as tendons and spider webs or drag lines, where several elements act in parallel (collagen fibres in the former, silk fibres in the latter) and where each element has its own "end-fitting" to the substrate (bone for tendon, twigs, leaves or other for the spider). Depending on the strain levels, which are acceptable, the materials may be more or less close to their breaking limits. Since it is more efficient to work at high stresses than low ones, provided that sufficient Young's modulus is available, tensile elements are generally made of high strength-high modulus fibres, in biology (silk, cellulose, chitin) as well as in engineering (high tensile steel for cables, glass, carbon and aramid fibres in composites).

When the loads are compressive and the structure needs to resist buckling the situation is dramatically different. Eq. (2.2) and (2.3) show that low density materials, such as cellular solids —wood and cancellous bone for example— have the advantage and that this advantage is greater for panel-like structures than for columns. From a design point of view it is now important to concentrate compressive loads in as few members as possible, to decrease the distance over which loads have to be carried and, all other things being equal, to increase the loads as much as possible. In fact the opposite strategy to tensile loads is required (this is due to some extent that structural elements loaded in compression do not need complicated end-fittings, if at all). Once again these rules find confirmation in the evolution of both natural and engineering structures. Compressive structures tend to be massive to increase the bending stiffness EI which governs buckling, and can be very expensive unless low cost materials are used. This is the reason for the success of stone, brick and concrete and also for the use of ceramic reinforcement in biology (mollusk shells, bones, and calcified tendons).

An interesting example of engineering compromises dictated by the need to design against buckling is to compare the tibia-fibula pair of bones with the radius-ulna pair in bipeds and quadrupeds. In bipeds, the high compressive loads associated with locomotion and the advantage of having foot rotation with respect to the knee joint have led to a much more massive tibia than fibula (as suggested by Eq. (2.2)). In contrast, the ulna and radius, also needed for the rotation of the forearm, are roughly of the same diameter since they do not carry direct compression, which may lead to buckling. In quadrupeds the pair of bones in all four limbs follow the same pattern as in the legs of bipeds, i.e. of one pair more massive than the other, concentrating the compressive loads in as few elements as possible and still allowing some rotation. More interesting is the case of jumping quadrupeds (rabbits, kangaroos) which, owing to the higher compressive forces in their hind quarters, have sacrificed limb rotation by fusing the fibula and the tibia to end up with a single compressive element.

In bending, where both tension and compression are present, the efficiency of a beam or plate in stiffness-controlled situations follows the same rules as for buckling of columns or panels since, in either case, lateral deflections are determined by the bending stiffness EI of the element. As a result, stiffness-controlled structures are rarely approaching strain levels close to the breaking limits of the materials used, except perhaps for extremely brittle solids. In general when the stiffness requirements have been met the strength requirements have also been satisfied. A good illustration of this can be seen in trees where the bending stiffness of trunk and branches is optimised to limit deflections (high $E^{1/3}/\rho$) and, the bending stresses due to self-weight and wind loads are well within the tensile and compressive strengths of wood.

The only situations where the ultimate strength of the materials becomes more important are pure tensile structures, working at relatively high strains, and compressive structures which cannot buckle and which may fail if the crushing strength of the material is reached. Among biological structures, tendons, muscles, skins, spider silks belong to the former category; the only examples of the latter, which come to mind, are very short bones such as vertebrae.

The efficiency of *strength-controlled structures* follows rules similar to that given in Eq. (2.1).

In tension:

$$Efficiency = \frac{P}{W} \propto \frac{\sigma_t}{\rho} \cdot \frac{n^{1/2}}{\ell n^{1/2} + kP^{1/2}\sigma^{-1/2}} \qquad (2.4)$$

where this time σ_t is the tensile strength of the material.

In compression:

$$Efficiency = \frac{P}{W} \propto \frac{\sigma_c}{\rho} \qquad (2.5)$$

where σ_c is the compressive crushing strength.

The concepts outlined in this section can be used to compare the relative performance of materials and structures in different roles and applications. They provide general ideas rather that specific solutions but they are extremely useful for studying the evolution of biological systems in mechanical engineering terms.

2.3. BIOLOGICAL FIBROUS COMPOSITES AND DESIGN OPTIMISATION

In addition to the approach outlined in the previous section, the fact that most biological materials are fibrous in nature and that fibre deposition and organisation during growth occur under stress, adds another dimension to design. As mentioned in Chapter 1, fibres in general and polymeric fibres in particular, are essentially very efficient in tension but rather poor in compression. Bending structures are very common in biology, leading to possible problems on the compression side of beams and plates. There are two main solutions, which have emerged in nature to deal with the weakness of fibres in compression: prestressing and lateral support of fibres.

Prestressing of fibres with high tensile strength in composites is a very efficient way of avoiding failure in compression. Load-bearing fibres are essentially very slender columns, limited in their compressive performance by premature buckling. This failure mode is quite common in wood, for example, where microbuckling of cellulose fibres in the cell wall initiates compression failure and also in antler (Dinwoodie 1968 and Watkins 1986). If the fibres can be prestressed in tension, then the onset of buckling can be delayed, achieving higher bending strength in the structure. This is the same principle used in prestressed concrete, except that, in this case, the prestressing is designed to offset the low tensile strength of concrete.

In biology prestressing of fibres in tension can come from two mechanisms: growth and internal pressure. Growth-generated prestressing is best illustrated by trees, simply because it is a phenomenon which has been studied very extensively (Archer 1986). When fibrous materials are deposited in the cell walls of new cells in the live cambium region of a tree trunk, just under the bark, they are highly hydrated. As the cells matures, water is expelled by drying and by the deposition and cross-linking of lignin, the matrix which binds the cells together. The new cells elongated in the grain direction, try to contract longitudinally but are prevented from doing so freely because they are bonded to the older, mature cells in the interior layers which partially restrain the contraction. The net result is that the peripheral new cells are prestressed in tension, at the expense of compression in the inner older ones. This process is a cumulative one and the amount of peripheral longitudinal prestressing increases with time, and hence with the age and diameter of the tree trunk.

This growth-related mechanism is probably also responsible for the prestressing which is observed in many "soft" biological fibrous tissues such as skin or blood vessels. It appears to be extremely common and it makes a great deal of sense from a design efficiency point of view. It is worth mentioning that nothing like this is possible in artificial fibre-reinforced composites, which suffer from the same lack of compressive strength as their natural counterparts, although it would be extremely desirable.

The other method of prestressing fibres in tension relies on having internal pressure as the source. This is the solution, which dominates in all non-lignified plant tissues and organs, in many invertebrates such as worms and tunicates, in mammalian cartilage and also in sharks. Parenchyma plant cells have non-lignified walls in their tissues; in order to resist the compression due to bending forces from gravity and wind, particularly in stems, they rely on high turgor pressure to prestress the cell walls in tension. The pressure is controlled by the difference in the chemical potential of water between the inside and the outside of the cells. In this way, so long as the internal pressure is mantained, the fibres in the cell wall are always in tension and failure requires the breaking of the cellulose fibres which are strong in tension (Hiller and Jeronimidis 1996; Jeronimidis and Liu 1998). The same osmotic mechanisms are responsible for the prestressing of collagen fibres in cartilage, allowing this tissue to take very high compressive loads in spite of its fibrous structure.

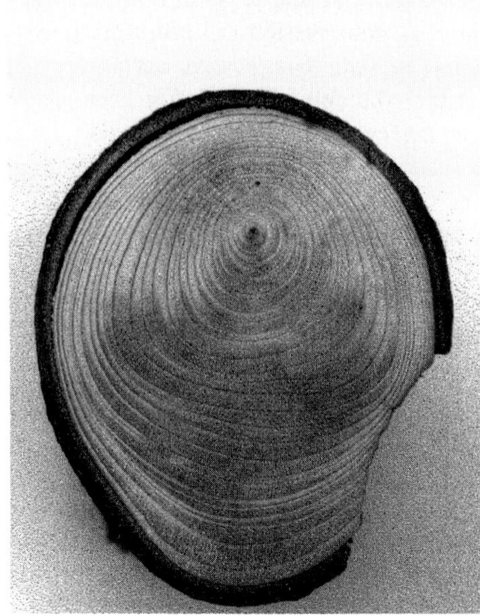

Fig. 2.6. Reaction wood formation on the underside of a branch of Lebanon Cedar (lower part of picture). Note also the eccentric growt.

Using internal pressure to prestress fibres in tension fits with the general rules for efficiency mentioned earlier. Diffuse tensile loads in as many tension elements as possible, i.e., the fibres (Eq. (2.1)) and concentrate compressive loads in as few elements as possible, i.e. the fluid under pressure (Eq. (2.2) or (2.3)). In invertebrates and sharks the fluid pressure needed to prestress the fibres is generated by muscle action and this provides them with efficient (i.e. low mass and hence low metabolic cost) semi-flexible structures for locomotion and swimming.

The alternative approach to prevent fibre buckling is to support the fibres laterally with stiff substances, increasing the interactions between fibres and fibres and matrix In plants, as mentioned earlier, this is mainly done by highly crosslinked phenolic substances (lignins); the same process is used to "harden" insect cuticles with chitin fibres. The main drawback of this approach is that the materials become extremely brittle. This is what happens in reaction wood of conifers, for example (Fig. 2.6). This tissue is called "compression" wood and it is a modification of the normal tissue located on the underside of branches, in compression, or on the compression side of the trunk of leaning trees. The cell wall structure is modified to resist increased compressive loads: the cell wall thickens (increased stability); the angle of the fibres becomes more perpendicular to the load direction (decreased axial load on fibres) and the lignification process is pushed further (increased lateral support of fibres). The net result is a tissue more adapted to resist compression but much more brittle in tension.

In bones and other stiff tissues, the supporting function to the polymer fibres (collagen) is provided by mineral substances. In order to be effective this solution requires that the mineralisation occurs at the level of the load-bearing fibres mineral unit, which becomes essentially a reinforced fibre within the composite. Depending on the extent and location of the mineralisation process, the mechanical properties of these type of tissues can be tailored for very high stiffness (but low fracture toughness), as in mammalian limb bones, or for high toughness but low stiffness, as in antler, which has to resist impact loads.

2.4. CONCLUSIONS

Design in nature offers many example of effective integration between efficiency attributes of the materials themselves and of the structures. Solutions are tailored to specific needs and requirements, which exploit the properties of the available materials as efficiently as possible. This is achieved by capitalising on the fibrous composite nature of most biological materials, on the hierarchical arrangements of fibre architectures, which allow to control and modify interactions between units, when needed, and by being able to offset weaknesses such as low compressive strength. Tissues can be modified continuously in living organism to adapt them and optimise them in different circumstances, as for example the formation of reaction wood in trees and resorption and redeposition in bone. Growth and especially growth under stress allows beneficial local and global modifications at all levels of structure, from the nano- to the macro- level. For the time being this processes are impossible to implement in man-made materials and structures. However, even though we cannot use these specific processes directly, we can learn a great deal from them by studying the results they have led to.

REFERENCES

Archer, R.R. (1986) *Growth Stresses and Strains in Trees* (Springer Series in Wood Science, Springer Verlag).

Ashby, M.F. and Jones, D.R.H. (1980) *Engineering Materials - An introduction to their Properties and Applications.* (Pergamon, Oxford).

Cox, H.L. (1965) *The Design of Structures of Least Weight.* (Pergamon, Oxford).

Dinwoodie, J.M. (1968) *Journal Inst. Wood Sci.,* **21**, 37.

Gordon, J.E. (1978) *Structures.* (Penguin Books, London).

Hiller, S. and Jeronimidis, G. (1996) *Journal of Materials Science,* **31**, 2779.

Jeronimidis, G. and Liu, J.H. (1998) in *Technische Biologie und Bionik 4. 4th Bionk Congress, Munchen,* ed. Nachtigall, W. and Wisser, A. (Gustav Fischer Verlag, Stuttgart) p. 65.

Jeronimidis, G. and Vincent, J.F.V. (1997) *Plant Biomechanics - Conference Proceedings, Reading, Vols I and II.* (The University of Reading, Reading).

Mattheck, C. and Vorberg, U. (1989) *Acta Botanica,* **104**, 399.

Rowe, N.P. and Speck, T. (1996) *International Journal Plant Sci*ence, **157**, 406.

Steven, G.P., Li, Q. and Xie, Y.M. (1999) in *Proc. NAFEMS World Congress 99 on Effective Engineering Analysis, Newport, Rhode Island,* (NAFEMS, Glasgow), p. 901.

Watkins, M. (1986) PhD Thesis, The University of Reading.

Worden, K. and Tomlinson, G.R. (1995) in *Proc. MIMR Conference, Sendai, Japan.*

Chapter 3

Structure and Mechanical Properties of Cortical Bone

Chapter 3

Structure and Mechanical Properties of Cortical Bone

M. ONTAÑÓN, C. APARICIO, M. P. GINEBRA and J. A. PLANELL

1. INTRODUCTION

Bone has been studied as a tissue for many years. It is however in the second part of this century that it has started to be analysed from a biomechanical point of view and as a material. This is why, at present it is possible to find many excellent reviews on the biomechanical aspects of bone. Books or chapters in books which can be recommended, amongst many others also excellent, include Cowin (1989), Currey (1990), Simon (1997) and in articles, the very recent by Weiner and Wagner (1998).

Bone is a living tissue and the structural feature which brings it into evidence is that it is interpenetrated by a complex network of blood vessels. Bone also undergoes continuous changes, it grows and it is modified by reconstruction processes, and all these transformations which take place during its life depend upon the stresses which act on it. Experience shows that when a bone remains immobile during a long period of time, it loses part of its mineral phase and becomes atrophied. On the contrary, its use leads to hypertrophy and to an increase in the bone mass. Wolff (1892) was the first to recognize that living bone changes according to the type of strains and stresses that it receives. These changes may be external, leading to superficial reconstruction and implying that new morphologies appear, or there may be internal changes, in terms of modification of porosity, mineral content or density of bone. These phenomena can be observed both in the growth process and also in a mature bone. In a review carried out by Evans (1973), the conclusion was reached that compressive stresses stimulate the growth of new bone. The process of reconstruction is the capacity of bone to adapt through a change of dimensions, shape or structure, to the mechanical requirements of its environment. These adaptations take place according to the so-called Wolff law: *the deposition of bone takes place when this is needed and resorption when it is not needed.*

The evolutionary process experienced by the skeleton has led to an optimum "design" of bone, to a biological solution better adapted to the mechanical requirements and limiting factors such as the nutritional reserves, muscular power and compromise between size and weight. This optimum design is based on two main premises: a) the presence of macroscopic and microscopic features which minimise the working stresses and b) an appropriate distribution of material with the aim of achieving a minimum weight (or volume). The skeleton performs two basic main functions, a mechanical function and a metabolic function. Some skeletal elements provide protection to vital internal organs such as heart, brain or blood-forming marrow, from external forces. It also provides internal support by offering insertion sites for muscles and tendons, which are essential for movement, providing also rigid levers for articular movement. Bone also plays a relevant role, together with other tissues, in the general metabolism of calcium, acting as the main deposit of calcium salts (97% of the total content of the body). An important difference between bone and cartilage is that bone is strongly vascularised and this means that calcium salts can be rapidly mobilised into the general circulation.

3.2. COMPOSITION OF BONE

Mineral ions, water and an organic matrix, approximately in equal proportions by volume, form bone as shown in Table 3.1. The precise composition varies with species, age, sex, the specific bone, and whether or not the bone is affected by a disease. The composition also depends on the type of bone tissue (cortical or trabecular), as shown in Table 3.2. Trabecular bone has a higher water content and a lower mineral content than cortical bone.

The main protein of the matrix is collagen type I, and it represents about 70 to 90% of the non-mineralised components of bone. The non-collagenic proteins, phosphoproteins, glycoproteins, sialoproteins, glaproteins and proteoglicans represent something ranging between 2 and 5% of the bone matrix and their role in the mineralisation process is unknown.

Table 3.1. Results of hydrated bone assays for 16 species using cortical bone from the tibia and the femur.

Species*	Specific Gravity	Water content, vol %	Mineral ash, vol %	Organic $+CO_2$, vol %
Fish (2)	1.80	39.6	29.5	36.9
Turtle (6)	1.81	37.0	29.2	40.1
Frog (4)	1.93	35.2	34.5	38.5
Polar bear (1)	1.92	33.0	26.2	40.1
Human being (15)	1.94	15.5	39.9	41.8
Elephant (1)	2.00	20.0	41.4	41.5
Monkey (3)	2.09	23.0	42.6	41.1
Cat (1)	2.05	23.6	42.2	40.5
Horse (3)	2.02	25.0	41.0	40.5
Chicken (4)	2.04	24.5	41.7	38.7
Dog (10)	1.94	28.0	38.7	35.5
Goose (2)	2.04	23.0	42.7	37.6
Cow (5)	2.05	26.2	42.6	36.2
Guinea pig (2)	2.10	25.0	43.5	37.0
Rabbit (2)	2.12	24.5	45.0	37.2
Rat (12)	2.24	20.2	49.9	38.3

* The number of adults of each species sampled is indicated in parentheses after the common species name. Table from Cowin *et al.* (1987) using data from Blitz and Pellegrino (1969). Reproduced with permission.

Table 3.2. Results of hydrated bone assays of cortical and trabecular bone for four species using cortical bone from the tibia or femur and trabecular bone from the vertebrae.

Species	Specific Gravity*	Water fraction, vol %	Ash fraction, vol %	Organic fraction, vol %	Volatile inorganic fraction, vol %
			Trabecular bone		
Human being	1.92	27.0	33.9	34.9	4.2
Monkey	1.89	27.1	32.9	36.1	4.0
Cow	1.93	28.1	33.5	34.2	4.2
Dog	1.91	28.8	32.6	34.5	4.2
			Cortical bone		
Human being	1.99	23.9	37.7	33.8	4.6
Monkey	2.04	23.7	38.2	33.7	4.7
Cow	2.00	25.2	36.6	33.6	4.6
Dog	2.00	22.3	36.8	36.3	4.6

*This is the specific gravity of the trabeculae, not the apparent specific gravity of the cancellous structure, which would be a number less than 1. Table from Cowin *et al.*. (1987) using data from Gong *et al.*. (1964). Reproduced with permission.

The collagen molecule is 300 nm long and 1.5 nm diameter, and it is formed by three chains of polypeptides (α) linked among themselves by a triple helix (see

Chapter 8). The fibres are joined by means of intra and intermolecular bonds and their preferential orientation is parallel to the main axis. Generally the collagen fibres provide the structure over which the mineral phase of bone is deposited. The existence of a molecule acting as a seed for the nucleation of apatite crystals is not considered, but in fact it is essential for the formation of bone.

Lipids and carbohydrates are related with the synthesis and the working of bone. Carbohydrates can be found in the proteoglicans and in the intracellular glycogen. The lipids are found mainly in the membranes and they present themselves as proteolipids and complexes Ca-acid phospholipid-PO_4. These seem to be the motors of hydroxyapatite deposition (Boskey 1981), and they control the flux of nutrients and electrolytes inside and outside the cell. They also determine the specific enzyme properties of the membrane. The rest of lipids are important in the development of bone acting as a nutrition source and keeping cellular integrity.

The enzymes and hormones are also involved as non-mineral components of bone. The enzymes act in the synthesis of the components of the matrix, in the reconstruction of bone and in the mineral deposition. The hormones play a role in all the processes which occur in the bone tissue.

The amount of water may vary, producing important changes in the mechanical properties of bone (Currey 1964; Lees and Davidson 1977). When the water is eliminated, the bone becomes stiffer and less tough. The presence of water has mechanical effects besides being the medium in which the transport of nutrients and products of the cellular metabolism takes place.

The mineral component of mature bone is made of calcium phosphates, the most important of which is hydroxyapatite, $Ca_{10}(PO_4)_6(OH)_2$, with a calcium deficiency ranging between 5 and 10% (Posner 1987). It contains a wide variety of calcium phosphates, including deficient apatites, witlockites, carbonated apatites, citrate and small quantities of fluorine, magnesium, sodium and chlorine (Driessens and Verbeeck 1986 and 1990). The bone apatite is characterised by carbonate substitutions and a certain degree of loss of crystallographic order.

The nature of the crystalline phase has been widely discussed. Certain authors defend the hypothesis of the existence of an initial phase of amorphous phosphate (Wuthier and Eanes 1975), whilst others consider hydroxyapatite as the first phase (Murphree *et al.*. 1982). The crystals are constantly resorbed and depositioned at a fast rate during growth and at a slow rate when the individual becomes mature.

The size and shape of the hydroxyapatite crystals have also been widely discussed. The literature is confused in this regard since factors such as the species, the age and the state of health of the individual determine changes in their structure. Studies by means of X-ray diffraction and direct measurements by means of transmission electron microscopy identify crystals shaped as plates, of a length ranging between 30 and 100 nm (*c* direction), a width between 20 and 40 nm and a thickness ranging between 4 and 6 nm (Voegel *et al.*. 1977; Posner 1969), although other studies have demonstrated the existence of even smaller crystals which may appear as amorphous when analysed by X-ray diffraction, and even some others which seem to be spherical with diameters ranging between 18 and 40 nm (Driessens and Verbeeck 1990; Boskey and Posner 1984).

A three-dimensional model showing the distribution of crystals in the bone matrix has been developed (Lees 1979). Most of the crystals are distributed with their *c*-axis parallel to the longitudinal axis of the collagen molecules and the rest of the crystals are distributed perpendicularly to it.

Moreover, the observation of a reversible and anisotropic contraction in compact bone when dehydrated in vacuum and at room temperature (Marino *et al.*. 1967; Lees *et al.*. 1979) has been interpreted in terms of the existence of a free space in the matrix, which accommodates the displacements of the crystals. In compact bovine bone a volume reduction of about 6.5% has been estimated. According to certain authors (Rougvie and Bear 1953) only the organic matrix is able to undergo such change when dehydrated. The variability of the mineral content also demonstrates the existence of such a free space in the mineralised tissue. Currey (1979a) obtained values for the ash content ranging between 59% for deer antler ad 86% for the whale bulla tympanica.

As reported in Table 3.1, Blitz and Pellegrino (1969) realised that there is a great inverse variation in the mineral volume fraction and in the water volume fraction for long bones in different species. They presented variations in mineral, which ranged from 29% in tortoise up to 50% in mice, and variations in water, which ranged from 37 % down to 20% respectively. The organic component for all the species ranged between 36 and 42%. Apparently, the mineral substitutes water in the mineralised tissue (Robinson and Elliott 1957), whilst the volume fraction of the organic component does not change.

In this three-dimensional model the weakest part of the structure seems to be the intermolecular space. The hydroxyapatite crystals have a very high elastic modulus. Katz (1971) gave a value of 114 GPa. The axial Young's modulus of the collagen molecule has been estimated to be 1.41 GPa (Lees and Davidson 1977, Enomoto and Krimm, 1962). Considering that the intermolecular bonds are individual chains in relation with the triple helix of the structure of the collagen molecule (Ramachandran and Reddi 1976), it can be concluded that these bonds break more easily than any of the other two elements, even being partially surrounded by mineral crystals (Lees 1979).

It has been noticed that when bone is considered as a composite material, its behaviour is not so clear as in other materials. The basic problem lies in the observation levels at which it can be structured. The cortical can be considered as a solid hierarchically organised, and formed by elements that have a discrete structure (Katz 1980a; Lakes 1993; Park 1979).

At different scales (Table 3.3) the structure of the cortical can be characterised as *particulate* (crystals of hydroxyapatite), *fibrous* (fibres of collagen and osteons), *porous* (vessels and lacunae of the osteocytes) and *lamellar* (lamellae) (Lakes 1993), being difficult to discern at which level it has to be studied. Fig. 3.1 rationalises this hierarchical organisation.

Table 3.3. Hierarchical structure of cortical bone.

Hierarchic level	*Structure*	*Scale*	*Method* (resolution)
Bend specimen	Compact bone	3.6 x 3.6 x 40 mm	Bending test (>1mm^2)
Osteons and laminae	Fibres and laminae	250 μm	Acoustic microscopy (30-50 μm)
Haversian channels	Pores	50-100 μm	Microhardness (30-50 μm)
Lacunae	Pores	5-15 μm	Microhardness (10-30 μm)
Lamellae	Laminar	5 μm	SEM* and spectrometry (5-10μm)
Fibres of collagen	Fibre	1-2 μm	Histology (optical microscopy 100-200X) (1-5 μm)
Crystals HAP**	Particles	5-50 nm	TEM*** (1-10 nm)

The most usual resolution for each one of the experimental techniques is shown in brackets.
* SEM: scanning electron microscopy,
** HAP: Hydroxyapatite,
*** TEM: transmission electron microscopy. Adapted from Park (1979), Katz (1980a) and Lakes (1993).

The dependence of the mechanical behaviour of cortical bone upon the size of its phases and their distribution starts at an elemental level (< 0.005 μm) and goes on to the microstructural (1-10 μm) which can be observed by SEM (Frasca *et al.* 1981).

At the next hierarchical level (10-50 μm), the mechanical behaviour of cortical bone may be analysed by means of microhardness tests (Amprino 1958), which allow one to quantify the physical effects of the changes in mineral content at a small scale (Evans *et al.*. 1990) and the relations with the elastic modulus and the ultimate strength (Currey and Brear 1990, Hodgskinson *et al.*. 1989). The microhardness has been combined with ultrasonic tests in order to evaluate the intrinsic homogeneity of the cortical (Yoon and Katz 1976). The acoustic scanning microscopy technique has been used to evaluate the changes in the local properties of the cortical as for the mineral content (Peck and Briggs 1987), the acoustic impedance and the stiffness (Meunier *et al.*. 1988), with a resolution ranging from 4 up to 100 μm.

At a more macroscopic scale, (> 1mm), the physical characteristics and the mechanical behaviour are function of the structure and the combination of the properties of the different phases like the volume fraction, the distribution and the bonds between the different phases (Bundy 1985; Lees 1979; Less and Davidson 1977).

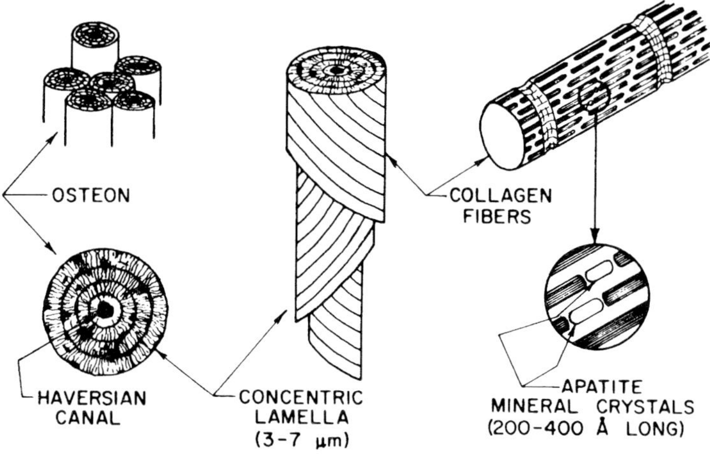

Fig. 3.1. The detailed structure of an osteon. From Cowin *et al.*. (1987). Reproduced with permission.

3.3. INTEGRATION AND ORGANISATION LEVELS

The study of bone may be carried out considering different levels of observation or hierarchical levels. The possibility of specifying the stage in which the work is being carried out is of great importance in order to interpret adequately the results obtained.

3.3.1 Macroscopic level

The bone architecture presents two categories which can be seen easily: *the compact bone* (or *cortical*) and *the spongy (*or *trabecular cancellous) bone.* The compact bone is a dense tissue. Its aspect is that of a continuous solid mass in which the only empty spaces are meant for blood vessels and bone cells or osteocytes. The trabecular bone consists in a network of septa or trabeculae intercommunicated and occupied by bone marrow. The main difference between the two types of bone is their porosity. The ratio between the volume of bone tissue and the volume occupied by pores is large in compact bone. The inverse relationship applies to spongy bone.

3.3.2 Microanatomic level

Long bones such as femur or tibia are the kind of morphologies that will be described in the present analysis. They are characterised by a long cylindrical shape and they are aligned in relation to a main axis. They are structured in three characteristic regions, which are sketched in Fig. 3.2 and listed below:

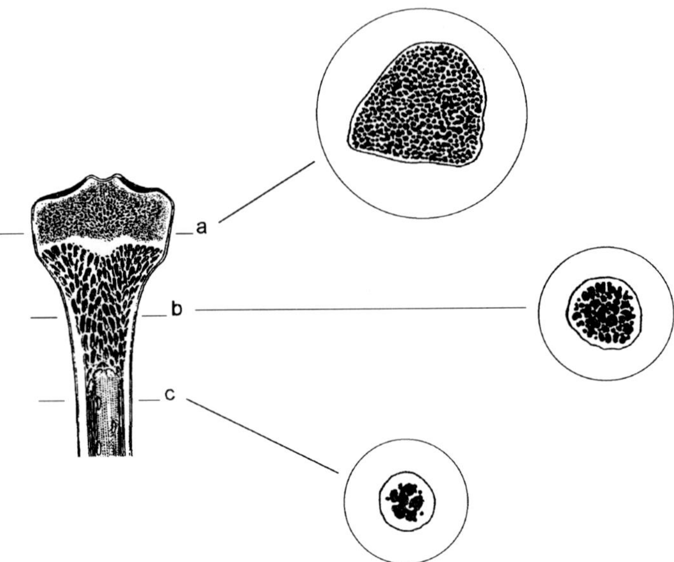

Fig. 3.2. Rational of the microanatomic organization of a long bone. Epiphysis, b) Metaphysis, and c) Diaphysis. Transversal cuts are shown inside of the circles where it can be observed the cortex or cortical region with a thick wall of compact bone (a), and the medullar region (b). Adapted from Lessertisseur and Saban (1967) and Ricqlès (1975).

- *Epiphysis*. Extreme parts of a long bone, which are mainly formed by trabecular bone covered by a thin layer of compact bone. A layer of specialised hyaline cartilage persists on the articular surface.

- *Metaphysis*. Region of transition between the epiphysis and the diaphysis. It is the region where the cartilaginous epiphysary plate or the cartilage of growth can be found, that together with the adjacent trabecular bone constitute a zone of longitudinal growth in the young bone. The ossification of the plate determines the fusion of the epiphysis and the diaphysis meaning the end of the period of active growth of bone.

- *Diaphysis*. Cylinder of compact bone, the internal surface of which closes the medullar cavity. This cavity is covered by the endosteum, a thin cellular layer highly vascularised. Externally the diaphysis is covered by the periosteum, a layer of conjunctive tissue with osteogenic capacity or with the ability to form bone.

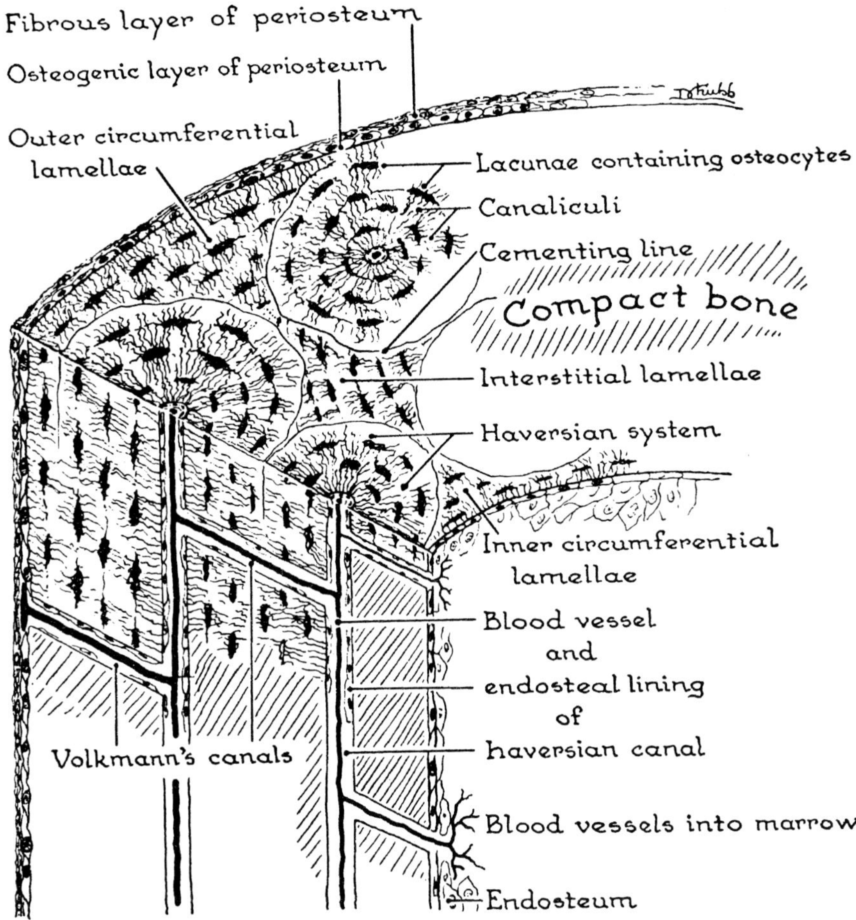

Fig. 3.3. The basic structure of compact bone. From Ham (1969). Reproduced with permission.

Before introducing the histologic level and in order to assist in further descriptions, a few previous concepts are necessary, and some of them are represented in Fig. 3.3 where the basic structure of compact bone is shown, and in the micrograph reproduced in Fig. 3.4:

- *Lamellae.* In mature bone, the collagen fibres run parallel to each other to form laminae called lamellae. The fibers in successive lamellae are about at right angles to the fibers in the previous one. The lamellae can be arranged in concentric cylindrical layers, in osteons, or parallel, like in the interstitial lamellae or in the outer circumferential lamellae.

- *Lacunae.* Array of ellipsoidally shaped cavities contained in the interfaces between the lamellae, which contain bone cells (*osteocytes*). The osteocytes are living cells physiologically active, which are mutually connected through cytoplasmatic prolongations inside very thin channels called *canaliculi.*

- *Simple primary vessel.* Thin vascular channel that does not present lamellar bone around it. The vessel is submerged in a mineralised matrix of bone of new formation.

- *Primary osteons.* Vascular channel surrounded by concentric lamellar bone of centripetal deposition and without previous resorbtion at the periphery of the channel.

- *Secondary osteons = Havers system.* Structures originated from a process of erosion initiated from the vascular channel towards the periphery, and followed by a later centripetal deposition of concentric lamellar bone. The secondary osteons are surrounded by a cement line as the result of bone resorption. The vascular channel of the centre of the secondary osteon is called haversian channel, and it has a diameter, which varies depending on the amount of lamellar bone deposited.

- *Primary and secondary bone.* The primary bone corresponds to bone deposited in a zone where bone tissue has not existed. The secondary bone corresponds to bone deposited in areas where the initial bone tissue has been resorbed (the concepts “primary” or “secondary” do not indicate an ontogenetic or phylogenetic temporal sequence).

- *Haversian tissue.* In cortical bone, secondary osteons can be distributed either highly dispersed or tightly packed. In this later case successive generations of secondary osteons may substitute one another. Each one of these generations is called, 1st, 2nd, 3rd, … generation.

- *Interstitial systems.* They constitute residual fragments of haversian systems of previous generations, which have been destroyed by the process of internal reorganisation that bone undergoes during its life.

- *Volkman channels.* Primary vascular channels with radial orientation, which are present in compact bone. These channels mutually connect different osteons.

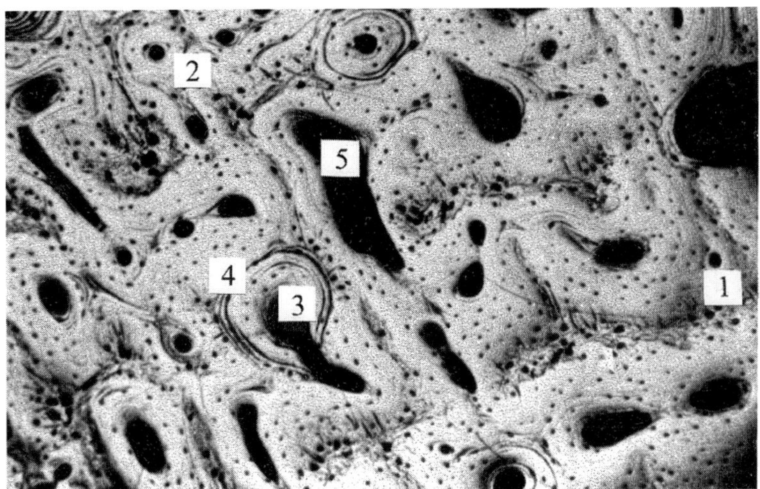

Fig. 3.4. Transversal section of the diaphysis of horse ulna. 1) Simple primary vascular channel, 2) primary osteon, 3) Haversian system, 4) Interstitial cement line, 5) Resorbtion cavity and 6) Lacunae.

- *Bone reconstruction.* It corresponds to a normal process more or less continuous of formation of new bone related with processes of morphogenesis during the initial stages of growth and with mechanical and physiological demands of the individual. The reconstruction includes two basic processes: the *resorbtion* and the *redeposition* of new bone.

- *Cement lines.* Irregular areas of approximately 1-2 μm in thickness which show the levels of discontinuity in the bone tissue. They are the result of a reconstruction process of bone and therefore they allow to differentiate the primary from the secondary bone, as well as the secondary osteons. These are weak regions from a mechanical point of view. When observed in the optical microscope under normal and polarised light, they appear bright and refringent respectively. They contain a low amount of collagen fibres and a high degree of mineralisation.

- *Acellular bone tissue.* It does not show osteocytes as such, but only cytoplasmatic extensions inside long and thin canaliculi coming from the bone cells.

3.3.3 ***Histological level***

The cortex or cortical region is characterised by the presence of different types of tissue. Tissues are associations of cells specialised in performing a specific function. Their classification has been confusing during a very long time because different authors had been using terminology that was ill defined and lacked precision.

From a general point of view, three basic criteria have been taken for the classification of biological tissues (Ricqlès 1975, Francillon-Vieillot et. al. 1990).

A first classification (A) is centred in the organisation of the bone matrix formed mainly by collagen fibres. The second category (B) does it from the bone vascularisation models. The third category and the less properly defined (C) uses the criterion of the ontogenetic models of formation of bone tissue. At present, the basic idea is to combine all these criteria in a single biological classification, which defines each of the bone tissues and allows their functional interpretation.

3.3.3.1 Organisation of the bone matrix. This classification criterion is mainly based in the orientation of the collagen fibres in the bone matrix. The three bone matrices, which will be defined, are related at the same time by other classification criteria such as the vascularisation, the shape of the bone cells or the degree of mineralisation, among others.

a.- *Fibrous bone matrix*
The collagen fibres that constitute it are of variable size and are randomly distributed. The bone cells or osteocytes are globular and with a high density of canaliculi. Under polarised light the fibrous matrix does not transmit light. This matrix, deposited in compact bone mainly from the periosteum is associated to a rapid ontegenia, which determines a poor degree of organisation and a dense vascularisation. The mineralisation degree may be high. This type of organisation is characteristic of embrionary bones and the majority of bones where ossification happens without going through a cartilaginous stage. Generally it may experience an erosion process during growth, or it may end its formation with the deposition of a thin lamellar matrix in the vascular spaces producing primary osteons. Whatever tissue that presents a matrix with such characteristics is called fibrous bone tissue.

b.- *Bone matrix of parallel fibres or pseudo-lamellar matrix*
The fibres of collagen are long and they mutually orient themselves parallel to each other. The osteocytes are flat and they are approximately randomly distributed. With polarised light a clear anisotropy is observed: dark phases and light phases depending on the orientation of the fibres (birefringence). The rate of deposition represents an intermediate degree between the fibrous matrix and the lamellar matrix. In this case, a tissue characterised by a matrix of collagen fibres mutually parallel is known as a bone tissue of parallel fibres.

c.- *Lamellar bone matrix*
In this case a high level of organisation is present. It is formed by fibrous layers or structural levels called lamellae positioned successively across the matrix. Each lamella shows a direction of the collagen fibres, which is inverse to the next lamella. Under polarised light the lamellae appear alternatively dark and clear. The osteocytes present flat shapes and they have very few canaliculi. This type of matrix is associated to a low ontogenic rate. Lamellar bone may present different origins giving rise to the lamellae in primary and secondary osteons and trabeculae of spongy bone in the medullar region. The bone tissue characterised by a matrix of fibres with alternate orientation in each consecutive lamella is known as lamellar bone tissue.

The next classification criterion is based on the models of bone vascularisation.

3.3.3.2 Vascularisation. Both the criteria of vascularisation and distribution of collagen fibres are strongly related. From a general point of view, two main types of tissues can be differentiated:

a.- *Non vascular bone tissue or avascular bone tissue*
Compact bone tissue without any type of intrinsic vascular network. The avascular primary bone does not contain either primary vascular channels or primary osteons. The description of the avascular bone can be carried out from the kind of extracellular matrix that can be fibrous, with parallel fibres, or lamellar. The osteocytes present in this type of tissue develop systems of canaliculi that substitute from a physiological point of view the lack of vascular channels, and they carry out the exchange of fluids between the bone and the body. The avascular bone forms the major part of the cortical bone tissue of snakes and lizards.

b.- *Vascular bone tissue*
Bone tissue that contains an intrinsic network of blood vessels. The classification of such tissues may be carried out according with the nature, the number and the orientation of the vascular channels and osteons, as well as the fibrilar organisation of the bone matrix.

If the two previously described criteria are combined, type of matrix and model of vascularisation, it is possible to generate a new typological classification which will give more information about the different bone tissues studied and which is represented in Fig. 3.5:

a.- *Laminar bone tissue.* This bone tissue is included in the complex named fibro-lamellar tissue. It is characterised by the presence of a fibrous matrix that surrounds the osteons, primaries or secondaries, made all of them by lamellar or pseudo-lamellar bone tissue. In this tissue the vascularisation is given by a large number of longitudinal primary osteons distributed in consecutive circumferential levels. The presence of many connections or anastomosis between the osteons of the different vascular levels is observed. A lamina will be defined as the thickness of bone centred at a vascular level and surrounded by fibrous matrix.

b.- *Plexiform bone tissue.* Very similar to the laminar bone but more densely vascularised. The vascular levels of each lamina are united by vascular channels oriented radially, producing a three-dimensional network. It is the characteristic tissue of animals that are growing very fast. The process of secondary reconstruction happens very slowly and depends on the maturation of the animal. In bovine bone this process is slower than in human bone in such a way that the cortex will present Haversian bone, only when the bull will be old (Carter *et al.* 1976; Wainright *et al.* 1976).

c.- *Radial fibro-lamellar bone tissue.* New variation, characterised by the abundance of primary osteons radially oriented. It corresponds to a process of rapid deposition of bone.

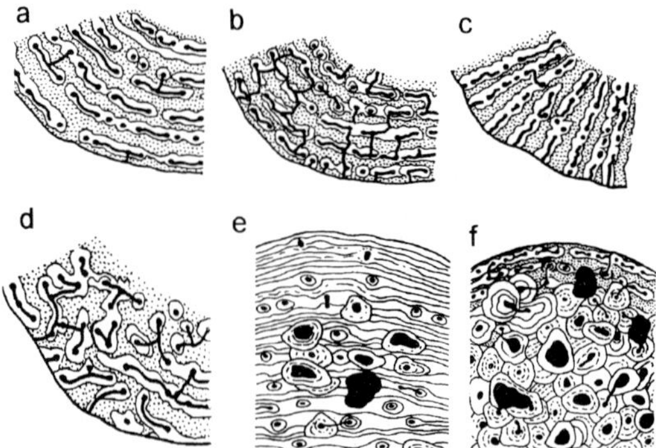

Fig. 3.5. Typological classification of primary compact bone tissues. a) Laminar bone tissue (fibro-lamellar bone tissue), b) Plexiform bone tissue, c) Radial fibro-lamellar bone tissue, d) Reticular fibro-lamellar bone tissue, e) Spread or diffuse haversian structure in a zonal-lamellar cortex, and f) Dense Haversian bone substituting a primary fibro-lamellar cortex. Adapted from Ricqlès (1975).

d.- *Reticular bone tissue*. New variation of the fibro-lamellar complex of the compact bone tissue. The primary osteons present an oblique orientation and irregular anastomosis between them. This tissue seems associated to a fast deposition of bone.

In a long bone the vascular network is formed by different points of arterial supply. The drainage takes place through venous channels, which abandon the bone through the surfaces not covered by the articular cartilage. One or two nutritional arteries cross the diaphysis obliquely. Once they arrive at the medullar cavity after crossing the cortical, they become ramified into ascendent and descendent branches, which go along the bone up to the extremes. These arteries are further subdivided (arterioles) and they penetrate into the endosteal surface in order to reach the cortex of the diaphysis where the Havers systems are found. In this region veins present a typical radial disposition.

3.3.4 Bone as a material

The previous ways in which bone can be described reveal the complexity and the structural diversity of this connective tissue which can dynamically adapt itself, in terms of its own structure, to the functions that it has to perform, both physiological and mechanical.

To organise all the available information referred to the hierarchical levels of Table 3.3 in terms of structural patterns allowing direct mechanical implications is not an easy task. However, Weiner and Wagner (1998) have managed to build up a rationale which starting from the nanometric level and ending at the macroscopic level, relates the seven levels of hierarchical organisation of bone tissue (Fig. 3.6) with the mechanical properties that every architectural distribution sustains.

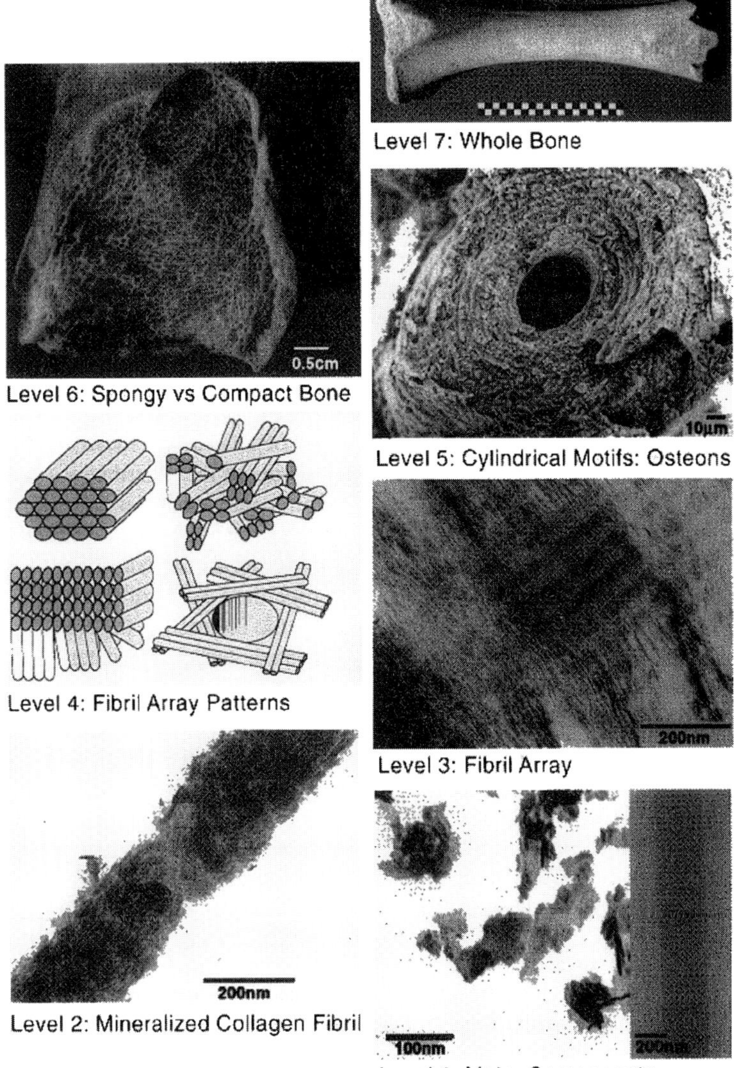

Fig. 3.6. The 7 hierarchical levels of organisation of the bone family materials. Level 1: Isolated crystals from human bone (left side) and part of an unmineralised and unstained collagen fibril from turkey tendon observed in vitreous ice in the TEM (right side). Level 2: TEM micrograph of a mineralised collagen fibril from turkey tendon. Level 3: TEM micrograph of a thin section of mineralised turkey tendon. Level 4: Four fibril array patterns of organisation found in the bone family of materials. Level 5: SEM micrograph of a single osteon from human bone. Level 6: Light micrograph of a fractured section through a fossilised (about 5500 years old) human femur. Level 7: Whole bovine bone (scale: 10 cm). From Weiner and Wagner (1998). Reproduced with permission.

The main constituents of the tissue are placed at the first level, i.e. the crystals of the mineral phase (apatite), the fibrils of type I collagen and the water. The composition of each one of the components, their different mechanical properties and the different relative proportions of each component make the bone a true composite material.

The basic structural unit of bone tissue is found at the second level: the mineralised collagen fibril. The position and organisation of the mineral phase and the water within the triple helix of type I collagen molecules are the decisive factors in the description of this level, in which a platelet reinforced fibril structure is found. This structure is highly orthotropic, due mainly to the shaped and distribution of the apatite crystals inside the fibril.

The third level of organisation corresponds to the mutual arrangement of fibrils, which takes place as arrays or bundles all along their length. This arrangement implies a great anisotropy, both structural and mechanical. This is the reason why at the next level the structural diversity becomes rationalised in order to achieve different structure with isotropic and anisotropic properties.

The different organisation patterns of the groups of fibrils are found at the fourth level. This level is from different points of view the key to understand the adaptability of the tissue to the different mechanical requirements. It is by varying such organisation patterns that the tissue may specialise and respond to a specific mechanical function. A pattern corresponding to a parallel array of fibrils, as in the case of the bone matrix with parallel fibers, will give a better response to the mechanical tension. Alternatively, a pattern of aligned fibrils as in the lamellar bone, i.e., with alternated inversely oriented fibrils, is meant to sustain forces in any direction. The pattern constituted by a radial alignment of fibrils allows compressive loading in a preferential direction. The main difficulty for a thorough study of the specific mechanical properties of the different organisation patterns of fibrils is that it is almost impossible to make macroscopic specimens containing only a single structure to be tested. In spite of these great difficulties, a great effort is being made in order to gain a deeper knowledge about the relations between structure and function. In this sense, novel testing techniques are being developed by designing and making specimens with dimensions even below one millimetre in some of them (Rho *et al.* 1999; Liu *et al.* 1999).

The fifth level of organisation corresponds to the remodelation structures such as the osteonal structure. At this level it is difficult to stablish good correlation between the cylinder structure of osteonal bone and the corresponding mechanical implications, mainly when compared with the planar organisations of the lamellae. In this sense this type of structures seem to be developed attending mainly the function of vascularisation of the bone than any mechanical function.

Finally, levels six and seven of the hierarchical organisation correspond to the macroscopic levels. The sixth level differentiates between trabecular and compact bone, while the seventh refers to the shape and design of the bone.

This brilliant description of the hierarchical organisation of the bone tissue made by Weiner and Wagner (1998) allows a good understanding of bone as a complex material. However, since bone is a living tissue in a constant remodelling process, vascularisation and cell activity will produce a constant evolution of local microstructures, which keep changing in time and space.

3.4. MECHANICAL PROPERTIES OF THE CORTICAL OF BONE

In this part the main mechanical properties of bone are described, the types of loads at which it has to work, and the factors which affect its strength and stiffness, as well as its fracture and fatigue behaviour. The aim of this description is to give a general idea of the mechanical behaviour of bone in normal conditions.

3.4.1 Factors affecting the mechanical behaviour of cortical bone

A simple approach to the mechanical properties of bone which provides information of important parameters such as stiffness and strength can be made through a tensile test which will give a stress-strain curve such as that shown in Fig. 3.7. The stress-strain curve presents two parts: a region linear elastic where the loads do not cause a permanent deformation and where the Hooke's law is valid ($\sigma = E\ \varepsilon$), and a plastic region in which the load increases more slowly with strain, up to fracture which takes place approximately at a deformation of about 1.5%. The trabecular bone can be deformed up to 7%. It seems that its porous structure gives to it a better capacity for storing energy (Carter *et al.*. 1976). According to Currey and Brear (1974) and Mauch *et al.*. (1992), the behaviour after the elastic limit is due to the damage caused by small cracks that have not propagated initially. According to these authors, bovine bone with a relatively high mineral content is unable to admit deformations larger than 0.0005 without suffering irreversible harm. If the load, which produces this deformation, continues to be applied, the produced damage will continue as well. The less mineralised bone, such as the deer antler seems to be able to experience larger deformations before suffering damage.

The stiffness of the material is evaluated from the linear elastic region of the stress-strain curve. The stored energy can be measured as the area under the stress-strain curve.

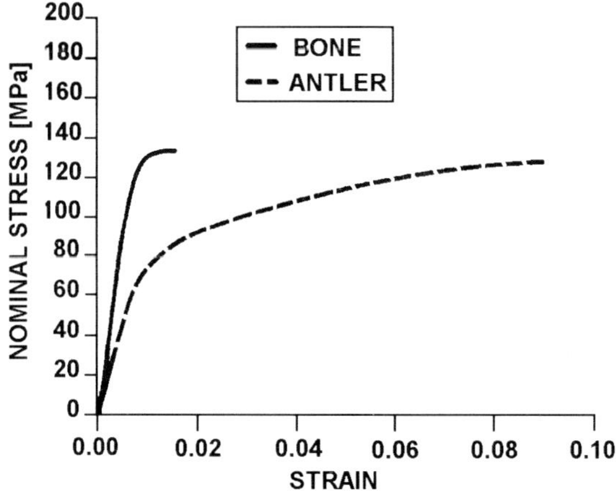

Fig. 3.7. Stress-strain curves for bovine cortical bone and antler in a simple pull to failure. Adapted from Zioupos *et al.*. (1996b).

The mechanical behaviour of bone is strongly influenced by the fact that bone is a viscoelastic material. The combination of elastic and viscoelastic interactions in the material implies that the stress or the strain in the material depends strongly upon the rate of deformation or the rate of loading respectively (Fig. 3.8).

A difference from the elastic materials where the deformation energy is stored during loading and it is recovered during unloading, in materials linearly viscoelastic the energy is dissipated as viscous flow. Stress and strain vary out of phase. It is observed that bone is stiffer and stronger at high deformation rates. It has been also seen that the deformation at fracture and toughness vary with the deformation rate. Carter and Hayes (1977a) found that both the strength and the elastic modulus are proportional to the 0.06 power of the deformation rate. This relation was considered for all bones of the skeleton. The effect of density and the deformation rate upon the compressive strength or ultimate stress of bone can be expressed as:

$$\sigma_{ult} = 68\ \rho^2\ (d\varepsilon/dt)^{0.06} \tag{3.1}$$

where σ_{ult} is the compressive strength or ultimate stress in MPa, ρ is the density in g/cm^3, and $d\varepsilon/dt$ is the deformation rate expressed in s^{-1}. Fig. 3.9 represents this relationship. It can be observed that the strength of bone depends strongly on density and more weakly on deformation rate.

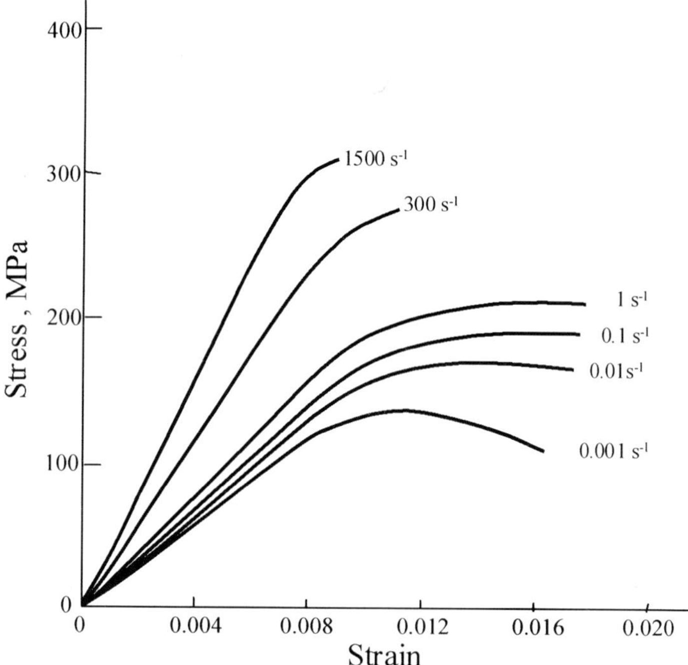

Fig. 3.8. Influence of strain-rate on the stress-strain behaviour in bone. Adapted from McElhaney (1966).

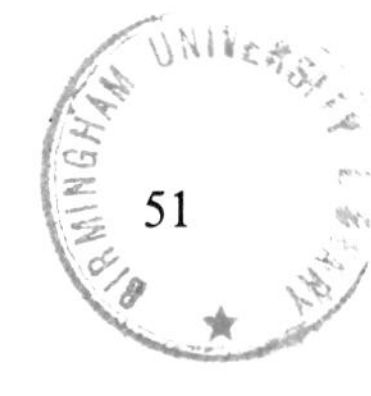

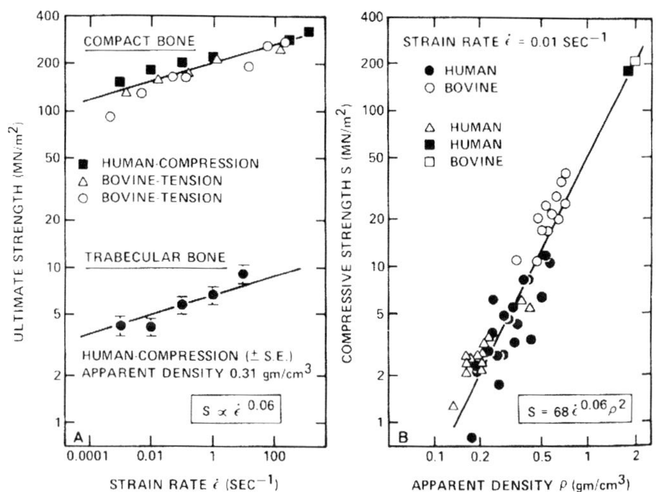

Fig. 3.9. (A) Influence of strain rate on the ultimate strength of compact and trabecular bone tested without marrow in situ. Data denoted by filled circles are from this study (±S.E.), filled squares are from Mc Elhaney and Byars (1965), open triangles from Crowninshield and Pope (1974), and open circles from Wright and Hayes (1976). (B) Influence of apparent density on the compressive strength of trabecular and compact bone. Data denoted by filled and open circles are from this study, open triangles are from Galante *et al.*. (1970), filled and open squares from Mc Elhaney and Byars (1965). From Carter and Hayes (1976a). Reproduced with permission.

The deformation rate at which a bone may be working in normal conditions ranges between 0.001 s^{-1} for slow walking and 0.01 s^{-1} for a more intense activity.

An important factor to take into account when considering the mechanical properties of bone is its anisotropy. Based on its structure, long bones have been supposed to have transversely isotropic symmetry. The plane of isotropy is the transverse plane of the long bone, and the unique direction is the axis of the bone. Tables 3.4 and 3.5 show this effect of anisotropy on the tensile and compressive properties of bovine and human bone respectively. The strengths in tension and compression in the axial direction are denoted by σ_0^+ and σ_0^- respectively. The strength in tension and compression in a direction making an angle of θ° with respect to the long axis of the bone will be denoted by σ_θ^+ and σ_θ^-.

Many other factors exist that produce variations in the strength of bone: age and sex of the animal, the location of the bone, the orientation of the load, the conditions of the tests carried out (dry or wet), the preservation state and the physiological conditions.

It has been found that both the tensile and compressive strength, the elastic modulus and the hardness become higher when the measurements are carried out in dehydrated bone (Fig. 3.10).

The shear strength in the direction perpendicular to the bone axis, and its capacity for absorbing energy, decrease also when bone is dry (Evans and Lebow 1951; Sedlin 1965). The dry bone is more brittle than the humid bone, breaking respectively at deformations of 0.4% and 1.2%.

Table 3.4. The yield stress, ultimate stress, and ultimate strain for bovine bone tissue.

Notation for yield stress*	Yield stress**, MPa	Ultimate stress**, MPa	Ultimate strain or rotation***
σ_o^+	141 (17.1) [58]	156 (23.5) [66]	0.0324 (0.0161) [66]
σ_o^-	196 (18.5) [25]	237 (38.6) [49]	0.0253 (0.0096) [49]
σ_{30}^+	....	109 (9.0) [21]	0.0118 (0.0025) [21]
σ_{30}^-	....	190 (12.6) [14]	0.0250 (0.0038) [14]
σ_{60}^+	....	60 (9.8) [12]	0.0075 (0.0019) [12]
σ_{60}^-	....	148 (2.6) [2]	0.0320 (0.0006) [2]
σ_{90}^+	....	50 (12.6) [52]	0.0067 (0.0024) [52]
σ_{90}^-	150 (30.7) [22]	178 (31.1) [26]	0.0517 (0.0199) [26]
τ	57 (8.4) [21]	73 (9.6) [49]	0.3910 (0.0908) [21]

* See text for explanation.
** The first number is the yield or ultimate stress in MPa, the number in parentheses is the standard deviation, and the number in brackets is the number of specimens.
*** The first number is the ultimate strain or the ultimate rotation in radians, the number in parentheses is the standard deviation, and the number in brackets is the number of specimens. Table from Cowin *et al.*. (1987) using summarised and condensed data from Reilly and Burstein (1975) and Cezayirlioglu *et al.*. (1985). Reproduced with permission.

Table 3.5. The yield stress, ultimate stress, and ultimate strain for human tissue.

Notation for yield stress*	Yield stress**, MPa	Ultimate stress**, MPa	Ultimate strain or rotation***
σ_o^+	115 (11.2) [202]	133 (14.1) [202]	0.0293 (0.0094) [202]
σ_o^-	182 (14.4) [19]	195 (19.6) [114]	0.0220 (0.0057) [114]
σ_{30}^+	....	100 (10.4) [23]	0.0198 (0.0083) [23]
σ_{30}^-	....	173 (13.8) [5]	0.0280 (0.0052) [5]
σ_{60}^+	....	61 (12.2) [19]	0.0069 (0.0022) [19]
σ_{60}^-	....	133 (15.0) [7]	0.0311 (0.0010) [7]
σ_{90}^+	....	51 (10.1) [31]	0.0072 (0.0016) [31]
σ_{90}^-	121 (9.2) [3]	133 (16.7) [13]	0.0462 (0.0260) [13]
τ	54 (5.2) [19]	69 (4.4) [31]	0.3299 (0.0890) [19]

* See text for explanation.
** The first number is the yield or ultimate stress in MPa, the number in parentheses is the standard deviation, and the number in brackets is the number of specimens.
*** The first number is the ultimate strain or the ultimate rotation in radians, the number in parentheses is the standard deviation, and the number in brackets is the number of specimens. Table from Cowin *et al.*. (1987) using summarised and condensed data from Reilly and Burstein (1975) and Cezayirlioglu *et al.*. (1985). Reproduced with permission.

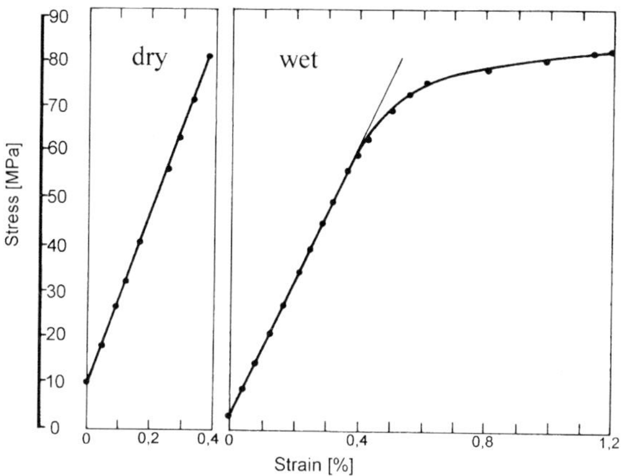

Fig. 3.10. Effect of humidity on the stress-strain curve of human femur. Adapted from Evans and Lebow (1951).

Studies on bone preservation show that fixation with alcohol produces a significant and irreversible reduction of mechanical properties in the human tibia (Sedlin 1965; McElhaney *et al.*. 1964). No significant differences have been found when the samples have been frozen at -20°C. This last technique is the most commonly used at present, and the samples are usually preserved with humid cloths in Ringer's solution, simulating the physiological environment (Hodgkinson *et al.*. 1989, Mauch *et al.*. 1992).

The age, sex and general state of the individual are factors that determine also the differences in mechanical behaviour of bone. The ultimate strength in tension, compression, shear and bending decreases with age. The same thing happens with the percentage of deformation and hardness. The elastic modulus increases up to the age of 40 and then it decreases (Burstein *et al.*. 1976). The fatigue endurance shows a low correlation with this variable (Evans 1973). The factor determined by the sex of the individual is closely related with the amount of bone present. Lindahl and Lindgren (1968) demonstrated that with age the density of the cortical of bone in the human humerus and femur increases gradually in men and decreases in women.

Another factor that has an influence on the mechanical characteristics is the origin of the bone samples. When comparing values of the human cortical, it can be observed that the radius shows the highest tensile and bending strengths; the fibula exhibits the largest deformation both in tension and in compression, the longest fatigue life and the highest elastic modulus; the femur has the largest compressive and shear strength in the direction perpendicular to the axis of the bone, and it is the hardest. If a long bone is divided in three parts, a proximal region (the closest to the body), a median region and a distal region, it is found that the largest values for the tensile strength are measured at the median region of the humerus, the femur and the tibia. The lowest values are found at the proximal fraction. The largest compressive strength is obtained at the median region of the tibia. In the femur the largest torsional strength has been measured at the median zone of the diaphysis and the smaller at the distal region (Evans 1973).

3.4.2 Behaviour of bone under the action of different forces

The application of loads and momenta in different orientations of bone may generate forces of tension, compression, bending, shear, torsion, and a combination of all or part of them.

Tension. The tensile strength is not as crucial, from a functional point of view, as the compressive strength. The tensile loads may be generated from structural elements of the body itself like ligaments and tendons. The skeletal system is designed with the objective to minimise such stresses (Currey 1984); in such a way that in the insertion zones, bone increases its section forming tubercles or tuberosities. It is well known that the larger the section, the greater are the strength and the stiffness. Other situations in which tension is important are under torsion and in bending. From a clinical point of view, fractures generated by tensile forces are mainly detected in the trabecular bone. An example is the calcaneum fracture close to the zone of union with the Achilles tendon. A large contraction in the *triceps surae* muscle may produce abnormally high tensile loads. In general, tensile fracture is structurally revealed by the separation of the cement lines and the extraction or lifting of osteons. The fracture is usually perpendicular to the bone, respecting the imposed planes of maximum stress.

Compression. The strength in compression is the key to the behaviour of bone *in vivo*. The compressive loads produce fractures mainly in the vertebrae and in the femur head. The most usual cause that creates the occurrence of such forces is an anomalous and strong contraction of the muscles adjacent to the affected bones. Generally the fracture is produced by the appearance of oblique cracks in the osteons, following planes of maximum shearing stress oriented at an angle of 30-35° in relation to the axis of the bone.

The fact that an inorganic phase is incorporated seems to be more important in the compressive than in the tensile strength. Mineralisation is a fundamental factor. The qualitative loss of mineral results in an increase of the risk of fracture, whilst an increase in the mineral density seems to increase the compressive strength (Kaplan *et al.*. 1985, Lotz *et al.*. 1990).

Shear. The load is applied parallel to the surface of the structure. The deformation takes place by the variation of angles. This type of fracture appears, usually, in trabecular bone. An example is the fracture produced at the femoral condyles and at the intercondylar face of the tibia. The studies carried out in the bone cortical show that the ultimate strength of human bone is different when tested under compression, tension or shear (Fig. 3.11). Both the ultimate stress and the ultimate deformation under compression are always higher than the corresponding values under tension. At variance, the yield stress is always higher in tension than in compression.

Bending. When a bone is loaded in bending, tensile forces are generated at the convex surfaces and compressive forces at the concave surfaces. The value of these forces will depend on the distance to the neutral axis, in such a way that the greater the distance the greater the force or the deformation. In an adult bone the fracture is initiated at the face of the bone which is under tensile loading producing a transversal fracture. The path of the fracture continues obliquely at 30-35°, respecting the planes of maximum

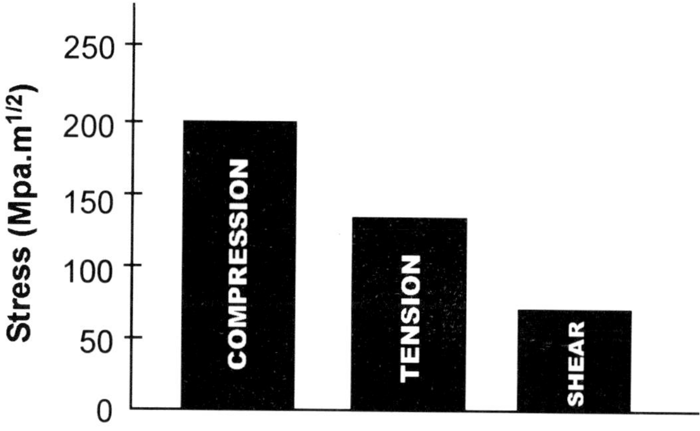

Fig. 3.11. Differences in the ultimate strength of human cortical bone when tested in compression, tension and shear. Adapted from Really and Burstein (1975).

shear stress. The face under compression may suffer two oblique fractures. Fracture may start under compression in an immature bone.

Torsion. Apart from being loaded in bending, many skeletal structures are loaded in torsion. This is mainly due to the range of mobility needed between joints in order to support certain elements. In torsion shear stresses are distributed over the entire structure. The maximum shear stresses act on planes parallel and perpendicular to the neutral axis whilst maximal tensile and compressive stresses act on planes diagonal to the neutral axis. Generally the torsion loads act in combination with bending, tension and compression giving rise to a complex distribution of stresses and deformations. The model of fracture in a bone loaded in torsion suggests that breaking takes place under shear observing the formation of a crack parallel to the neutral axis of the bone, and later a crack will form along the plane of maximum tensile stress.

The fatigue fracture of bone takes place by a slow repetition of large loads or by the rapid repetition of normal loads. This fracture cannot be visualised macroscopically. The energy absorbed by bone is determined by the breakage of bonds between the matrix and the particle and the formation of small microcracks (Forwood and Parker 1989). It has been suggested that part of the energy used in breaking these bonds may be responsible for the degradation of the mechanical properties observed with age and under different pathologies (Bundy 1985).

Even having individualised the different loads acting on bone, it is very clear that the real situation is much more complex. Bone presents a highly irregular geometry and it has to endure many different loads during quotidian activities. The clinical study of a great number of fractures shows that the great majority of them are the result of a combination of different types of loads.

3.4.3 Bone as a composite material

A great number of biological structures can be classified as composite materials. These materials are formed by two or more components that interact and give rise to specific mechanical properties. These properties depend not only on their composition but also on their structure (geometrical shape of the components, bonds between matrix and filler, etc.).

Bone is formed by collagen fibres and hydroxyapatite. The mineral phase is rigid and strong. The Young's modulus along its axis is about 165 GPa, although in the literature values of about 114 GPa (Katz and Ukraincik 1971) are also found. Its Poisson ratio is 0.22. The tangential modulus of collagen is 1.47 GPa (Currey 1969), and its Poisson ratio ranges between 0.13 and 0.35. The elastic modulus of bone is 18 GPa in a human femur in tension, which is a value in between that of hydroxyapatite and that of collagen. As a result of this combination, bone shows a strength higher than that of the components. The softer component avoids that the rigid component breaks under brittle fracture, whilst the stiff component avoids plastic deformation.

The study about how the two components are combined and the final mechanical result has generated a wide variety of models of bone based, most of them, in theoretical models obtained for composite materials. The first author to approach bone as a two phase composite was Currey (1964). In his work he considered that the modulus was calculated as the proportional mean of each one of the phases constituting bone. This model was adequate for materials with unidirectional continuous fibres, but not for bone (Katz 1971, 1980a,1980b, 1981). A new model as a fibre-reinforced composite was constructed where osteons were long and hollow fibres, and the interstitial lamellae were the solid fibres placed inside a matrix (amorphous substance). These osteons were oriented longitudinally and were packed in an hexagonal pattern in a transversal section. The collagen fibres presented characteristics associated with polymeric materials, and the mineral phase to a behaviour similar to ceramic materials. It had been observed that the different structures, which formed the laminar and Haversian bone, determined different mechanical consequences (Wainright *et al.*. 1976). The Haversian bone was structurally the same and as a consequence of this, the mechanical properties were the same in the directions radial and tangential. On the other hand, laminar bone presented different characteristics. Later on, considering a molecular level of study, Mammone and Hudson (1993) performed some work taking bone as a filled polymeric composite formed by a collagen matrix and crystals of hydroxyapatite. The relations between structure and function were considered at an extracellular matrix level.

Many authors think that the complex nature of the microstructure of bone may require the combination of different mechanical models. Moreover, a better understanding of the molecular level may provide useful information for further models based in the histology of bone.

3.4.3.1 Ultimate tensile strength models. Mammone and Hudson (1993) did evaluate the ultimate tensile strength incorporating new parameters such as the dimension of the mineral particles, the bonding between phases, the elastic constants between the two phases and the volume fraction of mineral or the degree of mineralisation:

$$\sigma_u = [(12\gamma\ E_0/d)\ (1/[E_C] + \Phi)]^{1/2} \tag{3.2}$$

where σ_u is the ultimate strength, γ is the work of adhesion between the particles, E_0 is the elastic modulus of the organic matrix, d is the dimension of the particles, E_C is the longitudinal elastic modulus of the composite and Φ is the volume fraction of mineral. The results of ultimate tensile stress obtained by these authors are shown in Table 3.6, together with the results obtained by other authors.

The prediction of Mammone and Hudson (1993) about the tensile ultimate strength based on a model of a polymeric composite reinforced by an inorganic phase is much higher than that experimentally observed for cortical bone. According to these authors this can be explained by the presence in bone of a great number of pores which act as defects that determine a reduction in the measured strength. According to these same authors, this variability in the data can be attributed to the inherent anisotropy of bone in relation to its properties and its heterogeneity generated by a biologically complex structure. The effects of the specimen preparation, the introduction of defects and the testing procedures are also parameters, which may affect when obtaining the fracture data.

Table 3.6. Values of the tensile ultimate stress for cortical bone.

Study	Ultimate tensile strength (MPa)	Specimen
Mammone and Hudson (1993)	1700	Shape factor of 10 Mineralisation of 0.65
Martin and Ishida (1989)	106	Bovine femur
Vicentelli and Grigorov (1985)	162 133	Human tibia
Currey (1975)	125	Bovine femur
Really and Burstein (1975)	133	Human femur
Burstein *et al.*. (1972)	175	Bovine femur

From Mammone and Hudson (1993). Reproduced with permission.

3.4.2.1 ***Elastic modulus models.*** Currey (1964) and Bonfield and Li (1967) considered that bone was a material constituted by two phases and that its modulus would behave according to the theory of mixtures:

$$E_b = V_o E_o + V_m E_m \tag{3.3}$$

where E and V represent the Young's modulus and the volume fraction and the subscripts b, o and m stand for bone, organic phase (collagen) and mineral phase (hydroxyapatite), respectively. This equation is also known as the Voigt model or the model of isodeformation. The Reuss model or the model of isostress has been also considered in two different studies (Katz 1971; Piekarski, 1973) and in this one E_b is evaluated from:

$$\frac{1}{E_b} = \frac{V_0}{E_0} + \frac{V_m}{E_m} \tag{3.4}$$

The microstructural analogy, which can be applied, is that of a plate formed by two alternate phases in the form of bands, which are stressed in tension and in compression either in a direction parallel to the bands or perpendicularly to the bands. These simple models provide respectively the upper and lower limit of the elastic modulus of the composite material.

When these models are applied to compact bone a whole set of contradictions appear. Taking the Eq. (3.3) for compact bone, Currey (1964) calculated the stresses in both phases starting from a reasonable value of stress. He found that the stress in tension in the mineral phase is much higher than that expected for a ceramic material, without the presence of fractures. Similarly, from Eq. (3.4) the paradox is reached were the modulus of bone depends only on E_o and V_o and that the elastic properties of hydroxyapatite did not matter at all.

A new model, which represents a combination of Eqs. (3.3) and (3.4), was proposed by Hirsch (1962) and Dougill (1962):

$$\frac{1}{E_b} = x\left[\frac{1}{V_o E_o + V_m E_m}\right] + (1-x)\left[\frac{V_o}{E_o} + \frac{V_m}{E_m}\right] \tag{3.5}$$

Where x and $(1\text{-}x)$ represent the respective weights of each one of the two models. Piekarski (1973) estimated a value of $x = 0.925$ for bone. This same author, together with Katz (1971) applied a more rigorous model based on an approximation by Hashim and Shtrikman (1963):

$$E_b^U = \frac{9K_b^U G_b^U}{3K_b^U G_b^U} \tag{3.6}$$

and

$$E_b^L = \frac{9K_b^L G_b^L}{3K_b^L G_b^L} \tag{3.7}$$

where E_b^U and E_b^L represent the upper and lower limits of the Young's modulus.

The upper limit of the volumetric modulus, K_b^U and the upper limit of the shear modulus, G_b^U, can be expressed as:

$$K_b^U = K_m + \frac{V_0}{\dfrac{1}{K_0 - K_m} + \dfrac{3V_m}{3K_m + 4G_m}} \tag{3.8}$$

$$G_b^U = G_m + \frac{V_0}{\dfrac{1}{G_0 - G_m} + \dfrac{6(K_m + 2G_m)\ V_m}{5(3K_m + 4G_{mm})\ G_m}} \tag{3.9}$$

Interchanging the subscripts o and m in the Eq. (3.8) and Eq. (3.9) will give the expressions for K_b^L and G_b^L respectively.

There are now some aspects to be discussed. In the first place, none of these models leaves a role for porosity in the material. In all of them it is assumed that $V_o + V_m = 1$. This is a relevant point since it is well known that even in compact bone, porosity ranging from 5 to 10% has to be expected.

On the other hand, when typical values for the constituents are taken into the equations, it can be noticed that the range of Young's moduli obtained is too wide to be useful. Taking $E_o = 1.2 \times 10^3$ MPa (Currey 1964), $E_m = 1.14 \times 10^5$ MPa (Katz, 1971), $V_o = V_m = 0.5$ (Wainright *et al.*. 1976), $\nu_o = 0.35$ and $\nu_m = 0.27$, the results shown in Table 3.7 are obtained.

Table 3.7. Values of Young's moduli calculated according to the models of particulate composite materials

Model	E_b (MPa)
Voigt model-Upper limit	5.76×10^4
Reuss model-Lower limit	2.38×10^3
Combination Voigt-Reuss with x = 0.925	2.10×10^4
Hashin-Shtrikman model-Upper limit	4.01×10^4
Hashin-Shtrikman model- Lower limit	6.83×10^3

When the anisotropy of the phases constituting the material is taken into account, other models can be proposed. For uniform stress on the components Paul (1960) proposed his model whilst for the case of uniform deformation Ishai and Cohen (1967) propose the corresponding model, being:

Paul model
$$E_b = E_0 \frac{1+(m-1)\,V_m^{2/3}}{1+(m-1)\left(V_m^{2/3} - V_m\right)} \tag{3.10}$$

where m is the ratio between the modulus of the mineral particle (E_m) and the modulus of the organic matrix (E_0).

Ishai and Cohen model
$$E_b = E_0\left(1+\frac{V_m}{\dfrac{m}{m+1} - V_m^{1/3}}\right) \tag{3.11}$$

The model by Kachanov *et al.* (1994) predicts the modulus of porous solids in terms of the pore density and shape, accounting for the anisotropy introduced by random orientations and the mixture of pores with different shapes. This model was used recently by Sevostianov and Kochanov (1998) to calculate the effective anisotropic elastic moduli of cortical bone in terms of the microstructure. Bone has been modelled in terms of three main systems of pores: the *Haversian canals* (around 50 μm) associated with pores parallel to the osteonal cylinder; the network of *canaliculi* and *Volkman's canals* (around 1μm) randomly distributed on planes perpendicular to the Haversian canals and the *lacunae of the osteocytes* (around 5 μm) which are randomly distributed in the whole bone. They also considered that, although with different sizes, the three types of pores represent similar volume fractions, i.e. the partial porosity of each kind of pore is similar. They also assumed an aspect ratio of the oblate cavities (the third type) of about 1/5, i.e. $a_1=a_2=5a_3$.

The elastic and shear moduli evaluated by Sevostianov and Kachanov (1998) agree rather well with the experimental results within the statistical dispersion found in the literature. However, the agreement fails for the Poisson ratios because being these constants sensible to the pore shape, in the model used the pore shape selected is different from the real ones.

However, the interesting all these models are, none of them takes seriously into account that the structure of collagen is a very relevant variable, very difficult also to be taken mechanically into account. A recent publication highlights the role of collagen in the declining mechanical properties of ageing human cortical bone (Zioupos *et al.* 1999). In fact, it should be thought that both the chemical bond within the collagen fibres and their architecture must play a leading role that most of the models seem to overlook, and specifically the last one referred.

As an alternative to these particulate models, *fibre models* can be introduced. The first model considering bone as a fibre reinforced material was applied by Currey (1969), following the theory first developed by Cox (1952). The resulting model is

$$E_b = E_o V_o + E_m V_m \left[1 - \frac{2}{\beta\, L} \tanh\left(\frac{\beta L}{2} \right) \right] \tag{3.12}$$

and

$$\beta = \left[\frac{2\pi G_o}{E_m A_m \cdot \ln(a/a_m)} \right]^{1/2} \tag{3.13}$$

where L is the length of the hydroxyapatite needle, G_o is the shear modulus of the organic matrix, A_m is the cross-sectional area of an individual hydroxyapatite crystallite, a_m is the radius of the hydroxyapatite crystal and a is the mean separation distance between the crystallites.

Alternative models for unidirectional composites have also been developed, such as that of Halpin and Tsai (1967):

$$E_l = E_m \frac{1 + ABV_f}{1 - BV_f} \tag{3.14}$$

where E_l is the Young's modulus in the longitudinal direction of the fibre, the subscript f indicates the fibre, and B is:

$$B = \frac{E_f - E_m}{E_f + AE_m} \tag{3.15}$$

where A depends on the different characteristics of the reinforcing phase, such as shape and aspect ratio, and it has to be determined experimentally.

Since these models predict the Young's modulus of a unidirectional fibre composite, Currey (1969) tried to elucidate its prediction as a function of the angle between the fibres and the axis of tensile loading:

$$\frac{E''}{E_\Theta} = \cos^4\Theta + \frac{E''}{E_\perp}\sin^4\Theta + \left(\frac{E''}{G} - 2\nu_{12}\right)\cos^2\Theta\sin^2\Theta \qquad (3.16)$$

where E_Θ= the Young's modulus of the composite measured along an axis at an angle Θ with the fibre axis; E'' = the Young's modulus measured at Θ = 0°; $E_\perp$ = the Young's modulus measured at Θ = 90°; G = shear modulus of the composite and ν_{12} = the major Poisson ratio of the composite. When the results yielded by this model are confronted with experimental results, the agreement is very poor.

In order to correct the fact that bone is not really a unidirectional fibre composite, and that actually the hydroxyapatite crystal are oriented in different directions, a randomly oriented fibre composite has been supposed and the model by Nielson and Chen (1968) has been proposed, where the modulus of the Eq. (3.16) is averaged over all orientations:

$$E_\Theta = \frac{\int_0^{\pi/2} E_\Theta d\Theta}{\int_0^{\pi/2} d\Theta} \qquad (3.17)$$

Katz, (1981) following the ideas of Krenchel (1964), proposed a model, which takes into account the composite nature of bone:

$$E_b = \frac{E_o V_o (1 - \nu_o \nu_b)}{(1 - \nu_o^2)} + \sum_n E_m V_m g(\Theta_n)\left(\cos^4\Theta_n - \nu_b\cos^2\Theta_n\sin^2\Theta_n\right) \qquad (3.18)$$

where ν_o and ν_b are the Poisson's ratios of the organic phase and bone respectively.

Models of osteons and from there models of Haversian bone have also been proposed, but they show important weaknesses.

Another approach has been to try to adjust an empirical model starting from experimental data. In this sense, Currey (1988) proposed several models but one of them seemed to agree quite well with experimental values in a wide range of microstructural parameters:

$$log\ E = -6.30 + 3.17\ log\ Ca + 3.52\ log\ V_f \qquad (3.19)$$

where Ca is the calcium content in mg.g^{-1}, and V_f corresponds to (1- % porosity).

On the other hand, Ontañón (1997) proposes a linear and a quadratic model depending on the number and type of animal species analysed. Such empirical models can be written as:

$$E = X\rho + Y V_{fm} \qquad (3.20)$$

and

$$E = S\rho V_{fm} - T\rho^2 + Z \qquad (3.21)$$

where ρ is the density of bone, V_{fm} corresponds to the volume fraction of mineral, and X, Y, S, T and Z are constants found empirically when adjusting the functions statistically determined. It is convenient to point out that the term density will include organic matrix, mineral phase, porosity and water content.

The main problem with these models is that they are not anisotropic. It seems that if it were possible to introduce a parameter accounting for the orientation of collagen fibres or at least the lamellar orientation, it would be possible to develop a better model which would take into account the anisotropic properties of bone. Unfortunately, the observation of the collagen fibre orientation is carried out in a microscope using polarised light and it provides two-dimensional information, and the technique is totally destructive in relation with the initial sample. The problem is then the lack of reliable quantitative three-dimensional models.

3.4.4 Fracture properties

3.4.4.1 Fracture mechanics. Fracture mechanics describes the fracture process in a material by relating the stress field close to the crack tip with the resultant extension of the crack length. This allows to describe the resistance of a material to rapid crack propagation in terms of two basic parameters: the critical stress intensity factor, K_C, also known as fracture toughness, and the critical strain energy release rate, G_C. This is the reason why the evaluation of K_C or G_C are so important for the design of structures with materials, in this case skeletal bones.

The tests which have to be conducted for the evaluation of K_C and G_C need to be carried out using pre-cracked specimens with a sufficient thickness in relation to length and width in order to guarantee plane strain conditions. Moreover, the specimen configuration must also allow sufficient homogeneity of the material structure throughout the gauge region of the specimen. This is the main reason why G_C evaluation cannot be reasonably conducted: every evaluation requires several specimens, which cannot come from the same region of a given bone. The structural and microstructural differences among the possible specimens would not allow to reach a reasonable value of G_C. Apart from these considerations it has been well established that single-edge-notched (SEN) specimens or compact tension (CT) specimens are useful for studying bone fracture toughness (Kobayashi, 1973). It has to be pointed out that only K_{IC} values (tension opening mode crack) can be found in the literature.

The different factors affecting the fracture process such as the influence of bone density or age in terms of the material and the influence of the strain rate, crosshead speed or thickness and type of specimen in terms of the test have been studied by different authors. Table 3.8 gives with detail the fracture toughness values obtained by different researchers together with the most relevant testing conditions. It should be pointed out that the meaning of K_{IC} for slow and stable crack propagation is doubtful since LEFM (linear elastic fracture mechanics) conditions are not properly followed, and consequently other methods for the extension of LEFM to elastic-plastic or even fully plastic conditions should be considered, such as the *R*-curve or the *J*-integral respectively. Although these comments should be kept in mind, only values of K_{IC} or G_{IC} are provided in the literature and they will be summarised and discussed here.

Table 3.8. Average values of K_{IC} (standard deviation) obtained by different authors where different testing features are provided.

Bone	Direction	K_{IC} ($MPa \cdot m^{1/2}$)	Specimen	Speed	Reference
Bovine femur	Longitudinal	3.21 (0.43)	SENT	Low	Melvin and Evans (1973)
Bovine femur	Longitudinal	5.05 (0.51)	SENT	Rapid	Melvin and Evans (1973)
Bovine femur	Transversal	5.58 (0.52)	SENT	Low	Melvin and Evans (1973)
Bovine femur	Transversal	7.69 (0.77)	SENT	Rapid	Melvin and Evans (1973)
Bovine femur	Transversal	2.2-4.6	SENT	Low	Bonfield and Datta (1976)
Bovine femur	Longitudinal	3.62 (0.73)	CT	Low	Wright and Hayes (1977)
Bovine femur	Transversal	5.7 (1.4)	3-PT	Low	Robertson *et al.*. (1978)
Bovine femur	Longitudinal	2.4-5.2	CT	Low	Bonfield *et al.*. (1978)
Bovine tibia	Longitudinal	2-5.6	CT	Low	Behiri and Bonfield (1984)
Bovine tibia	Longitudinal	6.3	CT	Rapid	Behiri and Bonfield (1984)
Human tibia	Longitudinal	2.4-5.3*	CT	Low	Bonfield *et al.*. (1984)
Bovine tibia	Transversal	11.2 (2.6)	SENB	Low	Moyle and Gavens (1986)
Bovine tibia	Transversal	6.5 (1.2)	CT	Very Low	Behiri and Bonfield (1989)
Bovine tibia	Longitudinal	3.2 (0.5)	CT	Very Low	Behiri and Bonfield (1989)
Human tibia	Longitudinal	3.7*	CT	Low	Norman *et al.*. (1991)
Bovine tibia	Longitudinal	7.2	CT	Low	Norman *et al.*. (1991)
Bovine tibia	Longitudinal	8.04 (1.4)	CT	Very Low	Norman *et al.*. (1992)
Human tibia	Longitudinal	2.88-3.28*	CT	Low	Norman *et al.*. (1995)
Bovine tibia	Longitudinal	6.2-6.7	CT	Low	Norman *et al.*. (1995)
Human femur	Transversal	6.4 (0.34)	SENB	Low	Zioupos and Currey (1998)

Direction: propagation direction of the crack; speed: propagation speed of the crack; CT: compact tension; SENT: single edge notched, tension; SENB: single edge notched, bending; 3-PT: three-point bending with a single notch. * Values which have been corrected for the specimen thickness. Compiled data by Currey (1998) and Melvin (1993).

Some authors pointed out that an increase in the loading speed increases the values of K_{IC} if the crack propagation is stable and slow (Melvin and Evans 1973; Bonfield *et al.* 1978; Behiri and Bonfield 1984). Behiri and Bonfield (1984) showed that for loading speeds above 0.1 cm/min the crack growth becomes very fast (more than 10 mm/s) producing the catastrophic fracture of the specimen. This latter effect upon fracture toughness seems to be contradictory since whilst Melvin and Evans (1973) established that K_{IC} increases by a 40 to 60 %, Behiri and Bonfield (1984) determined a decrease in fracture toughness by a 10 to 30 %, approximately.

When looking at the effect of the specimen thickness, Wright and Hayes (1977) and Behiri and Bonfield (1984), working with bovine bone, showed that values of fracture toughness, K_{IC}, are not affected when the thickness ranges between 0,5 and 3,8 mm. However, Norman *et al.*. (1991, 1995), studied specimen up to 9 mm in thickness and they showed that as the latter increases fracture toughness decreases. Moreover, they showed that for bovine bone, when the thickness is higher than 7 mm, the geometrical criteria of the ASTM 399 standard for CT specimens guarantee plane strain deformation for the determination of K_{IC}.

Most of the studies have been carried out by propagating the crack in the longitudinal direction, although this is not the usual way of bone fracture *in vivo*. This means that there is a lack of information about the transversal fracture process, which is clinically very relevant, taking into account the structural anisotropy of bone. Melvin and Evans (1973) determined for the first time that fracture toughness is higher when the crack propagates transversally, with a ratio K_C $(90^o)/K_C$ (0°) = 1,7. This ratio increased to 2 when calculated using the results obtained by Behiri and Bonfield (1989), that obtained values of K_{IC} for different angles between the longitudinal and the transversal direction. They noticed that K_{IC} increases gradually as the angle longitudinal to transversal increases. The fracture surface analysis revealed that for all the directions that have been tested, the pull-out of osteons was the failure mechanism. In this sense this results confirm that usually the cortical bone is stronger along its longitudinal orientation, which means when fracture takes place across the preferential direction of osteons, in other words, in the transversal propagation of the crack. It has been also shown that the stable and slow propagation of cracks follows the microstructure and the orientation of osteons, whilst for fast catastrophic propagation, the fracture surface is flat without any microstructural feature. In this last case the crack propagates catastrophically and it does not follow the preferential directions of osteons (Behiri and Bonfield 1989).

Other relevant parameters have been studied. In relation with the influence of the length of the initial crack, it has been recommended for CT specimens that the ratio a/W should be kept below 0.7 (Norman *et al.*. 1995), where a: length of the initial crack and W: the overall specimen width, in order to guarantee a K_{IC} value almost constant (Bonfield *et al.*. 1978). The degree of humidity is also very important and Melvin and Evans (1973) obtained a value of K_{IC} of about 60% when the test was performed with dry bone instead of humid bone. The value of the size of the critical defect have also been determined (Bonfield and Datta 1976; Robertson *et al.* 1978; Moyle and Gavens 1986) and the plastic zone ahead of the crack (Robertson *et al.* 1978), stablishing that the former is about the same order of magnitude of the vascular spaces (≈0,35 mm), rather than the lacunar spaces; and the latter (0,017 mm) leads to the conclusion that the crack propagation requires the localised disruption around the individual or small groups of lamellae.

The density of bone has a clearly positive correlation with K_{IC} values. Wright and Hayes (1977), as well as Behiri and Bonfield (1984) determined that the fracture toughness increased by 30 and 40 %, respectively when the density of bovine bone increased by 5%. Moreover, Behiri and Bonfield (1984) in the same study determined the influence of age upon fracture toughness and they obtained an inverse relationship. These results would agree with those by Currey (1979b) where it was shown that a significant drop of the energy absorbed by impact of human cortical bone takes place as its age increases. Only for bones over 60 years, the density affects the absorbed energy by weakening the bone as the density increases, independently whether there is porosity or not. Specially relevant is the conclusion which establishes that a great fraction of the decrease in the absorbed energy by impact can be attributed to the increase in the mineralisation of old bone, since it seems that the high content in mineral reduces the amount of plastic deformation of bone before the crack starts propagating. This last result would be in agreement with the fact that the hypermineralised phases of bone show more cracking (Boyce and Bloebaum 1993).

Up to now, very few fracture studies have been conducted with human bone (Bonfield *et al.* 1984; Norman *et al.* 1991; 1995; Zioupos y Currey 1998) and among these, only Zioupos and Currey (1998) have studied it with the transversal direction of propagation of the crack, which is the usual mode in which a bone breaks. The main problem associated with the study of the fracture toughness in human bone is the impossibility to obtain sufficiently thick specimens in order to ensure plane strain conditions for the test, being the maximum thickness obtained of about ≈ 3 mm. This is the reason why the different authors who have investigated human bone have calculated correcting factors which take into account the effect of the specimen thickness on the value of K_{IC} and G_{IC}. In this way, attempts were made to compare the values of fracture toughness of human bone, evaluated by applying the correcting factor, with the values obtained for other materials. However, these factors have been determined from the fracture results obtained with bovine bone, which makes them approximate (Bonfield *et al.* 1984), and it has not been possible to calculate homogeneous values of K_{IC} amongst the different authors. However, Norman *et al.* (1995) concluded that although human bone is significantly weaker than bovine bone in relation with its mechanical strength, their toughness is practically similar, although the data obtained were not sufficiently conclusive in order to determine which of them was tougher.

Although human bone is mechanically weaker in bending and tension than that of other animals, its osteonal structure seems to have adapted to prevent crack growth (Carter and Hayes 1976b; Martin and Burr 1989). Increased osteonal discontinuity increases toughness (Alto and Pope 1979), suggesting that although Haversian bone remodelling reduces bone strength it does not reduce bone toughness. The materials with a low shear strength often present good properties to impact and fatigue since larger displacements are possible along the shear planes before fracture. In this way, the weakness of the osteonal interface allows the bifurcation or the arrest of the crack due to the blunting of its tip and locking it in the lamellar structure. The deviation of the crack serves a double purpose of absorbing energy and making the crack to leave the plane of maximum stress, which in fact increases the fracture toughness (Norman *et al.*. 1995).

3.4.4.2 Fatigue. Bone is repeatedly cyclically stressed, and fatigue is one of the causes of bone failure reported in the literature (Griffiths *et al.* 1971; Hedlund and Lindgren 1986; Melton 1988; Krause and Thompson 1944). There have been a number of studies approaching the subject of fatigue failure of both; bone tissue and long bones.

In Fig. 3.12 conventional S-N diagrams, determined by cyclically stressing the bone tissue and determining the number of cycles to failure, obtained by different authors, with bone specimens from different species and applying different loading and environmental conditions are summarised (Currey 1998). As it could be expected, bending fatigue and torsional fatigue result in S-N curves that indicate a longer life for a given stress than life predictions generated from uniaxial tests, due to the stress gradients that exist in bending and torsion, but not in uniaxial loading (Caler and Carter 1989).

In all cases a highly significant negative correlation is observed between fatigue life and stress amplitude. Some factors that affect fatigue life of bone are the testing conditions (loading conditions, humidity of the specimen, etc.), the temperature, the density, or the microstructure. Whilst temperature negatively affects the fatigue life, a highly significant positive correlation between fatigue life and bone density is reported. On the other hand, it seems that primary compact bone has a longer fatigue

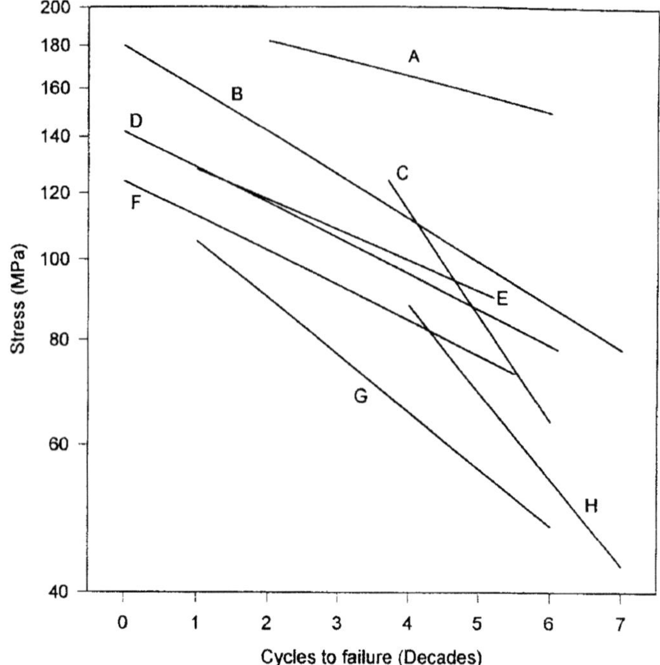

Fig. 3.12. A set of S-N curves for bone. The separate lines are the lines representing the equations produced by regression analysis. The lines are not extrapolated beyond the ends of the original data. In all cases the distributions were reasonably linear. The abscissa is measured in powers of ten. Taken from various experiments, with different loading conditions. A. Human four-point bending, room temperature, 2 Hz (Choi and Goldstein 1992). B. Human, compression, room temperature, 30 Hz (Gray and Korbacher 1974). C. Bovine rotating cantilever, room temperature, 30 Hz (Carter and Hayes 1976b). D. Bovine, tension, room temperature, 2 Hz (Zioupos *et al.*. 1996b). E. Human (27 years), tension, room temperature, 2 Hz (Zioupos *et al.*. 1996a). F. Red deer antler, tension, room temperature, 2 Hz (Zioupos *et al.*. 1996b). G. Human (69 years), tension, 37 °C, 2 Hz (Carter and Caler 1983). H. Human, rotating cantilever, room temperature, 70Hz (Swanson *et al.*. 1971). From Currey (1998). Reproduced with permission.

life that secondary Haversian bone (Carter and Hayes 1976b). In general, the age is also a significant factor affecting the fatigue life. Older bone tissue shows a lower fatigue strength than younger one (Zioupos *et al.* 1996a). However this effect can be related to the density and the microstructure of the tissue, which are dependent on the age. Fatigue life depends also on the species studied. In general, bovine bone shows higher fatigue life than human bone. This phenomenon can be explained by the fact that bovine bone has a higher density than human bone (Carter and Hayes 1976b).

Fatigue failure can be related to the microdamage accumulation. The amount of fatigue damage that bone can sustain just prior to failure is a parameter which can be measured as a function of the reduction of the elastic modulus of the material, and which can help to predict the fatigue life of bone, since it is observed that bone tissue is able to sustain about the same level of damage prior to failure. The accumulation of damage depends on the level of stress: damage develops much more slowly at lower stresses (Zioupos *et al.* 1996a, Zioupos *et al.* 1996b). However, it is not clear whether it exists an endurance limit, below which no damage accumulates (Zioupos *et al.* 1996b, Carter *et al.* 1981). Another feature to take into account is that the type of bone microdamage created by repeated loading is different in tensile and compressive loading. Whilst cyclic compression causes the accumulation of shear microcracks oblique to the loading direction, cyclic tension causes debonding of the osteons and separation of cement lines (Carter and Hayes 1977b).

However, it is necessary to be cautious when interpreting the practical significance of the results obtained by fatigue tests *in vitro*. It has to be kept in mind that in living bone it is alive and the matrix is in constant turnover. The matrix occupying any portion of the skeleton can be replaced before it has been exposed to sufficient cycles to cause fatigue failure. This is not the case when performing fatigue tests in the laboratory. *In vitro* data do not account for *in vivo* bone remodelling, which may act in different directions: for example, the initiation of a fatigue fracture in life can be presumed to evoke a healing response, and the crack propagation can be arrested by the healing response. In this case bone remodelling can extend the fatigue life (Swanson *et al.* 1971). Conversely, the remodelling cavities produced by bone resorbtion of the damaged tissue may intensify the local stresses and speed up the fatigue crack propagation (Zioupos *et al.* 1996a).

3.5. CONCLUSION

Nature has been able to produce a connective tissue with the appropriate properties to perform a life in service. When such a tissue is analysed from a material point of view, the properties, which define the mechanical performance, have to be understood in terms of the microstructure of the material. It has been seen that the microstructure is rather complex and that it varies with age, sex and processes such pathologies or healing. The mechanical properties will therefore be affected. A wide variety of measurements of mechanical properties have been carried out, and it is possible to find a great number of references in the literature where the mechanical behaviour of different bones of different species has been analysed. However, the main problem, from an engineering point of view, is that after such a great effort it does not seem possible to find a model which could predict the mechanical behaviour of bone. Although some models for the Young's modulus seems to work well, it is not so easy to find in the literature models for other mechanical properties and it does not appear that constitutive equations for bone similar to those existing for other materials could readily be proposed.

REFERENCES

Alto, A. and Pope, M. H. (1979) *Journal of Biomechanics*, **12**, 415.
Amprino, R. (1958) *Acta Anatomica*, **34**, 161.
Behiri, J. C. and Bonfield, W. (1984), *Journal of Biomechanics*, **17**, 25.
Behiri, J. C. and Bonfield, W. (1989) *Journal of Biomechanics*, **22**, 863.
Blitz, R. M. and Pellegrino, E. D. (1969) *Journal of Bone and Joint Surgery.*, **51**, 456.
Bonfield, W. and Li C. H. (1967) *Journal of Applied Physics*, **38**, 2450.
Bonfield, W. and Datta P. K.(1976) *Journal of Biomechanics*, **9**, 131.
Bonfield, W., Grynpas, M. D. and Young R. J. (1978) *Journal of Biomechanics*, **11**, 473.
Bonfield, W., Behiri, J. C. and Charambilides, B. (1984) in *Biomechanics: Current Interdisciplinary Research*, ed. Perrin, S.M. and Schneider, E. (Martinus Nijhoff, Dordrecht), p. 361.
Boskey, A. L. (1981) *Clinical Orthopaedics and Related Research*, **157**, 225.
Boskey, A. L. and Posner, A. S. (1984) in *Natural and Living Biomaterials*, ed. Hastings, G. W. and Ducheyne, P. (CRC Press, Boca Raton, Florida), p. 27.
Boyce, T. M. and Bloebaum, R. D. (1993) *Bone*, **14**, 769.
Bundy K.L. (1985) *Annals of Biomedical Engineering*, **13**, 119.
Burstein, A. H., Currey, J. D., Frankel, V.H. and Reilly, D. T. (1972) *Journal of Biomechanics*, **5**, 35.
Burstein, A. H., Really, D. T. and Martens, M. (1976) *Journal of Bone and Joint. Surgery*, **58A**, 82.
Caler, W. E. and Carter, D. R. (1989) *Journal of Biomechanics*, **22**, 625.
Carter, D. R. and Hayes, W. C. (1976a) *Science*, **194**, 1174.
Carter, D. R. and Hayes, W. C. (1976b) *Journal of Biomechanics*, **9**, 27.
Carter, D. R., Hayes, W. C. and Schurman, D. J. (1976) *Journal of Biomechanics*, **9**, 211.
Carter, D. R. and Hayes, W. C. (1977a) *Journal of Bone and Joint Surgery*, **59A**, 954.
Carter, D.,R. and Hayes, W.,C. (1977b) *Clinical Orthopaedics and Related Res*earch, **127**, 265.
Carter, D. R., Caler, W. E., Spengler, D. M. and Frankel, V. H. (1981) *Acta Orthopaedica Scandinavica*, **52**, 481.
Carter, D. R. and Caler, W. E. (1983) *Journal of Biomechanical Engineering*, **105**, 166.
Cezayirlioglu, H, Bahniuk, E., Davy, D.T. and Heiple, K.G. (1985) *Journal of Biomechanics*, **18**, 61.
Choi, K. and Goldstein, S. A. (1992) *Journal of Biomechanics*, **25**, 1371.
Cowin, S.C., Van Buskirk, W.C. and Ashman, R.B. (1987) in *Handbook of Bioengineering*, ed. Skalak, R. and Chien, S. (McGraw-Hill, New York), p. 2.1.
Cowin, S. C. (1989) *Bone Mechanics* (CRC Press, Boca Raton, Florida).
Cox, H. L. (1952), *Journal of Applied Physics*, **3**, 72.
Crowninshield, R. D. and Pope, M. H. (1974) *Annals of Biomedical Engineering*, **2**, 217.
Currey, J. D. (1964) *Journal of Bone and Joint Surgery*, **46B**, 356.
Currey, J. D. (1969) *Journal of Biomechanics*, **2**, 477.
Currey, J. D. and Brear, K. (1974) *Calcified Tissue Research*, **15**, 173.
Currey, J. D. (1975) *Journal of Biomechanics*, **8**, 81.
Currey, J. D. (1979a) *Journal of Biomechanics*, **12**, 313.
Currey, J. D. (1979b) *Journal of Biomechanics*, **12**, 459.
Currey, J. D. (1984) *The Mechanical Adaptations of Bones* (Princeton University Press, Princeton).
Currey, J. D. (1988) *Journal of Biomechanics*, **21**, 131-139.

Currey, J. D. (1990) in *Biomechanics of Diarthrodial Joints*, Ed. Mow, V.C., Ratcliffe, A. and Yoo, S. L. Y. (Springer-Verlag, New York).
Currey, J. D. and Brear, K. (1990) *Journal of Materials Science: Materials in Medicine*, **1**, 14.
Currey, J. D. (1998) in *Proceedings of the Institution of Mechanical Engineers.*, **212**(Part H), p. 399.
Dougill, J. W. (1962) in *Proeedings of the American Concrete Institution*, Vol. **59**, p. 1363.
Driessens, F. C. M. and Verbeeck, R. M. H. (1986) *Zeitschrift für Naturforschung*, **41c**, 468.
Driessens, F. C. M. and Verbeeck, R. M. H. (1990) *Biominerals* (CRC Press, Boca Raton, Florida).
Enomoto, S. and Krimm, S. (1962) *Biophysical Journal*, **2**, 317.
Evans, F. G. and Lebow, M. (1951) *Journal of Applied Physiology*, **3**, 563.
Evans, F. G. (1973) *Mechanical Properties of Bone* (Charles C. Thomas Publisher, Springfield, Illinois).
Evans, G. P., Behiri, J. C., Currey, J. D. and Bonfield, W. (1990) *Journal of Materials Science: Materials in Medicine*, **1**, 38.
Forwood, M. R. and Parker, A. W. (1989) *Calcified Tissue International*, **45**, 47.
Francillon-Vieillot, H., De Buffrénil, V., Castanet, J., Géraudie, J., Meunier, F. J., Sire, J. Y., Zylberberg, L. and Ricqlès, A. de (1990 in *Skeletal Biomineralisation: Patterns and Evolutionary Trends, I*, ed. Carter, J.G. (Van Nostrand Reinhold, New York), p. 471.
Fraca, P., Harper, R. A. And Katz, J.L. (1981) *Scanning Electron Microscopy*, **3**, 339.
Galante, J., Rostoker, W. and Ray, D. (1970) *Calcified Tissue Research*, **5**, 236.
Gong, J. K., Arnold, J. S. and Cohn, S.H. (1964) *Anatomical Record*, **149**, 325.
Gray, R. J. and Korbacher, G. K. (1974) *Journal of Biomechanics*, **7**, 287.
Griffiths, W. E. G., Swanson, S. A. V., Freeman, M. A. R. (1971) *Journal of Bone and Joint Surgery*, **53B**, 136.
Halpin, J. C. and Tsai, S. W. (1967) Environmental factors in composite materials design. Technical Report, AFML-TR-67, Air Force Materials Laboratory.
Ham, A. W. (1969) *Histology* (Lippincott, Phipadelphia).
Hashin, Z. and Shtrikman, S. (1963) *Journal of the Mechanics and Physics of Solids*, **11**, 127.
Hedlund, R. and Lindgren, U. (1986) *Acta Orthopaedica Scandinavica.*, **57**, 423.
Hirsch, T. J. (1962) in *Proceedings of the American Concrete Institution*, **59**, 427.
Hodgkinson, R., Currey, J. D. and Evans, G. P. (1989) *Journal of Orthopaedic Research*, **7**, 754.
Ishai, O. and Cohen, L. J. (1967) *International Journal of Mechanical Sciences*, **9**, 539.
Kachanov, M., Tsukrov, I., Shafiro, B. (1994) *Applied Mechanics Reviews*, **47**, S151.
Kaplan, S. J., Hayes, W. C. and Stone, J. L. (1985) *Journal of Biomechanics*, **18**, 723.
Katz, E. P. (1971) *Journal of Biomechanics*, **4**, 221.
Katz, E. P. and Ukraincik, K. (1971) *Journal of Biomechanics*, **4**, 221.
Katz, E. P. (1980a) *Nature*, **283**, 106.
Katz, E. P. (1980b) in *Mechanical Properties of Biological Materials*, ed. Vincent, J. F. V. and Currey, J. D. (Cambridge University Press, London), p. 137.
Katz, E. P. (1981) in *Mechanical Properties of Bone*, ed. Cowin, S. C. (American Society of Mechanical Engineers, New York), p. 171.
Kobayashi, A. S. (1973) *Experimental Techniques in Fracture Mechanics* (SESA, Westport, CT).
Krause, G. R. and Thompson, J. R. Jr. (1944) *American Journal of Roent*genology, **52**, 281.
Krenchel, H. (1964) *Fibre Reinforcement* (Akademisk Forlag, Copenhagen).

Lakes, R. (1993) *Nature*, **361**, 511.
Lees, S. I. and Davidson, C. L. (1977) *Journal of Biomechanics*, **10**, 473.
Lees, S. I. (1979) *Calcified Tissue International*, **27**, 53.
Lees, S. I., Cleary, P. F., Heeley, J. D. and Gariepy, E. L. (1979) *Journal of the Acoustical Society of America*, **66**, 641.
Lessertisseur, J. and Saban, R. (1967) Généralités sur le squelette, **16**, p. 334-404 ; Squelette axial, **16**, p. 585-708 ; Squelette appendiculaire, **16**, p. 709-1078 ; in *Traité de Zoologie, Mammifères, Téguments et Squelette*, ed. Grassé, P.P. (Masson et Cie., Paris).
Lindahl, O. and Lindgren, A. G. H. (1968) *Acta Orthopaedica Scandinavica*, **39**, 129.
Liu, D., Weiner, S. and Wagner, H. D. (1999) *Journal of Biomechanics*, **32**, 647.
Lotz, J. C., Gerhart, T. N. and Hayes, W. C. (1990) *Journal of Computed Assisted Tomography*, **14**, 107.
Mammone, J. F. and Hudson, S. M. (1993) *Journal of Biomechanics*, **26**, 439.
Marino, A. A., Becker, R. O. and Bachman, C. H. (1967) *Phyics in Medicine and Biology*, **12**, 367.
Martin, R. B. and Burr, D. B. (1989) *Structure, Function and Adaptation of Compact Bone* (Raven Press, New York).
Mauch, M., Currey, J. D. and Sedman, A. J. (1992) *Journal of Biomechanics*, **25**, 11.
McElhaney, J., Fogle, J., Byars, E. and Weaver, G. (1964) *Journal of Applied Physiology*, **19**(6), 1234.
McElhaney, J. and Byars, E. F. (1965) *ASME Publ. 65-WA/HUF-9*, p. 1-8.
McElhaney, J. (1966) *Journal of Applied Physiology*, **21**, 1231.
Martin, R. B. and Ishida, J. (1989) *J. Biomechanics*, **22**,419.
Melton, L. J. III (1988) in *Osteoporosis*, ed. Riggs, B. L. and Melton, L. J. III (Raven Press, New York), p. 133.
Melvin, J. W. and Evans, F. G. (1973) in *ASME Biomechanics Symposium* (New York, NY), p. 87.
Melvin, J. W. (1993) *Journal of Biomechanical Engineering*, **115**, 549.
Meunier, A., Katz, J. L., Christel, P. I. and Sedel, L. (1988) *Journal of Orthopaedical Research*, **6**, 770.
Moyle, D. D. and Gavens, A. J. (1986) *Journal of Biomechanics*, **19**, 919.
Murphree, S., Hsu, H. H. and Anderson, H. C. (1982) *Calcified Tissue International*, **34**, S62.
Nielson, L. E. and Chen, P. E. (1968) *Journal of Materials*, **3**(2), 352.
Norman, T. L., Vashishth, D. and Burr, D. B. (1991) in *Advances in Bioengineering, Vol. 20 BED*, ed.Vanderby, R. (ASME, New York, NY), p. 361.
Norman, T. L., Vashischth, D. and Burr, D. B. (1992) *Journal of Biomechanics*, **25**, 1489.
Norman, T.L., Vashischth, D. and Burr, D. B. (1995) *Journal of Biomechanics*, **28**, 309.
Ontañón, M. (1997) Ph.D. Thesis, Universitat Politècnica de Catalunya, Barcelona.
Paul, B. (1960) *Transactions of the Metal Society.*, AIME, **218**, 36.
Park, J. B. (1979) *Biomaterials: An Introduction* (Plenum Press, New York).
Peck, S. D. and Briggs, G. A. D. (1987) *Advances in Dental Research*, **1**, 50.
Piekarski, K. (1973) *Internactional Journal of Engineering Science*, **11**(6A), 557.
Posner, A. S. (1969) *Physiological Reviews*, **49**, 760.
Posner, A. S. (1987) in *Bone and Mineral Research*, ed. Peck, W.A. (Elsevier, Amsterdam), p. 65.
Ramachandran, G. N. and Reddi, A. H. (1976) *Biochemistry of Collagen* (Plenum Press, New York).
Reilly, D. T. and Burstein, A. H. (1975) *Journal of Biomechanics*, **8**, 393.

Rho, J.-Y., Roy II, M. E., Tsui, T. Y. And Pharr, G.M. (1999) *Journal of Biomedical Materials Research*, **45**,48.
Ricqlès, A. de (1975) *Annales de Paléontologie (Vertébrés)*, **61**, 51.
Robertson, D. M., Robertson, D. and Barret, C. R. (1978) *Journal of Biomechanics*, **11**, 359.
Robinson, R. A. and Elliott, S. R. (1957) *Journal of Bone and Joint Surgery*, **39A**, 167.
Rougvie, M. A. and Bear, R. S. (1953) *Journalof the American. Leather Chemists Association*, **48**, 735.
Sedlin, E. D., (1965) *Acta Orthopaedica Scandinavica*, **83**, 1.
Sevostianov, I. and Kachanov, M. (1998) *International Journal of Fracture*, **92**, L3.
Simon, S. R. (1997) *Ciencias Básicas en Ortopedia* (American Academy of Orthopaedic Surgeons, Medical Trends, Barcelona).
Swanson, S. A.V., Freeman, M. A. R. and Day, W. H. (1971) *Medical & Biolocial Engineering*, **9**, 23.
Vicentelli,R. and Grigorov, M. (1985) *Journal of Biomechanics*, **18**, 201.
Voegel, J. C. and Frank, R. M. (1977) *Journal of Biologia Buccale*, **5**, 181.
Wainright, S. A., Biggs, W. D., Currey, J. D. and Gosline, J. M. (1976) *Mechanical Design in Organisms* (John Wiley, New York).
Wolff, J. (1892) *Das Gesetz der Transformation der Knochen* (Hirschwals Verlag, Berlin).
Weiner, S. and Wagner, H. D. (1998) *Annal. Review of Materials Science*, **28**, 271.
Wright, T. M. and Hayes, W. C. (1976) *Medical & Biological Engineering*, **14**, 671.
Wright, T. M. and Hayes, W. C. (1977) *Journal of Biomechanics*, **10**, 419.
Wuthier, R. E. and Eanes, E. D. (1975) *Calcified Tissue Research*, **23**, 135.
Yoon, H. S. and Katz, J. L. (1976) *Journal of Biomechanics*, **9**, 459.
Zioupos, P., Wang, X.T., Currey, J. D. (1996a) *Clinical Biomechanics*, **11**, 365.
Zioupos, P., Wang, X.T., Currey, J.D. (1996b) *Journal of Biomechanics*, **29**, 989.
Zioupos, P. and Currey, J. D. (1998) *Bone*, **22**, 57.
Zioupos, P., Currey, J. D., Hamer, A. J. (1999) *Journal of Biomedical Materials Research*, **45**, 108.

Chapter 4

Structure – Properties of Soft Tissues Articular Cartilage

Chapter 4

Structure – Properties of Soft Tissues Articular Cartilage

DAN BADER and DAVID LEE

4.1. INTRODUCTION

Soft tissues are biological composite structures. In all cases they contain, in various amounts, the ubiquitous biological macromolecule, *collagen*, in fibrous form. The building block of collagen fibres is the tropocollagen molecule, 300 nm long and 1.5nm wide, with a molecular weight of approximately 300kDa. Its molecular form is ideally designed to support tensile loads, to which the structural composites are subjected. However, its precise role in the biological composite largely depends upon the nature of loading, which is present when performing the various functions of the individual soft tissues. Thus tendons and ligaments contain collagen as the main structural component arranged in the form of fibres approximately parallel to the long axis of the tissues. Thus their mechanical properties are largely determined by those of the collagen fibres. This design is ideal to support the tensile forces during normal physiological activities. Soft tissues such as spinal ligaments and skin are subjected to mixed loading modes, involving a combination of tension, torsion, shear and compression. In these tissues collagen is associated with other structural proteins such as *elastin*, which confer distinct mechanical properties such as an ability to permit large extensions even at relatively low applied tensile stresses. Other soft tissues, such as intervertebral disc and articular cartilage, contain collagen fibres closely associated with macromolecular gels. Their interaction provides mechanical integrity for theses tissues to support compression loading during the normal loading at synovial joints. This chapter will concentrate on the unique tissue, *articular cartilage*, which has traditionally attracted much research interest in the field of biomechanics and biomaterials.

4.1.1 General properties of articular cartilage

There are three types of cartilaginous soft tissues found in the body, namely *elastic cartilage*, *fibrocartilage* and *hyaline cartilage*. Articular cartilage, which is located in synovial joints, is a type of hyaline cartilage and is the focus of the present chapter. It is the soft tissue, which covers the articulating ends of the bones, which terminate at a synovial joint.

In this position cartilage is subjected to the forces which pass through the joint. Thus, the main functions of articular cartilage are to reduce the contact stresses to safe values, thereby protecting the subchondral bone from damage and to provide the joint with low-friction and low-wear bearing surfaces. Indeed, articular cartilage in conjunction with its lubricant, synovial fluid, produce a coefficient of friction in normal healthy joints, which is lower than can be achieved with any man-made engineering system.

The resultant forces, which are transmitted through the major load-bearing joints of the lower limb, are largely compressive and the cartilages, with their inherently low frictional properties, are subjected mainly to compression perpendicular to the articular surface. The magnitude of the resultant forces regularly attain five times body weight, equivalent to approximately 3500 N, during the period just after the heel-strike of the gait cycle. In some cases, involving vigorous sporting activities, joint forces can exceed 10,000 N. Taking into account the surface area of the supporting cartilage in major load bearing joints, contact stresses of the order of 5 MPa are common in normal walking.

The thickness of cartilage varies from joint to joint and with location on a joint surface. Cartilage thickness in major load bearing joints is generally between 1.5 and 3.5 mm, although cartilage located on the lateral facet of the patella can be 5 mm thick. The surface of articular cartilage demonstrates directional properties, when examined by a pinpricking technique to induce directional splits. The resulting split direction is pronounced and generally site specific.

Normal adult human articular cartilage does not contain any blood vessels and the mature subchondral bone/cartilage junction is generally believed to be impermeable to nutrients. Thus pathways must exist to supply its cells with the vital nutrients to maintain viability and remove waste products. In addition, articular cartilage is devoid of nerve endings. Therefore any perceived pain within the joint is probably a direct result of abnormal bone contact or other structural damage from within the joints.

4.2. STRUCTURE AND COMPOSITION

Articular cartilage may be considered to be a fibre reinforced polymer gel containing cells, known as chondrocytes. The approximate proportions of the major constituents are given in Table 4.1. The properties of these extracellular components and their interactions determine the physical and mechanical properties of the tissue.

Table 4.1. Relative proportion of non-cellular components in adult human articular cartilage.

	wet weight
Collagen	15-20%
Proteoglycan	3-15%
Water	65-80%
Non-collagenous proteins and glycoproteins*	1%

*e.g. cartilage oligomeric matrix protein (COMP), fibronectin, anchorin.

4.2.1 Chondrocytes

The chondrocytes are responsible for the synthesis and maintenance of the extracellular constituents of cartilage. Chondrocytes are reported to vary considerably in size with values between 7 to 30 μm in diameter and are contained within spaces called lacunae. The ratio of cell volume to tissue volume is lower than most tissues, accounting for between 1% and 10% of the tissue volume, with a reported mean chondrocyte density of 14,000 cells.mm^{-3} (Maroudas et al. 1975). The chondrocytes are most numerous near the articular surface.

The characteristics of chondrocytes change with depth from the articular surface. In normal adult articular cartilage, four cellular zones can be identified under the light microscope (Figure 4.1) namely:

- a superficial zone beneath the articular surface in which the cells are discoid and oriented parallel to the surface.
- a transition zone in which the cells are more ellipsoidal in morphology with their long axes at a range of orientations to the articular surface.
- a deep zone, which contains ellipsoidal or spherical cells in groups of four to eight arranged in columns perpendicular to the articular surface.
- a calcified zone beneath the uneven basophilic line, known as the tidemark, marking the transition to calcified cartilage, which contain hypertrophic chondrocytes

It is the cells in the transition and deep zone, with relatively large cytoplasmic volumes containing well-developed endoplasmic reticulum and golgi complexes, which produce the main synthetic activity in cartilage.

The chondrocytes in adult articular cartilage are supplied by nutrients in the synovial fluid, which are transported across the cartilage surfaces. Clearly the permeability of cartilage will affect cell nutrition via fluid transport and thus structural changes which occur with age and disease will affect these pathways.

The extracellular matrix (ECM) surrounding each chondrocyte can also be divided into three regions, known as the pericellular, territorial and interterritorial matrix.

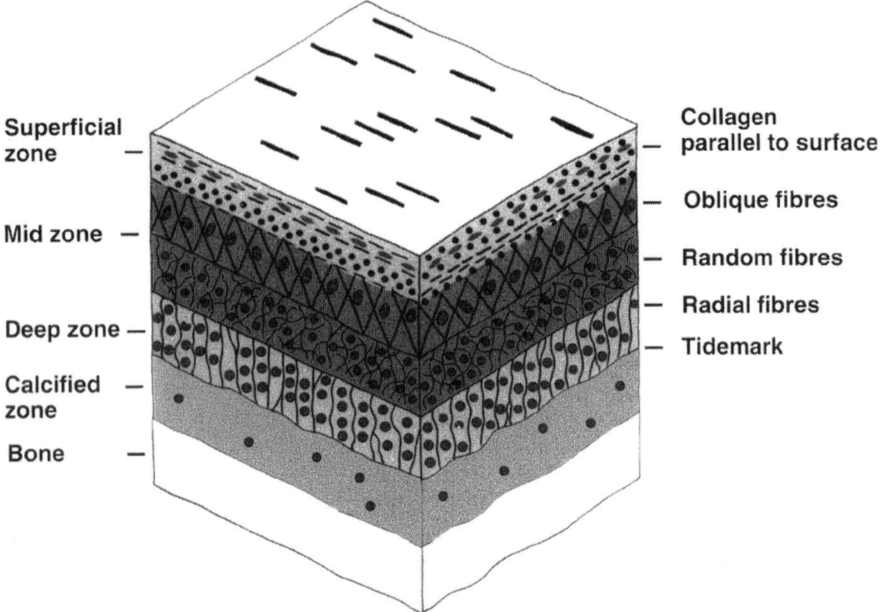

Fig. 4.1. Structural variation through the thickness of articular cartilage showing zonal arrangement of chondrocytes and collagen fibres.

These regions differ in both their proximity to the chondrocytes and their structure and organisation. The interterritorial region, comprising the majority of the tissue volume and is the main contributor to the mechanical properties of the matrix.

The behaviour of chondrocytes in a mechanical environment will form the basis of section 4.4 of this chapter.

4.2.2 Collagen

A large proportion of the non-aqueous ECM of cartilage is composed of a network of *collagen* fibrils (see also Chapter 8). The building blocks of collagen, the tropocollagen molecule, consists of three polypeptide chains, designated α chains, coiled together in a right-handed helical structure. Each α chain contains approximately 1000 amino acid residues. With the exception of the short non-helical sequences at the end of each chain, one third of the amino acid residues are composed of the small molecule glycine. Of the remainder, approximately 22% are either proline or hydroxyproline, which confer stability to the triple helix due to the inherent rigidity of their ring structures. The precise sequence of amino acids determines the type of collagen present. Collagens are conventionally classified according to the structures of the three α chains. Nineteen types of collagen have been identified and they are encoded by at least thirty genes (Thomas et al. 1994).

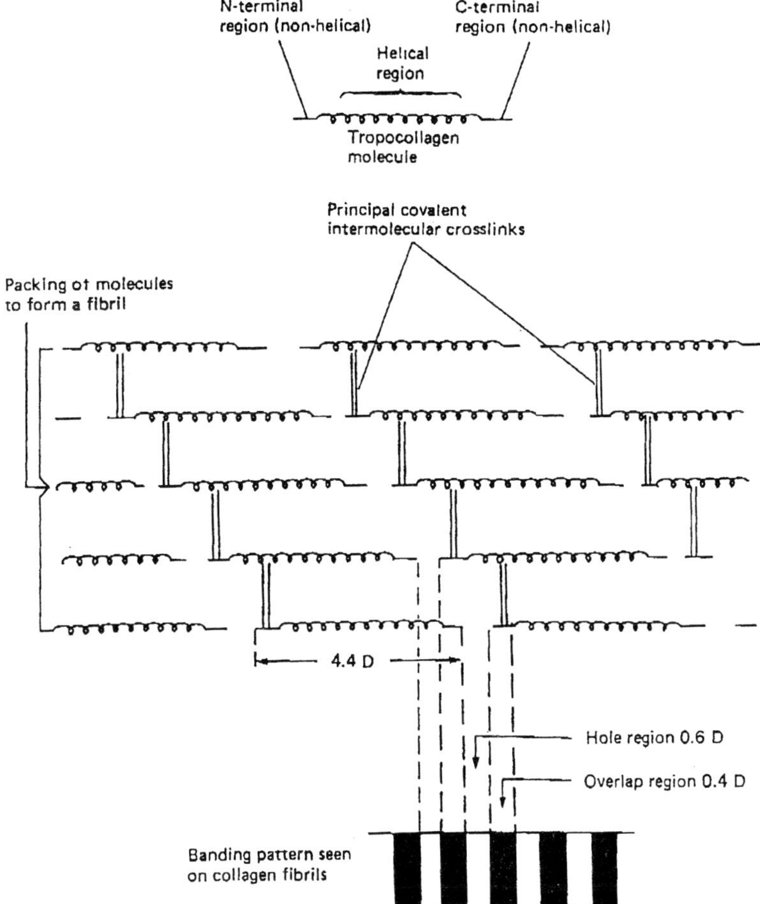

Fig. 4.2. Diagram of tropocollagen molecules and their packing arrangement in a collagen fibril
D indicates the periodicity seen in the native fibril

Articular cartilage contains predominantly type II collagen, in which each of three identical polypeptide chains contain a specific content of hydroxylysine residues and linked prosthetic groups. In the last decade other types of collagen have been reported within cartilage, namely types V, VI, IX, X and XI. These may have important roles in the overall structure of the tissue (Mayne 1989).

Collagen fibrils undergo a slow maturation process during which inter-molecular and intra-molecular cross-links are formed. The formation of these cross-links requires a degree of overlap between adjacent molecules, which is consistent with the 64 nm periodicity observed in the fibrils (Figure 4.2). Intermolecular cross-links may also be formed between residues located in the helical regions of adjacent molecules.

The reducible cross-links formed in immature cartilage are intermediate processes in the formation of more stable, non-reducible cross-links. There is also an increase in the intermolecular covalent cross-links with age in human tissues. Such observations are consistent with the marked increase in chemical stability of the collagen fibres in mature adult cartilage.

4.2.2.1 Collagen microstructure. Both the diameter and orientation of collagen fibres in articular cartilage vary with depth below the articular surface (Figure 4.1). These variations can be discussed with respect to the zones identified above.

The superficial zone, including the articular surface, extends to a depth of approximately 200 μm below the surface and contains fibrils of approximately 30 nm diameter. The fibrils are arranged in sheets, which lie parallel to the articular surface. In each sheet there is a range of fibrillar orientations (Kamalanathan and Broom 1993). In addition, the fibre orientation varies in subjacent sheets. Fibrils and fibre bundles are closely packed with little intervening proteoglycans when compared to the deeper zones (Weiss et al. 1968). At the surface of the superficial zone there is a thin layer composed of fine fibrils, approximately 5 nm in diameter associated with abundant proteoglycans (Weiss et al. 1968; Balazs et al. 1966).

The deep zone of cartilage occupies the remainder of the uncalcified tissue thickness. The collagen fibres surround the columns of cells and thus also tend to be orientated perpendicularly to the interface between the cartilage and the subchondral bone (McCall 1968; Bullough et al. 1968).

In the calcified region there are increasing deposits of calcium salts in the matrix surrounding the few cells. The collagen fibrils are radially aligned in this region, which occupies between 5 and 10% of the matrix volume.

4.2.3 Proteoglycan

The term proteoglycan describes molecules composed of a protein core to which at least one glycosaminoglycan chain is covalently attached. Glycosaminoglycans (GAG) consist of repeating disaccharide units comprising n-acetyl hexosamine linked to a hexuronic acid or hexose. Several GAGs exist in cartilage, namely chondroitin sulphate (CS), keratan sulphate (KS), heparan sulphate (HS), dermatan sulphate (DS) and hyaluronan. Their relative proportions vary with the type of cartilage and with age.

The most abundant proteoglycan in cartilage is *aggrecan*, which accounts for approximately 90% of the total content within cartilage. Aggregan, as represented in Figure 4.3, consists of a core protein to which both CS and KS chains and O-linked and N-linked oligosaccharides are attached. The core protein has three different globular domains, termed G1, G2 and G3. The G1 is situated at the amino-terminal end of the core protein, and acts as a binding site for hyaluronan (Figure 4.3). This interaction is stabilised by a link protein, with structural homology to the aggrecan G1 domain that binds to hyaluronan as well as to the G1 region of the aggrecan. Aggrecan and hyaluronan form multimolecular aggregates within cartilage matrix with molecular weights of the order of 50 million Da. The formation of aggregates acts to retain aggrecan within the matrix. When there is a large excess of proteoglycan over hyaluronan, as in cartilage, a large number of proteoglycan molecules interact with a single chain of hyaluronan, as shown diagrammatically in Figure 4.4.

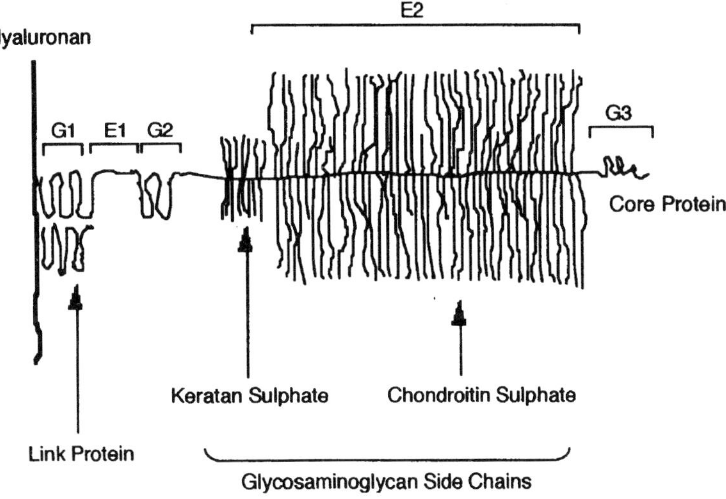

Fig. 4.3. Schematic representation of an aggrecan molecule bonded to hyaluronan via a link protein. (Reproduced with permission from Knight 1997)

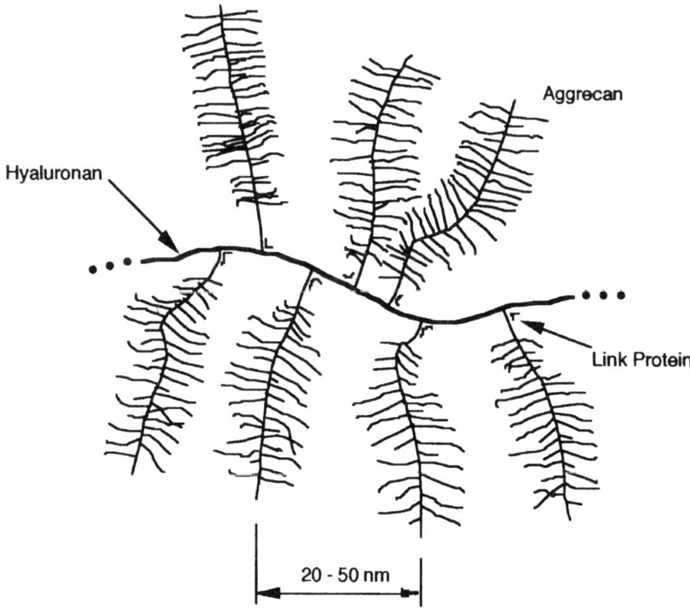

Fig. 4.4. Model of aggrecan-hyaluronan complex in articular cartilage. (Reproduced with permission from Knight 1997)

Other smaller leucine-rich proteoglycans, such as *biglycan*, *decorin* and *fibromodulin*, exist in articular cartilage. Their functions are largely unknown, but the latter two small proteoglycans are thought to be involved in collagen fibrillogenesis.

Proteoglycans are polyanions due to the negatively charged sulphate and carboxyl groups associated with KS and CS. These properties control the ability of proteoglycans to bind water osmotically and the polyelectrolyte gels may be considered as osmotic systems. The gel behaves like a solution in tending to dilute itself with solvent. In cartilage this process is limited by the extensibility of the collagen fibres with which the proteoglycans are enmeshed.

The proteoglycan content is inhomogeneously distributed throughout the depth of cartilage. In the superficial zone, there is very little hyaluronan present and as a consequence only small amounts of aggrecan. Instead the proteoglycan present in this zone are strongly associated with the densely packed collagen fibres. The content of proteoglycans increases significantly with distance from the articular surface attaining a maximum value in the middle and deep zones.

4.2.4 Interstitial water

Water is readily imbibed into articular cartilage because of the hydrophilic nature of the proteoglycans. The highest water content is found near the articular surface and it decreases towards the subchondral bone, attaining a value of approximately 65% in the deep zone (Maroudas 1979). Only a small proportion of the total water in cartilage is intracellular.

It is now well established that the interstitial water can exist in two distinct compartments. About 30% of the interstitial water is strongly associated with the collagenous network. The remaining water is associated with proteoglycan domains and is freely exchangeable during joint loading and unloading. It is this movement which is important for joint lubrication and chondrocyte nutrition and viability. Furthermore, the tissue fluid contains mobile charged ions, such as calcium, sodium and hydrogen, and can establish streaming potentials, which can alter cell metabolism.

4.2.5 Changes with ageing and clinical conditions

During ageing, changes occur in the composition of articular cartilage. This includes a decrease in total water content and an increase in the concentration of the proteoglycan (Wachtel et al. 1995). There are also alterations in the composition and size of aggrecan, in particular a decrease in the proportion of CS-rich region of the monomer and an increase in the proportion of the G1 domain (Wachtel et al. 1995). The composition of the smaller PGs also changes with maturation, with a marked increase in the ratio of decorin to biglycan. In addition, there is also a reported increase in the diameters of collagen fibrils with age.

Osteoarthritis is a degenerative condition, which affects the synovial joint. The prevalence of the condition increases with age, reaching a maximum in the sixth and seventh decades. However, there are a growing number of younger people who develop the disease subsequent to traumatic damage of major load bearing joints such as the knee. Some of the earliest detectable changes leading to osteoarthritis occur in the articular cartilage. Features of degenerative cartilage are a gradual softening and disruption of the articular cartilage. Small fissures appear in the superficial zone and the subsequent exposure and disruption of the collagen fibres is termed fibrillation. It should be noted that not all cartilage fibrillation will lead to a progressive form of degeneration - some mechanical weakening with age may be a direct result of the fatigue processes within the articular cartilage. Other manifestations of the disease condition include the formation of microfractures, subarticular cysts in the subchondral bone and gross geometrical changes.

These changes with age and disease will inevitably affect the mechanical properties and hence the functions of articular cartilage.

4.3. BIOMECHANICS OF ARTICULAR CARTILAGE

4.3.1 Load Carriage

It is the physicochemical interaction of the various components of the extracellular matrix, which is responsible for the mechanical properties of the healthy tissue. For example in articular cartilage, there is a physicochemical equilibrium between the osmotic swelling pressure ($P_{swelling}$) of the proteoglycan gel which is balanced by the hydrostatic pressures ($P_{elastic}$) due to the tensile stresses generated within the collagen fibre network. This balance exists even in unloaded articular cartilage, as indicated below.

$$P_{elastic} = P_{swelling} \tag{4.1}$$

The magnitude of $P_{swelling}$ is related to the concentration of the charged GAG, and has been estimated to be approximately 0.35 MPa in unloaded cartilage (Maroudas 1979). The balance is altered when the tissue is loaded in compression by an applied hydrostatic pressure ($P_{applied}$) resulting in a net pressure differential (Δp) and fluid flow away from the compressed tissue. This may be represented by:

$$\Delta p = P_{applied} + P_{elastic} - P_{swelling} \tag{4.2}$$

All these terms may be a function of time. This fluid flow will result in an increased proteoglycan concentration within the tissue and a change in the relative magnitudes of the stresses in the two solid components of articular cartilage. If the compressive load remains constant, the rate of fluid flow decreases with time and eventually reduces to zero at a new state of equilibrium, namely:

$$P'_{swelling} = P_{applied} + P'_{elastic} \tag{4.3}$$

Time dependent creep behaviour is characteristic of all viscoelastic soft tissues. If the applied force is suddenly released, the cartilage recoils almost instantaneously to a limited extent and then recovers gradually to its original thickness. This time dependent component of recovery occurs as water is re-imbibed into the cartilage matrix, until the original unloaded equilibrium position is reached. Cyclic loading produces similar behaviour, although the extent of the recovery within each cycle will depend on the form and frequency of the loading pattern.

The behaviour of the extracellular matrix may be modelled in terms of a biphasic material incorporating a *fluid phase* of interstitial water and a *solid phase*, the collagen-proteoglycan organic solid matrix to represent the fluid-filled porous-permeable medium (Mak et al. 1987; Armstrong and Mow 1982). Other phases have been recently introduced to accommodate the presence of interstitial ions within the matrix (Snijders et al. 1997). The movement of these ions in compressed cartilage establishes streaming potentials within the tissue, which may play a role in mechanotransduction pathways, as discussed later in the chapter.

4.3.2 *In vitro studies*

There have been a plethora of biomechanical studies over the last 35 years to investigate the *in vitro* characteristics of articular cartilage. These have been adequately reviewed in various publications (Mow et al. 1992; Kempson 1979). A range of loading modes has been employed, including shear, torsion, impact, compression and tension. However, in view of the mechanisms by which the extracellular components resist joint forces, most studies have concentrated on the tensile and compressive properties of articular cartilage. These have been examined commonly with relation to parameters such as age, state of cartilage surface and chemical composition. The latter may be investigated with the use proteolytic enzymes, which degrade, selectively, the structural components of articular cartilage.

4.3.2.1 Tension. Collagen fibres are the main tension resistant elements in connective tissues. Their presence in articular cartilage suggests that tensile stresses are present, even though the tissue is loaded predominantly in compression perpendicular to the articular surface.

Investigators have examined the tensile properties of thin slices of articular cartilage (Kempson 1979; Bader et al. 1981; Bader 1985). When an isolated dumbell-shaped specimen of cartilage is subjected to a tensile force in a plane parallel to the articular surface, the resulting stress-strain behaviour is non-linear in form, as illustrated in the curves in Figure 4.5.

The response can be regarded as a continuous progression of three phases of behaviour. Initially at low levels of stress the collagen fibres tend to become aligned in the direction of the tensile force. The tensile tangent modules in this phase depends on the initial orientation of the collagen fibres and the effective resistance of the proteoglycan gel to their alignment. With increasing alignment of the collagen fibres the component of the applied stress along the fibres increases and the stress versus strain curve increasingly reflects the mechanical properties of the fibres. With increasing stress, therefore, the tangent modulus increases until fracture of the specimen occurs within the gauge region.

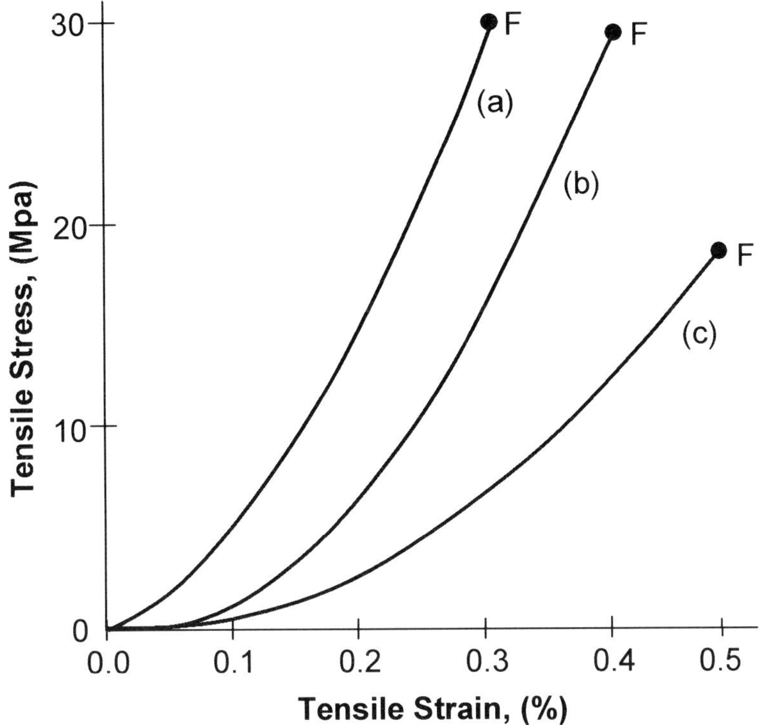

Fig. 4.5. Schematic representation of the tensile stress-strain behaviour of three specimens obtained from the superficial zone of human articular cartilage. Curves represent (a) untreated specimen (b) specimen with depleted levels of proteoglycan and (c) specimen with damage to collagenous network. F indicates fracture of specimen.

There is some variation in the tensile properties with orientation of the specimen. Superficial layer specimens have been shown to highly strain-limiting in tension, thereby implying least compliance, along the split-line direction and least strain-limiting across it. However, despite earlier reports to the contrary, a recent study has revealed no strong dependence of fracture strength on split-line orientation (Kamalanathan and Broom 1993). Tensile properties also decrease with respect to distance from the articular surface. These results demonstrate both the anisotropic and non-homogeneous nature of articular cartilage.

The dependence on the relationship between the two main structural components and tensile properties can be demonstrated by the incubation of cartilage specimens in proteolytic enzymes (Bader et al. 1981; Bader 1985). These studies demonstrated that the effect of proteoglycan degradation alone was limited to a reduction in the tensile stiffness in the initial phase of the stress-strain relationship, as seen with curve *b* in Figure 4.5. However, damage to the collagen network with associated release of proteoglycans from the matrix was sufficient to reduce both the tensile stiffness at all levels of stress and the tensile strength of cartilage, as shown with curve *c* in Figure 4.5. Indeed this response was evident with one specific enzyme, leukocyte elastase, despite no measurable release of collagen from the matrix. These results confirmed the importance of the covalent intermolecular cross-links, which elastase are known to disrupt (Starkey et al. 1977), on the overall mechanical properties of the collagen fibrils in articular cartilage.

In two related tensile fatigue studies by Weightman and colleagues (1976; 1978), it was demonstrated that human articular cartilage is prone to tensile fatigue failure *in vitro*. Tests on specimens from human femoral head cartilage revealed that the fatigue resistance decreased with age at a rate, which was faster than that which could be explained by normal usage. The decrease in fatigue resistance could not be related to either of the two major solid constituents of the specimens. By combining the observations the following model was produced:

$$S = 23 - 0.1a - 1.83 \log(N) \tag{4.4}$$

where S is the stress in MPa, a is the age in years and N is the number of cycles to failure.

In a recent *in vitro* study, the effects of partial fatigue on the tensile properties of articular cartilage were evaluated (McCormack and Mansour 1998). Cartilage specimens were repetitively loaded at a frequency of 0.75 Hz using a maximum compressive load of 65N for approximately 80,000 cycles. This procedure revealed no macroscopic damage to the surface of the cartilage specimen. Subsequent tensile tests produced a reduction in tensile strength, which was attributed a weakening of the interfibril connections which link collagen fibrils in the middle and deep zones of the cartilage matrix (Broom 1984).

4.3.2.2 Compression. Specific test methods have been developed for testing cartilage in compression. The two most common methodologies are the *indentation test* which uses an indenter to apply compression to discrete areas of the cartilage surface *in situ* and the *uniaxial compression test*, which involves the use of a platten or large indenter to compress isolated cylinders of cartilage perpendicular to the articular surface. This latter test has been performed with the cartilage specimen in either a confined state or an unconfined state. The confined state is achieved using porous platens to apply compression to the specimens, which are constrained by walls radially. This arrangement attempts to mimic the boundary conditions present *in situ*. However a recent paper has suggested that complete confined is impossible to achieve *in vitro* (Buschmann et al. 1998).

A critique of the two test methods is provided in Table 4.2. Both methods, however, will produce a similar response following the application of a rapid load to the cartilage surface, using a damped mechanical testing system (Armstrong and. Mow 1982; Kempson 1979). This is characteristic of a typical viscoelastic material, namely

Table 4.2. An appraisal of testing methods of articular cartilage in compression

Method	Advantages	Disadvantages
Indentation	Provides normal physiological constraints on deformation and fluid	Difficult to align indenter perpendicular to the cartilage surfaces.
	Permits assessment of properties across the joint surface	Complex stress distribution under the indenter makes it difficult to determine material constants.
Uniaxial Compression	Unidirectional stress allows the calculation of compressive stiffness.	Boundary conditions and fluid flow different from intact joint.
	Specimen size permits controlled tests with surrounding media of different concentrations or incubation with biochemicals.	

an initial elastic response, followed for a time-dependent creep response (Figure 4.6). Several studies have estimated the creep modulus 2 seconds after load application and related it to the chemical constituents of cartilage (Kempson 1979). Results indicated that this parameter, which as its name suggests includes a creep component, was significantly correlated to total glycosaminoglycan content, but was independent of the natural variation in the collagen content.

Stress relaxation tests using confined geometry have enabled the estimation of the material parameters, hydraulic permeability and aggregate modulus (H_A). The latter parameter reflects the intrinsic stiffness of the solid components of the ECM. A summary of representative values of derived stiffness for articular cartilage is presented in Table 4.3. This also shows some data from cartilage areas where the damage ranged from slight surface fibrillation to gross ulceration.

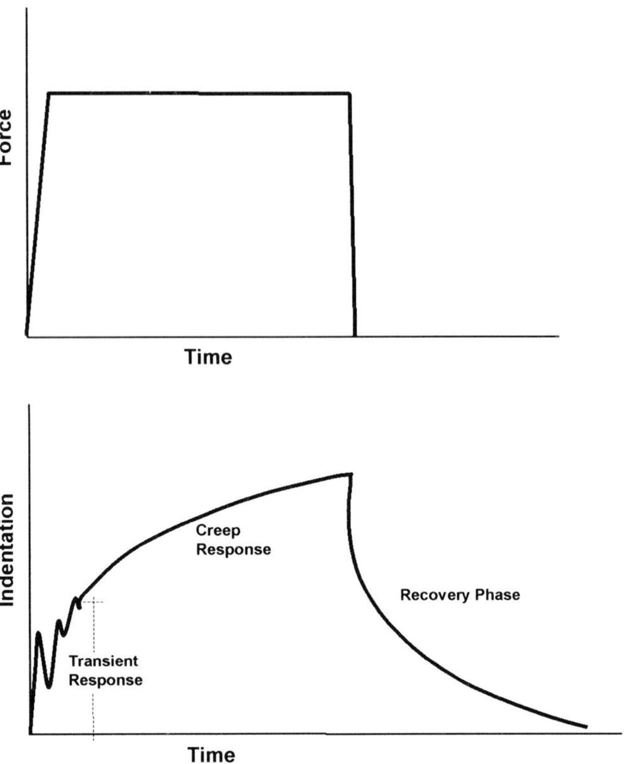

Fig. 4.6. Typical response of articular cartilage to a compressive step-load input, with transient response indicative of an underdamped mechanical loading system.(Based on Bader 1985)

In the above studies the short-term response of the tissue was partly determined by the dynamic characteristics of the overdamped test apparatus. This limitation was recognised by Woo and colleagues (1980) on finding that the initial elastic stiffness of articular cartilage continued to increase at very high loading rates and its measurement is thus limited ultimately by the response of the measuring equipment. Two separate studies both showed that when loaded rapidly in compression, cartilage displayed a transient oscillatory response, which decayed to a steady creep after less than one second following the point of loading (Woo et al. 1980; Coletti et al. 1972). The authors suggested that this initial transient oscillatory response of cartilage could be used to uncouple the elastic stiffness and the viscous damping in the tissue. This could be achieved by designing an underdamped test apparatus and using it to examine the damped free oscillatory response using standard dynamics analyses (Bader and Kempson 1994). This response is illustrated in Figure 4.6. A similar method employing free oscillations in shear has been used to test non-biological polymeric materials (Ferry 1970).

Table 4.3. Stiffness values for adult human articular cartilage.

Reference Test Model	Joint Surface	Stiffness Modulus (MPa)	Poisson's Ratio
G. Kempson (1979)			
Indentation	Femoral head	1.9 – 14.4	0.50
2 second creep	Normal areas (mean)	7.0 – 8.7	
Linear elastic	Damaged areas(mean)	3.1 – 6.4	
D. Bader (1985)			
Compression			
unconfined	Femoral condyles	6.1 – 14.9	—
0.6 second	Femoral head	5.3 – 19.7	
C. Armstrong and V. Mow (1982)			
Compression			
confined	Patella	$0.79 < H_A < 1.91$	—
Biphasic			
K. Athanasiou et al. (1991)			
Indentation	Femoral condyles	$0.59 < H_A < 0.70$	$0.07 < \nu < 0.10$
Biphasic			

To analyse the transient response it was assumed that the short-term viscoelastic properties of articular cartilage could be represented by a simple Voigt phenomenological analogue, in which elastic forces are linearly proportional to the compressive deformation and viscous forces are linearly proportional to the rate of compressive deformation. This model allows uncoupling of the elastic and viscous elements of the response and their separate determination.

A study was undertaken using such an underdamped mechanical system to test core specimens of human articular cartilage in unconfined compression (Bader and Kempson 1994). It examined the effects of two enzymes, cathepsin D and leukocyte elastase, on the two uncoupled parameters, which characterise the short-term compressive properties of cartilage. Both enzymes produced an increase in the amplitude of the oscillation. However whereas leukocyte elastase caused the frequency of the oscillation to decrease, as illustrated in Figure 4.7, there was no change in the frequency with cathepsin D. The results demonstrated that the collagen component of cartilage largely influenced the elastic stiffness. The damping term, however, was influenced by the proteoglycan constituents, as demonstrated by the statistically significant linear relationship in Figure 4.8. Examination of the data related to individual cartilage specimens revealed an inverse relationship between the elastic stiffness of cartilage and the specimen thickness, t, as illustrated in Figure 4.9. This statistically significant relationship is consistent with the expression for the stiffness of an elastic prism, k, of constant cross-sectional area, A, and constant Young's modulus, E, where:

$$k = \frac{EA}{t} \tag{4.5}$$

The result implies that the initial "elastic" modulus of cartilage in compression is fairly constant in healthy joints yielding a value of approximately 10 MPa.

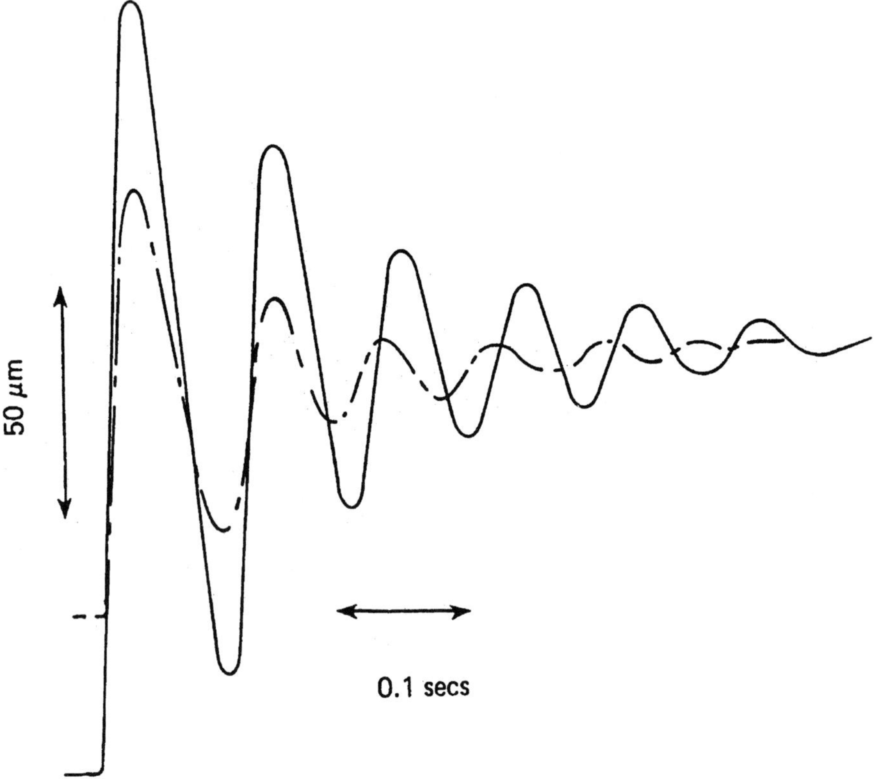

Fig. 4.7. Effect of leukocyte elastase on the transient oscillatory response of human articular cartilage to a compressive step load. _____ _ _____ Response of the untreated specimen ; _______ Response of the same specimen after incubation in leukocyte elastase for 72 h at 37 °C. (Based on Bader 1985).

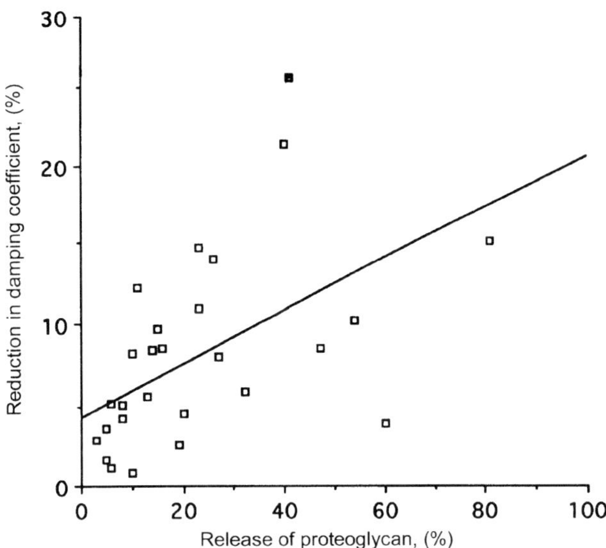

Fig. 4.8. Reduction in damping coefficient of human articular cartilage from the hip and knee joints with sequential release of proteoglycan after treatment with cathepsins B and D.

($y = 4.44 + 0.16x$; $r = 0.51$, $p < 0.001$)

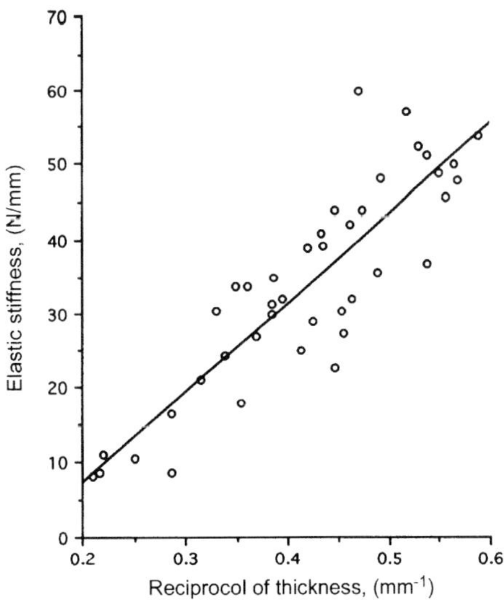

Fig. 4.9. Elastic stiffness of cartilage from the transient oscillations versus the reciprocal of specimen thickness.

($y = -16.9 + 121\ x$; $r = 0.88$, $p < 0.001$)

4.3.3 In vivo studies

The development of *in vivo* biomechanical techniques has been stimulated by the requirement to measure the stiffness of cartilage during clinical investigations. One of the few such instruments, which can be used during arthroscopic investigations, was based on an indentation method (Lyyra et al. 1995; Lyyra 1997). The device consists of a reference plate, which is placed against the cartilage surface and pressed gently with a constant force for a period of one second. This enables a small probe to be deformed by a fixed value of 300 microns and the resulting force can be used to estimate the structural stiffness of the localised region of cartilage. This system which is now commercially available (Artscan 1000 System, Finland) can be used to assess potential cartilage damage and cartilage repair following surgical procedures. However, in order to establish material properties of cartilage a measure of its thickness is required and an estimate of the stress distribution under the probe.

4.4. CELL SEEDED REPAIR SYSTEMS

4.4.1 Repair strategies

Degenerative disease and injuries to soft tissues are extremely common in hospital clinics. They involve all ages of the population. Indeed, soft tissue replacements amount to an estimated 35% of the world market for all medical devices, Materials Technology Foresight in Biomaterials (1995). However, the vascularity of many soft tissues are poor, as is the case of many tendons, or non-existent as with articular cartilage, and therefore the natural healing response is limited.

Many of the conditions causing partial and full thickness chondral and osteochondral defects, including trauma, osteochondritis dissecens, chondromalcia and tumours occur commonly in the younger population. Joint replacement arthroplasty is unsuitable in this group due to their physical demands and prolonged life expectancy, which can lead to early loosening and prosthetic failure. Even a successful prosthesis only lasts about 15 years before a revision is indicated and for a young patient, a series of revisions would be inevitable. There have been many options proposed for the repair of chondral and osteochondral lesions in Table 4.4.

Table 4.4. Options available in the biological resurfacing of cartilage defects

Pridie method
Synthetic materials e.g. carbon fibre
Allogenic materials
Xenograft materials
Infusion of growth factors
Cellular grafts e.g. periosteal cells
Cell engineered implants

It is beyond the scope of this chapter to detail all the options and the reader is referred to many excellent review articles on this topic (Buckwalter and Mankin 1997; Messner and Gillquist 1996). To review briefly the options generally involve synthetic materials, biological materials or a combination of the two. Synthetic solutions have generally been chosen due to their acceptability in biological environments. Such systems to repair cartilage lesions involve the use of porous polymers and carbon fibres, in designs varying from straight bundles to non-woven patches (Muckle and Minns 1990). However their instability in the body leads to relatively poor long-term performance.

Biological solutions traditionally involve autografts, allografts and xenografts (Shaghadi et al. 1991), depending on their source of tissues. Each of these options has proved to be less than ideal with, for example, xenografts proving difficult to position optimally in a defect and autografts inevitably resulting in donor site morbidity.

The relative failure of many synthetic and graft solutions, has led to the growing interest in the development of cell seeded repair systems for solving a number of clinical problems related to connective tissues, such as articular cartilage, menisci and ligaments. One approach is to use implants of isolated viable chondrocytes, but these have largely resulted in the formation of fibrocartilage, or cartilage surrounded by fibrous tissue, which functions in a different manner to articular cartilage. To avoid the morbidity associated with autologous grafts of articular cartilage, another approach involves grafts derived from periosteum and perichondrium tissues, both of which contain progenitor cells capable of chondrogenesis. In a specific methodology, Brittberg and associates (1994) utilise cultured chondrocytes and inject them under a peroiosteal flap sutured over a defect in the cartilage surface. The procedures, which are detailed in Table 4.5, have been employed in both animal models and an increasing number of human knees with cartilage defects, which do not extend to bone. This and other derivative techniques have been adopted by a growing number of tissue engineering companies, such as Genzyme Tissue Repair Corporation (Boston, USA) and Verigen Transplantation Service Ltd. (Copenhagen, Denmark). These companies are now offering their services for the processing of autologous cells. Some of the early clinical results are quite encouraging, although the mechanical integrity of this repair system at all times post implantation has not been confirmed.

Table 4.5. Stages followed in the chondrocyte transplantation into defects of the human knee

Stages
Treat partial thickness cartilage lesions of areas 1.6 - 6.5 cm^2
Biopsy from non-weight bearing area of healthy cartilage
Enzyme digestion
Cultivation for 11-21 days - 10 fold expansion
Trypsin treatment
Suspension of 2.6 - 5.0 x 10^6 cells
Periosteal flap, taken from the medial tibia, sutured over lesion
Injection of cultured chondrocytes under flap into lesion

Based on Brittberg et al. (1994)

A major design feature of for any cartilage repair is that the implant must be able to support normal dynamic joint forces immediately post implantation. This could be accomplished if the cells were contained within a construct with inherent mechanical integrity. Typically autologous or allogenic cells are isolated from a tissue biopsy removed from a low load-bearing site remote from the injury. The cells are expanded in cell culture and seeded in a suitable 3D resorbable scaffold material, which, on implantation, will elicit a biological repair. In addition, the biological nature of this so-called *tissue engineered repair system* can ensure maintenance and turnover of the repaired tissue in the long term. Success depends, however, on the ability of the cells to synthesise a functional matrix at a rate sufficient to balance the loss of the mechanical integrity of the resorbing scaffold material. On implantation, the tissue-engineered systems will be subjected to normal physiological forces. Thus, the associated mechanical environment will influence the cell response in a manner, which cannot be predicted in an unstrained cell culture environment. It is vital; therefore, to understand the effect of dynamic mechanical strain on cells within tissue engineered systems, in order to predict and optimise the device performance *in vivo*. Another important consideration is the general conditioning of the cell-seeded devices prior to implantation. Indeed, the use of bioreactor technology to produce cartilage cells on a production basis has already been established in the companies, Genzyme Corporation and Advanced Tissue Sciences, in the United States.

The choice of biomaterials has to date been largely empirical based on biocompatibility and the maintenance of cell morphology and function. Materials such as polyglycolic acid, collagen in various forms and alginates have been employed. The inclusion of bioactive molecules, such as growth factors, within the devices has often been deemed important for the successful elaboration of extracellular matrix. Most of the post implantation analysis has involved histological and biochemical analysis of repair tissue, with only a few reports assessing its mechanical integrity (Kim et al. 1994; Paige et al. 1996). However, the use of *in vivo* measurement systems, as described in section 4.3.3, is currently gaining popularity.

4.4.2 Cells in load bearing tissues

As has been previously stated the cells in articular cartilage, although occupying less than 10% of the tissue volume, are necessary for the synthesis, assembly, maintenance and degradation of the ECM. The cells are therefore crucial to the structural integrity and function of the tissue. It is known that the cells in all load bearing soft tissues, whether chondrocytes in cartilage, fibrochondrocytes in menisci or tenocytes and fibroblasts in tendon and ligament respectively, are able to alter their metabolic activity in response to applied load. Both the level of strain applied and the dynamic frequency are known to be important in determining response. These processes are believed to be major factors in determining cellular activity in tissues, such as articular cartilage. Indeed *in vivo* studies have shown that the mechanical environment will influence the structure and function of articular cartilage. Typically, moderate exercise leads to an increase in cartilage proteoglycans, whereas immobilisation of joints leads to a reversible release of proteoglycans (Kiviranta et al. 1988; Saamanen et al. 1987).

The mechanisms by which cells detect and respond to the mechanical environment are termed *mechanotransduction pathways* and are both complex and poorly understood. Mechanotransduction events in articular cartilage may be resolved into extracellular components including cell deformation, hydrostatic pressures, fluid flow and streaming potentials, followed by intracellular signalling events such as intracellular calcium fluxes, cAMP production and cytoskeletal alterations, which finally lead to altered effector cell response. It is unclear whether mechanotransduction is a universal process or whether various metabolic parameters are influenced by distinct intracellular signalling pathways, which are uncoupled. A better understanding of the link between initial application of load and effector cell response is necessary for the appreciation of metabolic control in normal and pathological tissues and will be of use in the development of tissue engineered repair systems. This goal is complicated by the need to investigate processes at the cellular level. This has been heightened in the last decade by the considerable developments in molecular biology.

4.4.3 Characterisation of model systems

There are two approaches which have been adopted to examine the response of cultured chondrocytes to biomechanical stimuli *in vitro*. One involves the use of cartilage explants in which the chondrocytes will be associated with ECM similar to that *in situ* (Gray et al. 1988; Sah et al. 1989). The alternative involves models using isolated chondrocytes maintained in various cultures systems including suspension cultures, monolayer cultures of either high or low cell densities, or homogenous gels, such as alginate or agarose (Lee and Bader 1997; Freeman et al. 1994). A critical appraisal of the two representative approaches is provided in Table 4.6. Explant systems have the disadvantage of not being suitable to examine one possible pathway for mechanotransduction such as cell deformation due to the coupling of mechanical and physicochemical processes in the ECM. For this and other reasons, the present authors have employed a physical model system involving chondrocytes embedded in agarose gel (Lee and Bader 1995).

In order to examine this hypothesis it is necessary to determine that an initial stimulus, such as cell deformation, can induce distinct responses in a number of metabolic parameters.

It is recognised that any model system is inherently non-physiological. Nevertheless, the authors and others have shown that the agarose/chondrocyte system exhibits several suitable features. These include :-

- The chondrocytes remain phenotypically stable over an extended culture period
- The model allows the investigation of the influence of cell deformation, as a single pathway, on the metabolism of cells subjected to mechanical loading.
- The model is relatively simple and reproducible
- The model can be characterised in mechanical terms. Thus both quasi-static and dynamic mechanical parameters have been reported at different culture periods (Knight et al. 1996).

Table 4.6. Two distinct systems to examine chondrocyte behaviour in compression

System	Advantages	Disadvantages
Explants	Provides normal extracellular environment for chondrocytes	Inherent coupling of mechanical and physicochemical processes will lead to complex response Inherent variability between explant sources e.g. different locations and joints
Physical model e.g. chondrocytes seeded in agarose gel	Homogeneous and simple Examine single parameters such as cell deformation Preparation of uniform specimens	Different physiological state than normal for cartilage Modulus considerably lower than articular cartilage

- The model permits chondrocyte deformation when gross strain is applied to the agarose, which may be visualised using confocal microscopy, as shown in Figure 4.10. Using simple mathematical analysis, it could be shown that at a gross compressive strain of 15% the resulting deformation was equivalent to a cell strain of approximately 15%, a level considered to be physiological in loaded cartilage (Broom 1984; Guilak 1994).

4.4.4 Mechanical conditioning of model systems

Conventional *in vitro* mechanical tests require the soft tissues to be kept in a moist environment and are either performed on a Universal test facility or on a specially designed test system. However, if tissue explants or cell containing biomaterial constructs are to be tested, viability must be maintained in a conventional incubator, whilst the system is subjected to static and dynamic loading. A common method to apply such loading is via a commercial strain unit (Flexercell, Flexcell Intl. Corp., Mckeesport, USA), in which cells are attached to a flexible substrate at the base of culture plates. Negative pressure is applied in a cyclic manner, to provide deflection of the base of the plate. This produces a non-uniform strain field across the substrate.

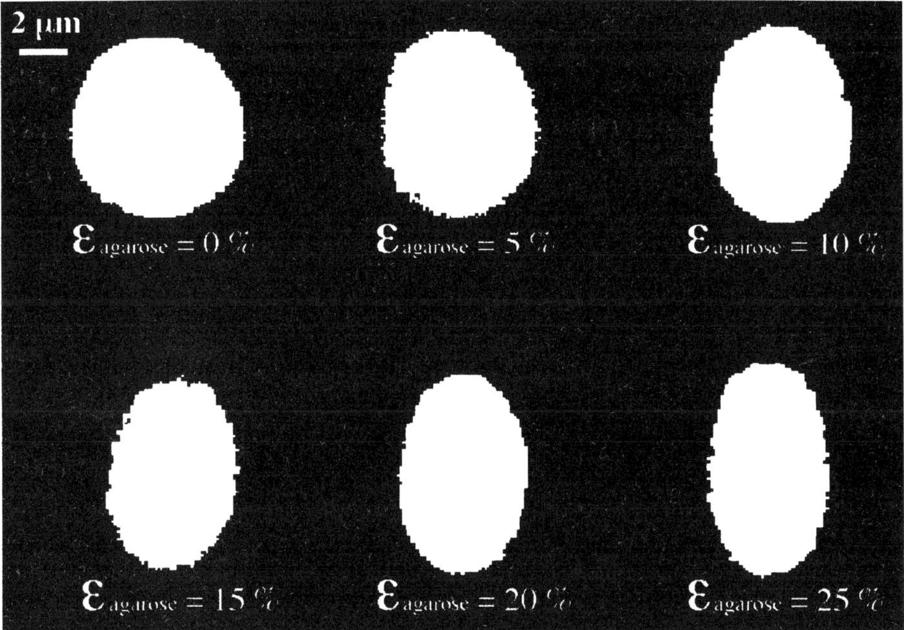

Fig. 4.10. Horizontal confocal sections bisecting the centre of a single chondrocyte, stained with calcein AM and seeded within an agarose construct subjected to compressive strains of up to 25%. (Based on Knight 1997).

Recent studies have used this system to apply cyclic strain to tendon cells and examine effects, in conjunction with growth factors, on the stimulation of DNA synthesis (Banes et al. 1995).

An alternative cell-straining apparatus (Dartec Ltd., Stourbridge, U.K.) was developed by the authors to apply static and dynamic compression to biomaterial constructs seeded with chondrocytes (Lee and Bader 1997). This apparatus, as shown schematically in Figure 4.11, consists of a conventional loading frame with an hydraulic actuator-controlled vertical assembly, which enters a tissue culture incubator (Heraeus Instruments, Brentwood, U.K.). The assembly is connected to a central rod which is attached to a mounting plate located within a perspex box which, in turn, is placed on a circular platter fixed to the base of the loading frame. The mounting plate holds 24 loading pins, half of which are unconstrained to move vertically in harmony with the loading assembly. Each loading pin incorporates an 11mm circular perspex indenter, which applies compressive strain to samples located within separate wells of a tissue culture plate. All appropriate components must be sterilised prior to setting up any culture experiments.

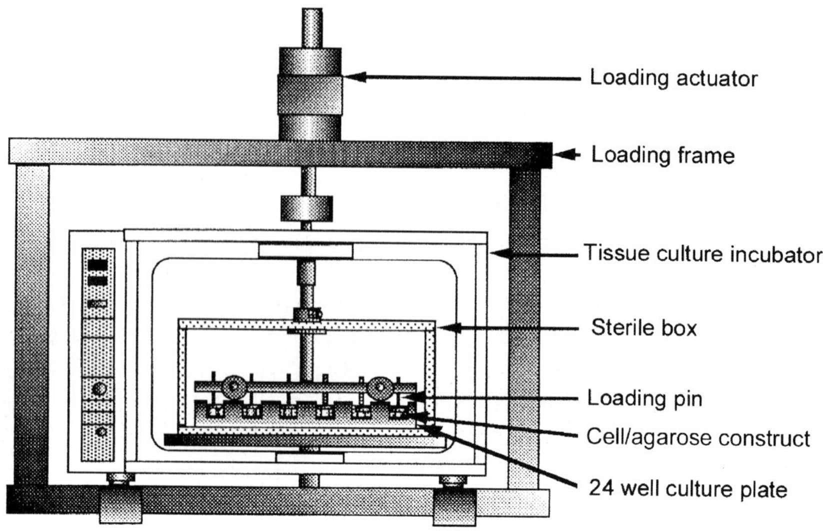

Fig. 4.11. Schematic of cell straining apparatus, which was used to apply compressive strain to chondrocytes seeded in agarose constructs.

The development of this apparatus has enabled the authors to perform a series of studies, which have examined the performance of chondrocyte-seeded agarose constructs when subjected to prescribed loading regimens. The motivation for these studies was to:-

- Gain an improved understanding of the role of cell deformation as an extracellular signalling pathway in mechanotransduction.
- Assess the current procedures employed in the tissue engineering of cartilage.
- Enhance the potential of tissue engineered implants by stimulating cell-seeded constructs to produce ECM *in vitro* and hence provide an implant with increased potential for long term stability post implantation.

The production of chondrocyte seeded agarose constructs have been detailed by the authors in previous reports (Lee and Bader 1995 and 1997). To review briefly, slices of cartilage were removed from the metacarpalphalangeal joint of 18 month-old steers, washed briefly in Earle's Balanced Salt Solution and then cultured at 37°C in 5% CO_2 for 16 hr in Dulbecco's minimal essential medium (DMEM)+20% foetal calf serum (FCS) (all Gibco, Paisley, U.K.). The chondrocytes were isolated by sequential enzyme digestion and embedded in 3% agarose. Cylindrical core constructs, approximately 5mm in diameter and 5mm in height, were cut from the gel and weighed to determine the number of cells. The cylindrical constructs were cultured in

1ml of DMEM+ 20% FCS at 37°C in 5% CO_2 for 16 hr to allow equilibration to culture conditions.

Individual constructs were then located in a 24 well tissue culture plate. For each experiment, 12 of the specimens are strained (experimental group), whilst the other 12 are unstrained except for a tare strain of 0.8% resulting from the mass of the loading pin (control group). One millilitre of DMEM + 20% FCS + 1 μCi/ml [^{3}H]-thymidine or 1 μCi/ml [^{3}H]-proline (Amersham International, Amersham, U.K.) was introduced to each well. The control electronics were set to produce a crosshead movement equivalent to a compressive strain ranging from 0% to 15%. For the dynamic strain conditions, a sinusoidal waveform was used at each of three frequencies, namely 0.3Hz, 1Hz and 3Hz. The static strain condition involved the application of 15% compression. All of the chondrocyte/agarose cylinders were incubated at 37°C in 5% CO_2 for 48 hr. Three metabolic processes were examined, namely the synthesis of GAG, incorporation of [^{3}H]-TdR into DNA and incorporation of [^{3}H]-proline into protein.

During the 48-hour culture period under strain, there was no significant difference in the viability of chondrocytes under static and dynamic strain compared with unstrained controls. Thus any differences in metabolism could not be attributed to alterations in chondrocyte viability.

A summary of the results are provided in Table 4.7. It can be seen that static strain reduced the level of [^{3}H]-TdR uptake, a marker of cellular proliferation, whereas dynamic strain at all frequencies induced an increase in chondrocyte proliferation. With respect to glycosaminoglycan, static and low frequency (0.3Hz) dynamic strain inhibited GAG synthesis, while a frequency of 1 Hz induced a significant stimulation of GAG synthesis. Although other studies have suggested an increase in GAG

Table 4.7. The effects of static and dynamic compression on the metabolism and proliferation of chondrocytes isolated from full depth cartilage and seeded in agarose constructs.

	Strain – Amplitude (0.0 — 0.15)			
	Static	*Dynamic*		
		0.3Hz	1.0 Hz	3.0Hz
GAG synthesis	—	—	+	nc
GAG released into medium	+	+	+	+
[^{3}H]-TdR incorporation	—	+	+	+
[^{3}H]-proline incorporation	—	—	—	—

+ (—) increased (decreased) ; *nc* no change

Values are compared to unstrained controls cultured for 48 hours in DMEM + 20% FCS within the test apparatus.

synthesis with frequency, no other studies have examined the response to frequencies exceeding 1 Hz. Thus the findings at the high frequency of 3 Hz in which GAG synthesis returned to unloaded control levels, suggest the presence of a cut-off frequency, which is probably associated with the nature of fluid flow within these constructs.

Although all loading regimens yielded an inhibition in protein synthesis, as measured using proline incorporation, the analysis of data revealed an association between the frequency rate and the level of inhibition. The results implied that the three main parameters were each influenced by dynamic strain regimens in a distinct manner, implying that the associated signalling mechanisms are uncoupled.

This study has been extended to investigate the effects of cell origin on compression induced alterations in proliferation and GAG synthesis. Chondrocytes within the superficial zone of articular cartilage are known to be morphologically and metabolically distinct from cells deeper within the tissue. Differences are maintained when the cells are isolated.

In a recent study of Lee et al. (1998), thin slices of cartilage representing the uppermost 20% of the tissue depth were removed from the bovine metacarpalphalangeal joint. The cells isolated from these slices were termed "superficial cells". The residual cartilage tissue was harvested taking care to avoid contamination with calcified cartilage. The cells isolated from these slices were termed "deep cells". Both superficial and deep cells were seeded into separate 3% agarose constructs and tested in an identical procedure to that adopted in the previous study (Lee and Bader 1997).

Results in Figure 4.12 indicate that proliferation of superficial cells was stimulated at all frequencies of dynamic strain. No such influence was observed with deep cells. With reference to GAG synthesis, there was a general inhibition by superficial cells. By contrast, deep cells produced a variable response to dynamic strain; at 1 Hz there was a significant stimulation of glycosaminoglycan synthesis, whereas at 0.3Hz there was a significant inhibition (Figure 4.13). These results strongly suggest that the two metabolic processes occur in different subpopulations of chondrocytes within the full-depth cell isolate. In particular it appears that

In current work, the authors are pursuing the identification of intracellular pathways and signalling molecules activated during mechanical stimulation. They are also examining the various stages associated with the current tissue engineering approach for cartilage defects (Table 4.5). In particular, investigations are underway to assess the performance of chondrocytes following monolayer expansion *in vitro*.

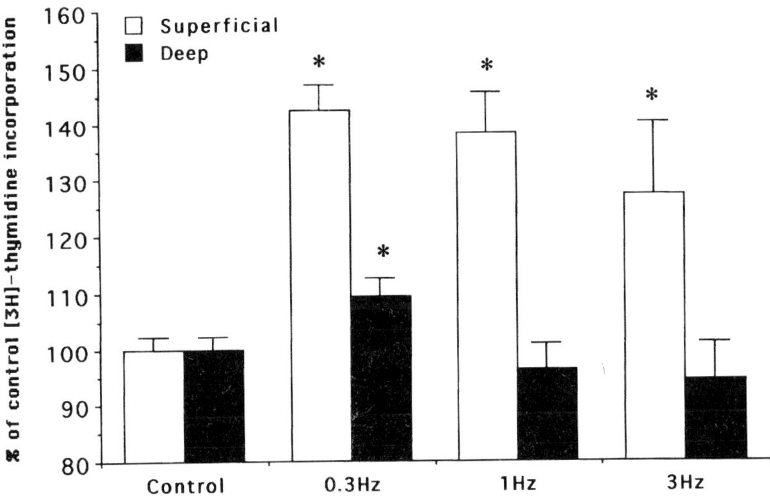

Fig. 4.12. [^{3}H] thymidine incorporation, as a marker for cell proliferation, for both surface and deep chondrocytes embedded in agarose and subjected to 15% gross compressive strain at various frequencies for 48 hours. The values are normalised to unstrained control values. Each value represents the mean and SE of at least 16 replicates.

* Unpaired student's t-test indicate significant differences at the 5 per cent level.

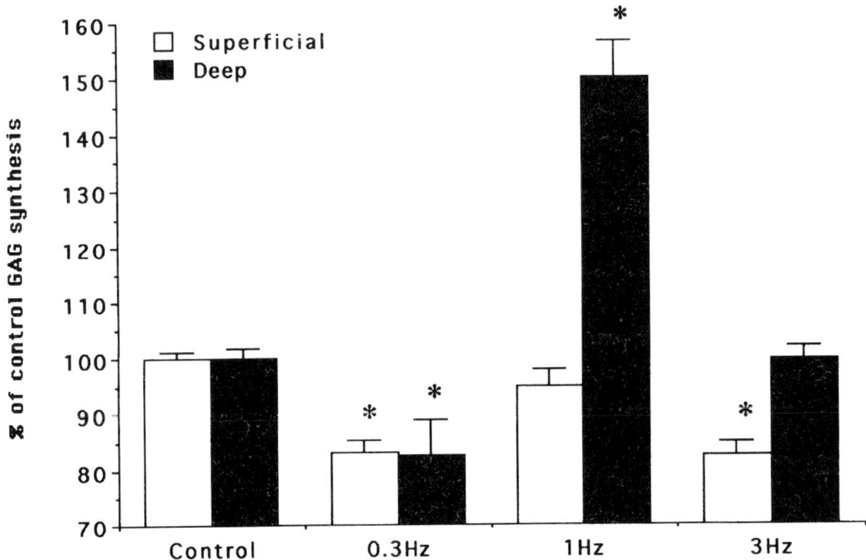

Fig. 4.13. Glycosaminoglycan synthesis by both surface and deep chondrocytes embedded in agarose and subjected to 15% gross compressive strain at various frequencies for 48 hours. The values are normalised to unstrained control values. Each value represents the mean and SE of at least 16 replicates.

* Unpaired student's t-test indicate significant differences at the 5 per cent level.

4.5. FINAL COMMENTS

This chapter attempts to provide an insight in the biomechanical performance of articular cartilage at a range of hierarchical levels. However, despite the large research activity invested in tissue mechanics it is still very difficult to characterise the mechanical behaviour of normal and diseased/damaged articular cartilage in terms of discrete values for established material parameters. This limits the effectiveness of models, employing techniques such as finite elements (FE) to predict behaviour of the tissue in physiological loading conditions. The current interest in new technologies, involving molecular biology and tissue engineering, has led to the emergence of cartilage biomechanics at the cellular level. This may prove a viable opportunity to attract research funding at both national and international level.

ACKNOWLEDGEMENTS.

The authors would like to acknowledge the invaluable support of Drs Geoffrey Kempson and Martin Knight and other colleagues at the IRC in Biomedical Materials for various aspects of this work. Funding for the more recent studies was provided by the Engineering and Physical Sciences Research Council of Great Britain.

REFERENCES

Armstrong C.G. and Mow V.C. (1982) *J.Bone Jt. Surgery*, **64**(A), 88.

Athanasiou K.A., Rosenwasser M.P., Buckwalter J.A., Malinin T.I. and Mow V.C. (1991) *J. Orthop. Res.*, **9**, 330.

Bader D.L., Kempson G.E., Barrett A.J. and Webb W. (1981) *Biochim. Biophys. Acta*, **677**, 103.

Bader D.L. (1985) Ph.D Thesis, University of Southampton, U.K.

Bader D.L. and Kempson G.E. (1994) *Bio-medical Materials and Engineering*, **4**, 245.

Banes A.J. et al. (1995) *J. Biomech.*, **28**(12), 1505.

Balazs E.A., Bloom G.D. and Swann D.A. (1966) *Fed. Proc. Fed. Am. Soc. Exp. Biol.*, **25**, 1813

Brittberg M., Lindahl A., Nilsson A., Ohlsson C., Isaksson O. and Peterson L. (1994) *N. Eng. J. Med.*, **331**, 889.

Broom N. (1984) *Arthritis and Rheum.*, **27**, 1028.

Buckwalter J.A. and Mankin H.J. (1997) *J. Bone Jt. Surgery*, **79A**, 612.

Bullough P. and Goodfellow J.G. (1968) *J Bone Jt Surgery*, **50B**, 852.

Buschmann M.D., Soulhat J., Shirazi-Adl A., Jurkelin J.S. and Hunziker E.B. (1998) *J. Biomech.*, **31**, 171.

Coletti J.M., Akeson W., Woo S.L.-Y. (1972) J. Bone Jt. Surgery **54** (A), 147.

Ferry J.D. (1970) in *Viscoelastic Properties of Polymers,* ed. Ferry, J.D. (John Wiley. New York) p. 145.

Freeman P.M., Natarajan R.N., Kimura J.H. and Andriacchi T.P. (1994) *J. Orthop. Res.*, **12**, 311.

Gray M.L,, Pizzanelli A.M., Grodzinsky A.J. and Lee R.C. (1988) *J. Orthop. Res.*, **6**, 777.

Guilak F. (1994) *J. Microscopy*, **173**, 245.

Kamalanathan S. and Broom N. (1993) *Journal of Anatomy* **183**, 567.
Kempson G.E. (1979) in *Adult Articular Cartilage,* ed. Freeman (Pitman. London) p. 281.
Kim W.S. et al. (1994) *Plastic and Reconstructive Surgery*, **94**(2), 233.
Kiviranta I., Tammi M., Jurvelin J., Saamanen A-M. and Heliminen H.J. (1988) *J. Orthop. Res.*, **6**, 188.
Knight M.M. (1997) Ph.D Thesis, University of London, U.K.
Knight M.M., Lee D.A. and Bader D.L. (1996) *Cell Eng.* **1**, 97.
Lee D.A. and Bader D.L. (1995) *In vitro Cell Dev. Biol. Animal*, **31**, 828.
Lee D.A. and Bader D.L. (1997) *J. Orthop. Res.*, **15**, 181.
Lee D.A., Noguchi T., Knight M.M., O'Donnell L.B., Bentley G. and Bader D.L. (1998) *J. Orthop. Res.*, **16**, 726.
Lyyra T., Jurvelin J., Pitkanen P., Vaatainen U. and Kiviranta I. (1995) *Med Eng. Phys.*, **17**, 395.
Lyyra T. (1997) Ph.D Thesis, University of Kuopio, Finland.
Mak A.F., Lai W.M. and Mow V.C. (1987) *J Biomechanics*, **20**, 703.
Maroudas A., Stockwell R.A., Nachemson A. and Urban J.P. (1975) *J. Anat.*, **120**, 113.
Maroudas A. (1979) in *Adult Articular Cartilage* ed. Freeman (Pitman. London) p. 215.
Materials Technology Foresight in Biomaterials(1995) Institute of Materials, London.
Mayne R. (1989) *Arthritis Rheum.*, **32**(3), 241.
McCall G. (1968) Lancet **2**, 1194.
McCormack T. and Mansour J.M. (1998) *J. Biomech.*, **31**, 55.
Messner K. and Gillquist J. (1996) *Acta Orthop.* Scan., **67**, 523.
Mow V.C., Ratcliffe A. and Poole A.R. (1992) Biomaterials, **13**, 67.
Muckle D.S. and Minns R.J. (1990) *J. Bone Jt. Surgery*, **72B**, 60.
Paige K.T., Cima L.G., Yaremchuk M.J., Schloo B.L., Vacanti J.P. and Vacanti C.A. (1996) *Plastic and Reconstructive Surgery*, **97**, 168.
Saamanen A-M., Tammi M., Kiviranta I., Jurvelin J. and Heliminen H.J. (1987) *Connect. Tiss. Res.*, **16**, 163.
Sah R.L.Y., Kim Y.J., Doong Y.V.R., Grodzinsky A.J., Plaas A.H.K. and Sandy J.D. (1989) *J. Orthop. Res.*, **7**, 619.
Snijders J., Huyghe J. and Janssen J. (1997) *Int. J. Num. Meth. Fluids*, **20**, 1039.
Shaghadi B.F., Amis A.A., Heatley F.W., McDowell J. and Bentley G. (1991) *J. Bone Jt. Surgery*, **73B**, 57.
Starkey P.M., Barrett A.J. and Burleigh M.C. (1977) *Biochem. et Biophys. Acta*, **483**, 386.
Terrig Thomas J., Ayad S. and Grant M.E. (1994) *Ann. Rheum. Dis.*, **53**, 488.
Wachtel E., Maroudas A. and Schneiderman R. (1995) *Biochim. Biophys. Acta* **1243**, 239.
Weightman B. (1976) *J. Biomech.*, **9**, 193.
Weightman B., Chappell D.J. and Jenkins E.A. (1978) *Ann. Rheum. Dis.*, **37**, 58.
Weiss C., Rosenberg L. and Helfet A.J. (1968) *J. Bone Jt.Surgery*, **50A**, 663.
Woo S.L-Y., Simon B.R., Kuei S.C. and Akeson W.H. (1980) *J. Biomech.Eng.*, **102**, 85.

Chapter 5
Bioartificial Implants: Design and Tissue Engineering

Chapter 5
Bioartificial Implants: Design and Tissue Engineering

ROBERT A. BROWN

5.1. BIO-CENTRIC LOGIC IN BIOENGINEERING

Until recently, much of the thinking in bioartificial repair has been dominated by engineers and material scientists. This is often for good reason, since clinical imperatives and available technology tended to demand this type of approach. However, recent advances in our understanding of biological mechanisms have begun to feed into the concept of 'engineering' of true tissues: the construction of bioartificial grafts. The biomedical and the engineering approaches to these questions are distinct and the coming challenge is to construct effective fusion's of the two disciplines. Table 5.1 contrasts (not too seriously) the two approaches, in this case the incompatibility of automotive engineering and clinical logic as applied to 'repair'. The aim here is to explain this view and to discuss current attempts to achieve the fusion.

Table 5.1. Why repairing a Ford and repairing Aunt Sally's leg are different.

Ford Escort [1.6 GLS]	Aunt Sally's leg
If the repair fails you can always do another	In the repair fails you have to have a good story for the patient and the scar
… and another, and another	Patients come with limited blood, excess pain-receptors and legal rights
Ford will always supply more spare parts: including parts for old models	Patients only have 2 legs, often no relatives and are old: = poor spares supply
Second-hand spares can be cleaned, polished and reground as good as new	Used spares are soft, pink and very rare: NIL shelf-life; come with the previous owner's VIRUSES and are *completely* ruined by cleaning treatments
Tolerances in the handbook are defined	What tolerances, what handbook?
Fords have clones	Aunt Sally has devoted relatives
Cars can't hire lawyers	****

Tissues, which we may wish to (re-) construct, can fall into two groups; *structural/conductive* or *metabolic/processing*. Structural and conductive tissue would include the connective tissues (e.g. skin, tendon), nervous tissues (e.g. peripheral nerves, particularly in the hands and face) and blood vessels, such as coronary arteries or capillary beds in the leg. Metabolic/processing tissues would include organs such as liver, kidney, spleen and pancreas. There is much overlap in the engineering of each type of tissue, but the emphasis of the final function makes it better to deal with them separately. The majority of this review will be aimed at the structural/conductive class of application.

Figure 5.1 illustrates the spectrum of implants from *biological* grafts to *non-biological* prostheses. These devices, implants, grafts and engineered tissues, form a continuum span between the extremes of totally artificial implants, such as hip replacements and contact lenses, and classical surgical autografts like skin flaps and muscle. Not surprisingly, much of the historic success has been in the replacement of tissues of the structural and conductive types. This has been based on the use of traditional materials and conventional engineering concepts and techniques. It is possible to trace the parallel evolution of materials and implants from wooden legs and eyeglasses through to modern steel and plastic hip joints and fabric vascular implants.

Future progress in tissue engineering and implants will inevitably require a fundamental shift in the thinking and understanding of how tissues operate, particularly in the long-term. Traditional examples of implants (artificial hips or vascular implants) clearly never become part of the recipient's body or biological function; they do not age and are not replaced. Indeed they begin their process of

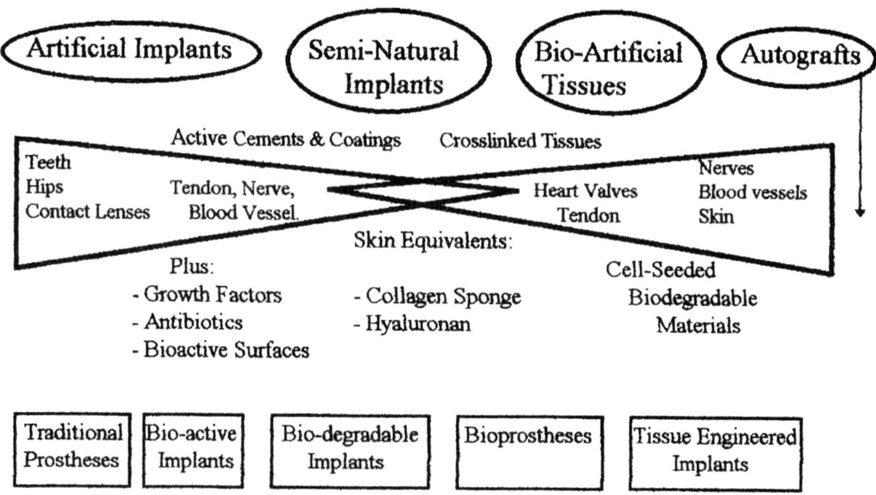

Fig. 5.1. Simplified scheme illustrating the spectrum of implantable devices from traditional, wholly engineered prostheses to tissue engineered, bioartificial grafts (ending with native tissue grafts, not regarded as devices). The progressive levels of biological interaction can be identified and are elaborated in the text.

wearing out and failure from the moment of implantation, in some instances this is accelerated by cellular action. Although such devices will continue to be useful, even dominant forms of implant for many years, future devices and materials will be based on fundamentally different logic.

Until recently even biologically enlightened designs for implants were based on the idea that the materials to be replaced (i.e. the biological connective tissues) behaved predominantly as conventional, synthetic polymer materials, though complex in nature. This appeared to be particularly applicable to tissues such as cartilage and tendon, which, in adults, have sparse cell populations. However, it is this cell content, no matter how small, which represents the difference in thinking. It is possible to use this as a definition to distinguish between *conventional* implants and *bioartificial* or tissue engineered implants.

To qualify as a bioartificial tissue by this definition, the final device must not only contain cells which remain in the material, but must achieve an environment in which those cells *manage* that support matrix in order to maintain the function of the tissue. The term *manage* refers to the ability of cells in a natural matrix to turnover the tissue, respond to external stimuli such as mechanical, electrical and chemical input and maintain the material in the face of wear and damage. This unity of cellular and material function and their interdependence is not found in conventional implants, even though local cells may populate the surfaces or pores of the implant structure. Such resident cells do not participate in the maintenance and upkeep of an implant and chemical/mechanical messages from the materials to such cells are ambiguous and inappropriate.

Clearly by this definition of interplay between the cell and extracellular matrix (ECM) the nature of the material must be amenable to cellular activity (deposition of new material and removal of existing materials). Since biological building blocks are proteins and polysaccharide aggregates, or combinations of the two, it is likely that the *final* bioartificial tissue will be made of these backbone components. Towards this end temporary templates, supports and guides for cell activity can use a diverse range of synthetic or modified biopolymers. Strategies to reach this end point include;

a.- provision of the initial material from protein and polysaccharide components

b.- provision of an initial supporting material made from bio-reabsorbable polymers which the resident cells will replace in time with their own extracellular matrix.

In both instances the long-term outcome is likely to be that resident cells have replaced all of the initial scaffolding supplied with the bioartificial implant, with their own ECM (e.g. after 1-2 years a future bioartificial tendon would be expected to consist almost entirely of the patient's own collagen).

This *bio-centric* approach to implants is a small revolution in design thinking, principally because of the central role which it places on the resident cell, rather than on the implanted material. Cells in a living adult tissue can occupy as little as 1 to 10% of its volume and yet transform the remaining 90%+ into a material for which there is no direct equivalent in non-biological systems. For example, the supporting matrix elements of a uterus are reduced in mass by many times immediately after birth by hormone-regulated resident cells (Woessner 1982). Alternatively, tendons of the arm grow many times their initial length between the ages of 1 and 18 years, but at *all* times they are under functional tensional load. Soft biological materials grow and repair by the insertion of new matrix *throughout* the entire structure (i.e. around each cell), rather than by addition of new material at the ends (without obvious cutting, splicing or loss of function, Birk et al. 1991; Byers and Brown 1990). In soft tissues this is referred to as interstitial growth. There are no synthetic material paradigms for these events. In engineering terms interstitial growth would only occur if new hemp fibres or steel wire could be inserted into rope or cable at (perhaps) 0.1mm intervals along its length such that the structures became longer. Cells carry out this process naturally and the current challenge is to produce bioartificial structures, which participate in this process.

5.1.1 Where to copy and where to adapt

So much for the dream. In terms of perfectly reproducing biological systems we are several hundred million years behind, and what is more, do not have the benefit of an *embryo bioreactor* (i.e. foetus-in-uterus) to fabricate the template of tissue structures in the first place. The biological basis for many events in developmental biology is still uncertain and poorly controllable. It would be ideal to be able to fabricate a new, fully functional cornea from a few autologous cells in a back room of your local ophthalmological practitioner. Sadly, with the present level of biological understanding this is *not* going to happen quickly. In the meantime we make the best use of pieces of glass and plastic which we understand how to make; cheaply, reliably and in mass batches. Conceptually, then, it is necessary to adapt our designs to mimic biological processes, using conventional materials and engineering processes, rather than attempting only to copy them faithfully, i.e. purely biologically. This means that designs need to adapt modern man-made materials and control techniques towards *bio-impersonation*. The aim of this impersonation is to deceive the cell. The conclusion then, is that tissue engineering presently aims to utilise adult tissue *repair* processes rather than embryonic tissue formation.

5.2. NORMAL STRUCTURE OF ADULT SOFT CONNECTIVE TISSUES

Before it is possible to rationally design materials, techniques and bioartificial constructs to replace human tissues, it is essential to understand the structure, function and limitations of those tissues. Firstly, we shall concentrate on *normal* and *adult* tissues. Realism and a degree of humility suggests that the constructs which are engineered will not be 'normal' tissues, but this at least can be the aspiration. The focus here is on soft/non-mineralised connective tissues, which excludes bone and teeth.

Production of bioartificial tissues for children, subject to growth periods, presents particular problems, In this case the implanted tissue must not only be capable of expansion in size, but must do so in proportion to surrounding tissues, (in terms of overall structure postnatal tissue is similar to adult, but embryonic connective tissues can be radically different). Extension of non-biological implants, particularly in bone, represents a relatively *simple* engineering problem and a number of examples of expanding orthopaedic implants have been described. In the case of soft tissue implants, the remaining sections of anatomically normal, growing tissue attached to the implant may helpfully make up *some* of the growth of surrounding structures. It is known for example, that grafted tissue such as skin will grow with the child. Our limited understanding of the processes of soft connective tissue growth and growth co-ordination represent recurrent biological impediments to successful tissue engineering (Woessner 1982; Byers and Brown 1990). However, the very process of developing more sophisticated tissue engineering implants and materials seems likely to improve this understanding.

Characteristic features of any given tissue are a result of their *composition* or *architecture*. There are numerous reviews on the composition of connective tissues both specifically and in general (Birk et al. 1991; Nimni 1988) and the reader is referred to key articles cited here.

5.2.1 Connective tissue composition

Most connective tissues have a similar composition, in terms of *basic* components. Alterations in the sub-types and proportions of these extracellular matrix (ECM) components contribute to the structural variability of tissues. In most cases the main tissue component is water (Comper 1996). Clearly, water is critical to function but is normally only considered as a special component in tissues such as articular cartilage. The overall dry compositions of representative connective tissues, in terms of protein and protein-polysaccharide complexes (collagen, glycosaminoglycans, proteoglycans, elastin etc.), are shown in pie charts in Figure 5.2.

5.2.1.1 Collagen. (See also Chapter 8.2.2). The main protein component in mammalian connective tissues, with few exceptions is collagen (reviewed in Bateman et al. 1996). Indeed it is the most common protein in the mammalian body, comprising up to 25% of the dry protein. It is a molecule primarily adapted to transmit and resist tensile mechanical loads. However, it is important to distinguish that it can function in the transmission of tensile load both at the tissue or macro-level (i.e. connecting bone to bone in the case of ligaments) and at the cellular or micro-level (i.e. transmitting tension between fibroblasts within a contracting dermal scar). The former is of course familiar to everyone through the gross structural properties of skin and ligaments, but its function (particularly minor collagen types such as types IV, VI & VIII) is to provide suitable anchorage and a source of mechanical stress for cells resident in ECM.

The collagens make up a family of structural proteins currently comprising over 20 forms (Bateman et al. 1996). However we need to consider only a very few of these. The main load bearing, architectural collagen within vascularised tissues (excluding the cartilages) is Type I collagen. In the cartilages its role is performed by Type II

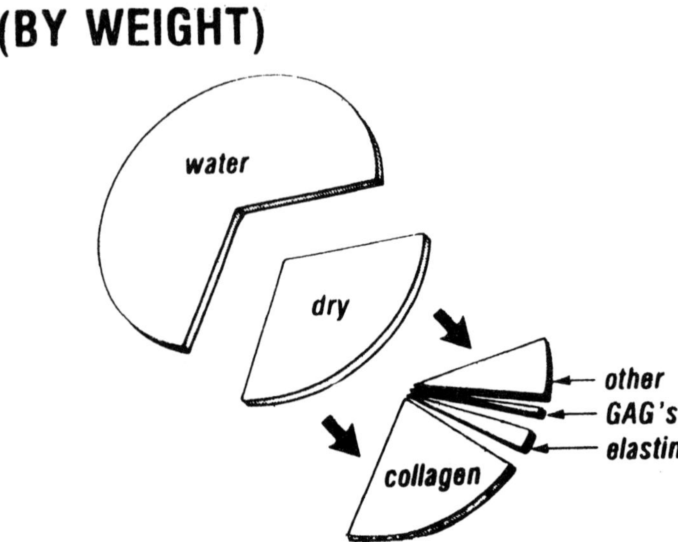

Fig. 5.2. Pie chart illustrating the approximate proportions of the major connective tissue components in normal ligament. Note the preponderance of collagen in the dry material. Much the same components (though with subtle differences) make up most connective tissues. Specific tissue properties are mainly due to different proportions and spatial organisation (architecture). GAG = glycosaminoglycans. (Frank et al. 1985)

Collagen. Type III Collagen forms fine fibrillar aggregates and is found in blood vessels and in mature tissue repair sites, whilst Type IV collagen is limited to basement membrane structures, for example beneath epithelial layers of the gut or endothelium of blood vessels. Types I, II and III form classical quarter-staggered, high tensile strength fibrils and fibre bundles, whilst type IV collagen forms more weakly structured fine meshwork aggregates, packed with proteoglycans.

The excellent mechanical properties of collagen in tension are a result of a highly specialised structure (reviewed in Nimni 1988; Bateman et al. 1996). The monomer consists of three polypeptide chains wound together into a tight triple helix, to give a fibre-type protein, 300 x 1.5nm. The helix is hydrogen bond stabilised into approximately 3.3 residues per turn. The distribution of glycine as every third residue, facing *into* the core of the helix gives the tightest possible coil with no capacity for deformation or extension, short of rupture. Fibril-forming collagens are synthesised as monomers with propeptide extensions at either end. The propeptides prevent spontaneous aggregation within the cell. Once outside the cell these propeptides are cleaved and the remaining tropocollagen, consisting almost entirely of the helical domain, spontaneously self-aggregates. This process of self-aggregation is critical to collagen structure and function. As a result of this rigidly controlled structure collagen monomers (tropocollagen) are able to pack laterally into semi-crystalline fibrils where each molecule packs precisely with its neighbours. It is driven solely by physico-

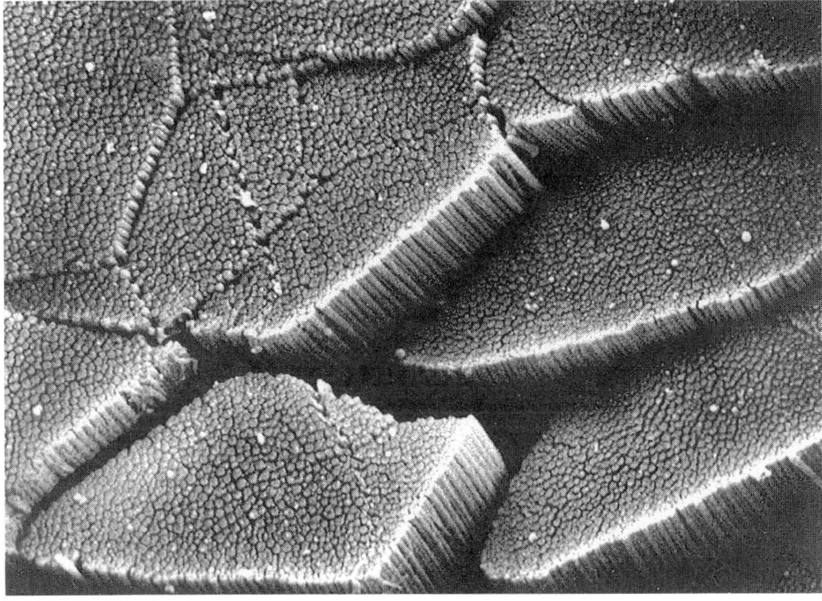

Fig. 5.3. Normal human tendon in cross section (scanning electron microscope image of freeze fractured specimen) showing collagen fibril aggregates in fibres which appear to glide over one another (Brown et al. 1997: x25k). Reprinted by permission of Blackwell Science, Inc.

chemical forces and occurs rapidly under physiological conditions. Fibrils can be identified by a characteristic banded staining pattern seen in the electron microscope, formed as a result of the rigid, repetitive ordering of charged amino acids exposed over the fibril surface. Molecules in such fibrillar aggregates are in a staggered array and crosslinked to give structures with great tensile strength. Molecular packing/aggregation can continue to give fibrils of between 20nm and 500nm diameter. Beyond this, fibrils are deposited together into fibres and then more extensive fibre bundles, transmitting loads across long distances through tissues. Figure 5.3 illustrates the type of tensile structure produced, in tendon.

5.2.1.2 Proteoglycans. (PG) are found in close association with collagen in many tissues, where their type and quantity vary from a few percent in tendon to up to 20% of the dry weight of cartilage. Proteoglycans are heterogeneous molecules due to the variable nature of their large polysaccharide component. They are composed of a protein core component carrying variable amounts of charged polysaccharides known as glycosaminoglycans (GAG). The GAG content can vary from one to many hundreds of chains, each of variable length, per protein core (Toole 1991). GAGs are characteristically highly negatively charged, frequently by extensive sulphation, examples being, chondroitin-, dermatan-, and keratan sulphates. Hyaluronan is an important form of GAG, which occurs free of protein and unsulphated (Lauren and Fraser 1992). The characteristic properties of these potentially enormous molecules are normally related to the large fixed charge they carry and their consequential osmotic activities (Hardingham and Fosang 1992).

Huge PG super-aggregates known as aggregan are characteristic of articular cartilage matrix (Tole 1991; Hardingham and Fosang 1992; Fosang and Hardingham 1996), dermatan sulphate PGs are found associated with collagen fibrils in dermis, whilst a specialised heparan sulphate PG, Pearlecan, is associated with type IV collagen and important to basement membrane function. In general, PGs are effective in holding water within the tissues, by virtue of their osmotic activity. In articular cartilage this swelling is essential to allow the collagenous network to effectively work under compressive and shear loading (Urban 1994). In other tissues PGs can generate and maintain swelling, characteristic of tissue turgor. The free, non-protein bound GAG, hyaluronan (formally known as hyaluronic acid -8) is widely distributed at the interfaces of gliding surfaces in the body, for example, around the synovial membrane in joints and between tendons and surrounding sheaths. Hyaluronan is important in cell attachment and motility in some situations and appears to be a biological lubricant between soft tissue surfaces (Toole 1991).

5.2.1.3 Elastin. Some tissues also contain dense, profoundly insoluble fibres of elastin (reviewed in Cleary and Gibson 1996). This is a highly hydrophobic protein which can be extended by the application of mechanical loads (in complete contrast to collagen fibrils) but which re-folds to its original size and shape on removal of the load. Hence, as its name implies, this component is responsible for much of the elastic recoil of tissues (e.g. in skin, in artery walls and in the elastic cartilage of the ears). The importance of elastic recoil of connective tissues is obvious in individuals with inherited disorders of elastin (such as cutis laxa and Marfan's syndrome), typically pendulous, folded skin and severe vascular disorders (Cleary and Gibson 1996; Ayad et al. 1994).

5.2.1.4 Cells. A small component of most adult connective tissues is the resident cell population. Unfortunately, the cellular compartment is probably also the least well understood. Even the naming of resident ECM cells is imprecise, the most common term in soft connective tissue being *fibroblasts*, or the specialist tissue forms of these. The matrix-producing stromal cells of bone are osteoblasts (or osteocytes), in tendon, tenocytes, they are dermal fibroblasts in skin and chondrocytes in cartilage. All of these forms of *matrix-managing* cells are of similar origin, share many properties and in some cases can switch between specialities. Even within these broad groupings there are different sub-types or populations of matrix-managers. For example, within articulating joints there are different types of chondrocyte in the surface and deep zones of the articular cartilage (Kuettner et al. 1993) giving way to fibrocartilage cell populations at the insertion point of ligaments and tendons.

In other soft connective tissues it has proved harder to identify sub-types of matrix-manager cells (except on the basis of tissue location) and the term fibroblast is more widely used. In the dermis there are known differences in behaviour between fibroblasts from the upper (papillary) zone, the deeper (reticular) zone and the subcutaneous adipose layer (Schor and Schor 1987). Likewise, tenocytes (tendon fibroblasts) from the surface of fascicles (epitenon) have distinct functions from those that are deeper (endotenon) and those in the surrounding sheath. Structural functions in peripheral nerves are served by epi- and endoneurial fibroblasts and perineurial cells. A further level of complexity is evident from the pronounced regional differences in the structure within even the same connective tissue. For example, skin from the foreskin, scalp, sole of foot and forehead are quite distinct (Burkitt et al. 1993). In each case different cellular/functional specialisations are apparent at that location (i.e. mucus secretory cell, hair follicle keratinocyte, keratinocyte stratum corneum and dermal fibroblast, respectively).

5.2.2 Connective tissue architecture

The biochemical nature of the principal molecular building blocks of soft connective tissues are considered mainly in their monomer form but these are far below the scale at which they can functionally operate in a structural matrix. Rather, it is the aggregation of the main matrix components, which is critical to the overall function of the whole tissue. Water in this case will not be considered in detail, though its role is important in some tissues functions (Comper 1996) normally related to macromolecular charge density.

5.2.2.1 ***Collagens.*** The most important connective tissue components with regard to architecture are the fibrous elements, principally collagen. This is an inescapable property of its anisotropic structure, as a long thin molecule, aggregating to give longer, thin fibrils and fibres. Clearly, the direction/plane/axis (if any) in which fibres are deposited will have profound effects of the architecture of the parent tissue.

The collagen molecule (and its larger aggregated forms) can essentially be considered as cylinders, radially symmetrical in cross-section but with a profound biaxial asymmetry in the longitudinal plane (figure 5.4). These fibrils can branch frequently, in some tissues, giving a near isotropic network or mesh structure with no apparent orientation, for example in mid-zone articular cartilage. Tissues such as skin and the annulus fibrosus of the intervertebral disc (figure 5.5) can be regarded as partially orientated networks of collagen. The dermis for example is a *basket weave* of collagen fibre bundles, though predominantly in a plane parallel with the surface. This structure has asymmetry and *local* fibril orientation. However, because orientation is predominantly short range (apparent at the microscopic level), the tissue itself is deformable; i.e. extensible in numerous planes over longer ranges, at the macroscopic level. Where there are long range macroscopic planes of fibre orientation (for example in areas of habitual uniaxial loading) the tissue also becomes more asymmetrical in behaviour. The third type of architectural asymmetry (maximal anisotropy) is found in tendon, ligament, parts of peripheral nerve and blood vessels. In these tissues collagen fibres and fibre bundles are highly orientated in a single plane, over long ranges. The obvious mechanical consequence of such pronounced orientation of inextensible fibres

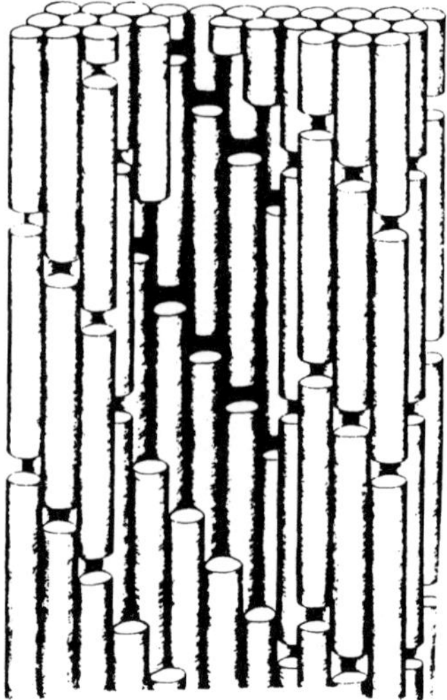

Fig. 5.4. Schematic diagram of the apparent arrangement of collagen molecules within a fibril. This 3D illustration attempts to combine the ideas of lateral packing, parallel orientation and quarter stagger of the molecules (each cylinder represents a collagen molecule: from Woodhead Galloway 1982).

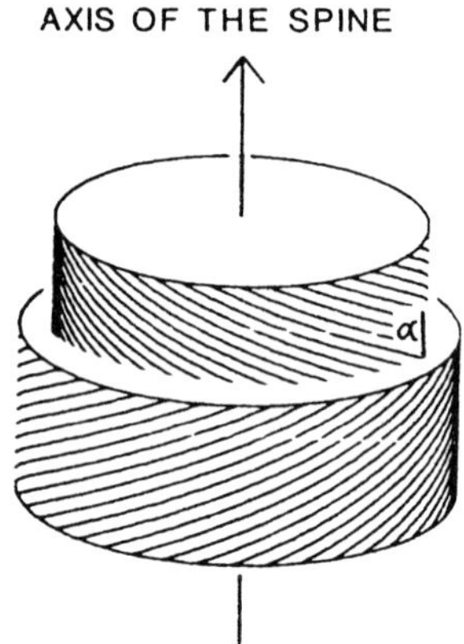

Fig. 5.5. Diagram illustrating the lamellar structure of the annulus from an intervertebral disc, showing the pronounced collagen fibre orientation in two adjacent lamellae. The inner nucleus pulposus of the disc is an aqueous gel restrained within these lamellae, through which axial loads on the spine are transmitted. Deformation of the angle of the collagen fibres (α), by gliding between the lamellae, permits compression of the nucleus and with it lateral dissipation of some of the load (from Hukins 1982).

is to give the tissue material great stiffness in the plane of fibre orientation. Significant local tissue anisotropy of this type also results in the formation of preferred planes of diffusion, fluid flow and cellular movement. Diffusion gradients are thought to be important in some biological control processes (new blood vessel formation and tissue degradation) mediated by inter-cellular signalling molecules. The effects and persistence of such gradients will also be dramatically altered by tissue anisotropy. Asymmetric tissue density can directly alter cell migration by limiting cell penetration (i.e. resistance to movement) and by influencing cell speed (section 5.3.1).

5.2.2.2 ***Proteoglycans.*** Although proteoglycans are important connective tissue components they do not have the rigidly anisotropic basic structure of the collagens. They are, in contrast, variable in structure and tend to take up random distributions. This absence of structural precision and ability of PG molecules to fold in many ways means that aggregates containing PG also have no determined size, structure or orientation and consequently, at the molecular and microscopic level, they contribute very little to tissue asymmetry. PGs can however contribute to higher levels of asymmetry and tissue organisation, in that the level and type of PG can differ between layers or planes and so affect tissue architecture. For example, the surface layer of normal articular cartilage contains low levels of PG whilst mid and deep zones contain very high levels with altered types of GAG substitution. Also, whilst tendon is poor in PG, at sites of tendon insertion to bones a transition occurs to produce *fibrocartilage*, rich in cartilage-like PG, which substantially alters its properties (Woo et al. 1988).

5.2.2.3 ***Elastin.*** A relatively minor component of many connective tissues but nevertheless critical for normal function. Since collagen fibrils are inextensible, tissue deformation is a result of the movement of fibres and fibre bundles relative to each other. Whilst directional extension of such structures under muscular tension is inevitable, there would be no automatic return to the initial tissue shape without the recoil properties of elastin, set between the collagen fibres. In skin, elastin networks have little obvious organisation, apparently facilitating multi-directional extension. In major blood vessel walls elastic recoil is an essential part of the tissue function and the stresses are in a predominant, radial orientation. The result is that elastin fibres take on an appropriate circumferential orientation, within a particular layer of the vessel wall, to generate a recoil tension as the vessel dilates under cardiac pressure (Burkitt et al. 1993).

5.2.2.4 ***Cells.***.Also important to the architecture of a tissue is the orientation of the cells present. Cells such as fibroblasts are frequently highly aligned and bipolar, giving an anisotropic structure. These cells can be aligned by environmental cues such as mechanical loading shown in figure 5.6 (Eastwood et al. 1998), or by contact guidance on a substrate using topographical features (fibres) or adhesive tracks (Dickinson et al. 1994; Wojciak-Stothard et al. 1997; Ejim et al. 1993; Clark et al. 1991). Once fibroblasts are aligned, the collagenous matrix, which they produce also,

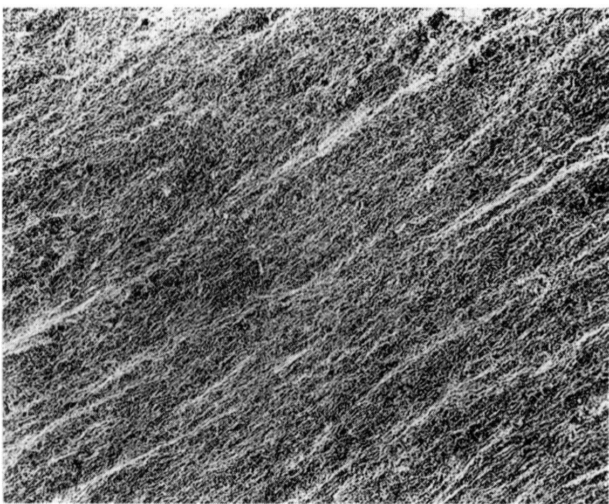

Fig. 5.6. Scanning electron micrograph of human dermal fibroblasts (long thin, bipolar dense white structures) embedded in a native collagen gel (the surrounding fine fibrous mesh). These cells were directed into a bipolar shape (from a multi polar stellate or rounded morphology) and a parallel alignment, by application of small, low frequency (1 cycle/hour) uniaxial mechanical loads (Eastwood et al. 1998). Cell alignment was parallel with the applied loading (which was between top right and bottom left corners).

appears to be aligned in the same axis (Birk and Trelstad 1980). Alignment of cells is important in smooth muscle layers, e.g. in major blood vessels where large numbers of aligned cells contract, producing forces in a particular plane. Endothelial cells lining blood vessels assume an elongate shape orientated parallel with the axis of blood flow (Levesque and Nerem 1985). Sheets of specialised epithelial cells are critical to tissue architecture at many boundary locations (skin, gut, urogenital tract) and this architecture is important to function, disruption of this architecture is a frequent problem. Lying over the external surface of the dermis is a keratinocyte layer attached basally through a basal lamina and anchoring filaments to the underlying dermis. Proliferation and differentiation towards the surface produces a constant supply of flattened, keratinised squaemal layers, providing a shedding, waterproof barrier. Epithelial (urothelial) cells lining the bladder and urothelium again form multi-layer barriers over the surface of supporting layers, in some areas forming highly specialised, expandable liquidproof sheets (umbrella cells). These sheets have characteristically sharp polarities, with distinct *surface and basal* functions and structures. In addition, they have distinct lateral functions, in that they are adapted to bind tightly to all their surrounding neighbour cells, i.e. forming stable sheets. Many of these spatial/architectural characteristics are innate behaviours of the differentiated cell types, but, critically, cells clearly require environmental cues to produce the appropriate orientation. These cues are precisely the features which become confused during injury and repair (i.e. scarring: Frank et al. 1985, Jackson 1982).

Hence we can see cellular architecture can originate either in a predominant shape and orientation of cells and support matrix or as layers of the cell components. This is made more complex in many tissues by structural adaptation of connective tissue architecture (particularly collagen and cells) along the length of a particular tissue. Examples of this (at both simple/gross and in more subtle forms) are common in the vasculature, skin and tendons, where matrix organisation appears to adapt to the predominant needs of the tissue environment locally. This is obvious in skin, for example, the soles of the feet, eyelids, scalp (Burkitt et al. 1993) and more subtle in tendons where fibre structure is adapted to the gliding, compression and insertion into surrounding tissues (Eastwood et al. 1998; Walbeehm and McGrouther 1995).

5.2.2.5 Tissues with no significant fibre orientation. There are few examples of isotropic organisation amongst the collagenous tissues, presumably due to the major role of collagen in resisting external tensional loading. The midzone of articular cartilage seems to contain a fibril network with little or no spatial organisation, though fibrils of the adjacent superficial zone have a distinct tangential orientation (to the plane of articulation, parallel to predominant shear). The nucleus pulposus of the intervertebral disc and the vitreous of the eye are gel-like tissues with little collagen content and apparently an isotropic organisation.

5.2.2.6 Tissues with multiple fibre orientation. A wide range of tissues require to deform in a number of planes under loading. These tend to have either weak, short range orientation (as in the dermis, described above) or different predominant fibre alignments in different planes, such as the annulus of the intervertebral disc, in figure 5.5, (Hickey and Hukins 1980) and the fibrocartilage menisci found in knee joints (Arnoczky et al. 1988). Both the annulus and meniscus redirect and dissipate forces, which are initially compressive, as multidirectional tensional loads. The cornea is a somewhat special example since it has one of the most rigidly anisotropic structures of all collagenous tissues, with alternative layers of near perfectly parallel fibrils arranged, with crystalline regularity, perpendicular to each other in a single plane (figure 5.7). This however, is not simply to produce particular mechanical properties but imperative for optical transparency.

5.2.2.7 Tissues with uniaxial fibre orientation (anisotropic). Examples of this form of organisation are relatively easy to identify, such as tendon and ligament, where very large muscular and gravitational loads must be transmitted in a single direction (i.e. between muscle and bone -themselves highly aligned tissues- or at an articulating joint between two bones). The fibre organisation in tendon and ligament is rope-like, producing strongly anisotropic structures, over very long ranges, as in figures 5.5 and 5.8. Other less obvious long, thin tissue structures can have comparable fibre organisations, such as peripheral nerves where collagen within the nerve core (endoneurium) is predominantly parallel with the long axis (Ushiki and Chizuka 1990). Whilst the tough surrounding epineurium has a generally similar orientation it is much more of a basket weave pattern. Large blood vessels at particular sites can have collagenous layers that, while not uniaxial, have predominantly circumferential

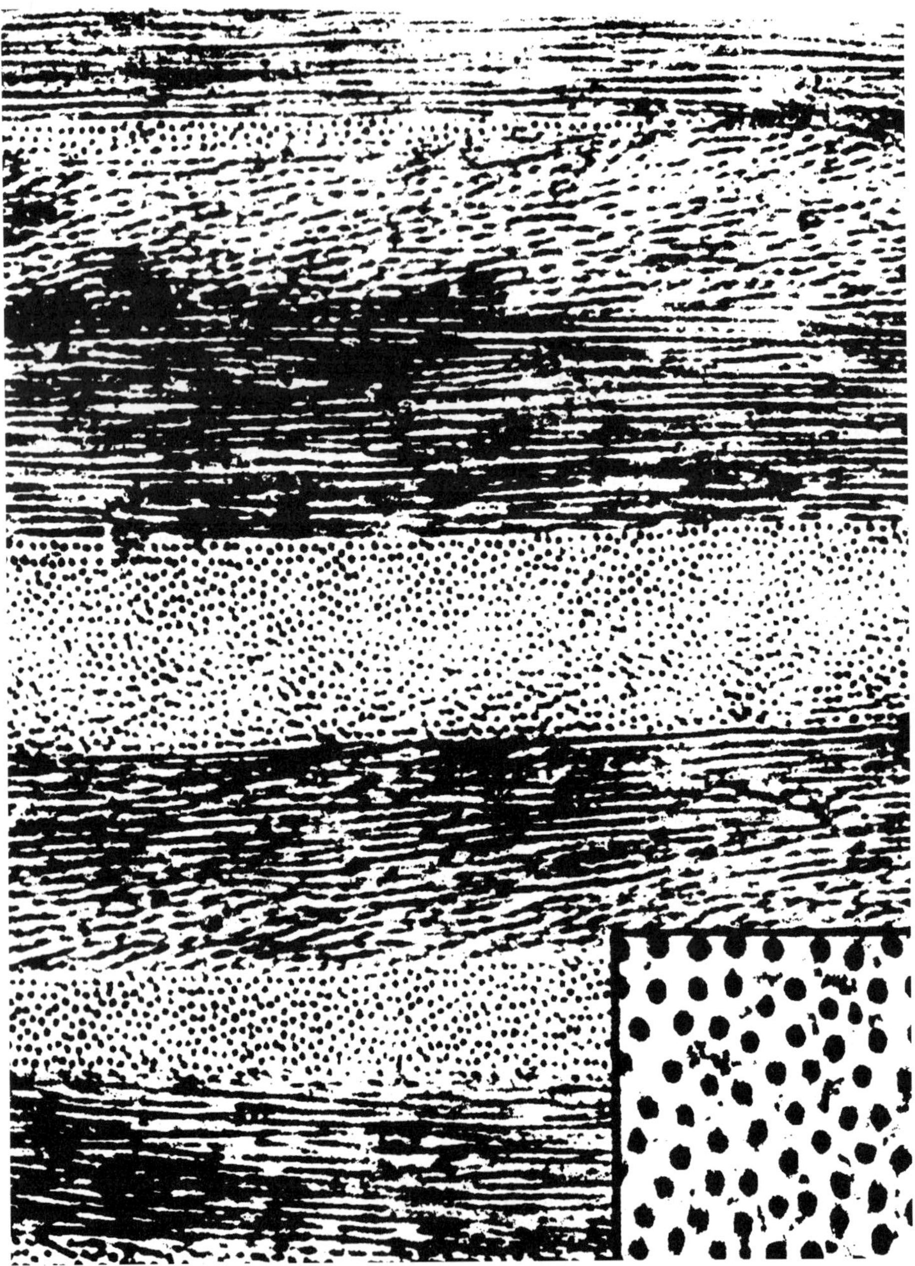

Fig. 5.7. Transmission electron micrograph of corneal collagen matrix showing the orthogonal pattern of collagen fibrils, arranged in parallel and perpendicular arrays. Note the precision of organisation and the consistency of fibril diameter (see inset).

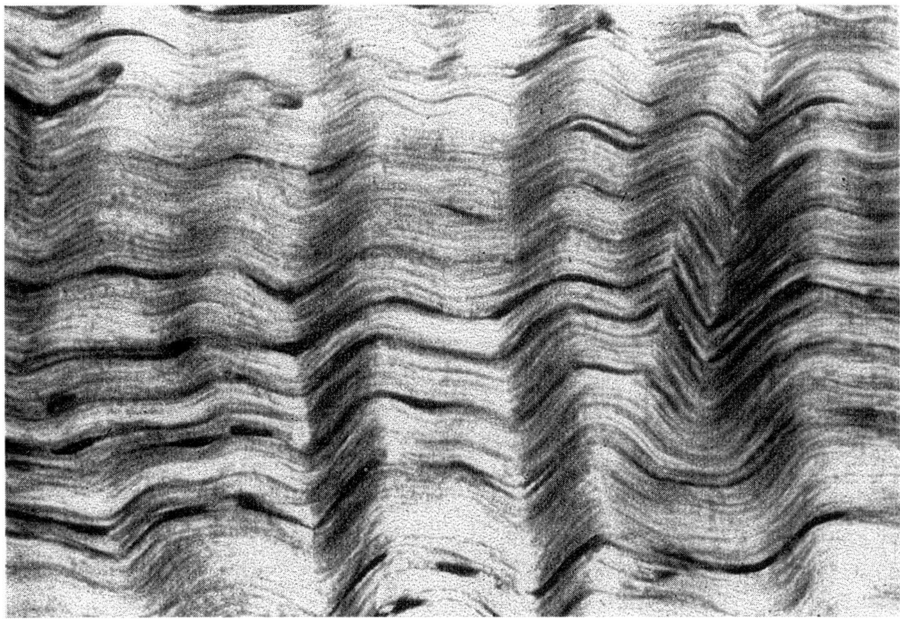

Fig. 5.8. Low power micrograph of normal ligament using birefringent illumination to show the predominant collagen fibre orientation across the section. Fibres are densely packed, with a single plane or orientation, disturbed only by the characteristic crimp pattern (from Frank et al. 1985).

5.3. GENERAL DESIGN OF BIOARTIFICIAL TISSUE AND CONSTRUCTS

Consciously or otherwise, the first stages of any design process must include a series of decisions on the important functions (imperatives) to be fulfilled by the final product. This axiom is no less true for designs of engineered tissues. The field of bioartificial tissues, though, is so complex that a completely new (biological) viewpoint is now being introduced and with it a new set of imperatives. This is fundamental since the suitability of one design or another relates to the compromises, which are made to reconcile opposing imperatives (e.g. weight, cost, strength, and ease of manufacture). Since these compromises are subordinate and consequential to functional level imperatives, the appearance of *new* imperatives tends to produce revolution in, rather than evolution of design.

In tissue engineering of implants new biological imperatives are being introduced together with the more familiar requirements of the surgeons, material scientists, engineers and patients. These imperatives draw on solutions based firmly in our knowledge of the biology of tissue repair, growth and maturation. Our first revolution, then, is that the growth and repair of tissues progresses through a series of stages, rather than as a single step, for example, in the fitting of a traditional prosthesis.

5.3.1 Design imperatives (primary and secondary stages)

For many conventional prosthetic implants the surgical imperatives are ease of fixation and minimal patient discomfort and the rapid restoration of function very shortly after implantation. Design is simplified since the device/material is not intended to change substantially post implantation, though resorbable sutures involve some evolution away from this. When a surgeon designs a graft procedure, most of the decisions are made in the operation and pre-treatment of the donor tissue. Once implanted there is little question of intervention. However, where the aim is to use controlled, natural, cell-based repair processes to produce the new tissue, it is appropriate to ask at what stage implantation should occur. Biological imperatives can lead us to culture more and more complex layers of cells on tailored materials in the laboratory, until tissues resembling the required graft have been produced. Whilst this is slow and expensive it is also controlled and predictable. However, the same imperatives can suggest that designs effectively use the patient's body as an incubator chamber by designing structures into the implant, which will control its development long after the first surgery.

In principle a cell engineering solution could be implanted at one of a number of stages in its *progression* from lab to functional tissue. A primary stage implant might consist of a smart material or template capable of guiding and controlling the formation of a new section of biologically functional tissue. A secondary stage implant in this series, then, would have appropriate cells grown (at suitable sites) within that material prior to implantation to seed the structure with resident *repair* cells which will subsequently form the final tissue. Finally in a tertiary stage implant, a complex, near-complete tissue would be formed entirely in culture, ready for implantation. This stage most closely resembles a graft.

The scheme in Table 5.2 illustrates the rationale behind this division into three possible stages for implantation. Implanted materials (matrices) might be based on collagen, fibronectin or synthetic resorbable polymers. Seeded cell types might be fibroblasts, endothelial cells, Schwann cells or keratinocytes, depending on the tissue. Control agents could be cell growth factors such as platelet derived growth factor - PDGF, transforming growth factor-beta -TGF-β (Heldin and Westermark 1996), antibiotics, chemotactic factors (e.g. fibronectin fragments, PDGF), fibre and pore dimensions, surface chemistry or shape and orientation (Brown et al. 1997).

The *primary, secondary* and *tertiary* stages, in Table 5.2, correspond to artificial divisions in the natural tissue repair sequence (i.e. 1. haemostatic fibrin/platelet blood clot; 2. granulation or provisional repair tissue; 3. mature scar tissue). This is a useful model for rationalising the design and staging of implants. Many attempts at tissue engineering would fit into either stages (1) or (2), depending on whether they were early stage *guide and control* constructs (e.g. for nerve regeneration) or tissue constructs with structure and form close to that of the final tissue (e.g. artificial skin, blood vessels). At present, tertiary stage (3) functional tissue implants, subverting much of the natural tissue repair process, remain largely an aspiration. Where immediate function is essential, for example in heart valve replacements, non-living prostheses would seem to be the likely solution for some time. One of the earliest and

Table 5.2. Three possible stages for implantation

Component	PRIMARY	SECONDARY	TERTIARY
MATRIX	Template Implants and Smart Materials	Repair Tissue + Support Material	Stable Natural Connective Tissue Matrix
CELLS	Non OR Temporary Feeder-cells, Genetically Engineered Cells	Native Repair Cells, Phagocytic and Stem Cells	Mature Tissue Resident Cells Population
CONTROL AGENTS	Inflammation Control Chemotactic and Mitogenic Growth Factors	Cell Segregation, Mitogenic Factors and Activators of Synthesis	Tissue Maturation and Homeostasis Factors

most important design decisions, then, is the stage at which the construct will act, primary template or a more functional provisional tissue, with functional donor repair cells.

Primary tissue-engineered constructs would, for example, be expected to be remodelled in vivo and replaced by secondary and eventually mature tissues as the repair and maturation process proceeds. In some cases, these downstream consequences of the primary implant are predictable and controllable by incorporation of suitable chemical/physical agents (such as growth factors or material surface topography). At the present level of biological understanding, however, the possibilities for precise, predictable control of such processes are limited. Forms of secondary stage implants serve to replace secondary, or provisional, repair material and cells, equivalent to granulation tissue stage, characteristic of vascularised tissue repair sites. For example in dermal repair, fibroblasts and endothelial cells rapidly accumulate and deposit a loose vascularised network of collagen (the granulation tissue). Under normal circumstances, this would mature to a *scar*, with increased collagen density and reduced cell population.

In the case of the artificial skin example, the aim would be (a) to implant a primary stage bioartificial implant, comparable in role to the haemostatic fibrin based clot, to control the structure/composition of the secondary and tertiary phase tissues. This template could take the form of a synthetic or semi-natural support matrix (e.g. polylactate/glycolic acid or collagen sponge) with localised fibre diameter and alignment for cell guidance, containing depots of cell selective growth factors, chemotactic agents to promote the recruitment of suitable cells (fibroblasts and keratinocytes) from surrounding skin. Longer term control may be achieved by seeding with limited life feeder cells (often not from the patient) or cells transfected to overproduce required growth promoter or regulatory growth factors. Alternatively (b) a secondary stage tissue implant could be constructed, with two or more layers, seeded with the patients own (autologous) keratinocytes and fibroblasts. One particular imperative in dermal repair is to reduce and regulate the exuberant secondary stage of the natural repair, which produces many of the undesirable effects of scarring (Frank et al. 1985; Jackson 1982; Heldin and Westermark 1996). A primary stage implant would be likely to address this through features of the support matrix and regulators that it contained. A secondary stage implant might concentrate on selection of suitable cell populations to minimise scarring.

Design factors for control of tissue engineered constructs

Biological design imperatives can be divided into four general groups. A fifth catch-all category comprising tissue and site-specific features could also be described as clinically driven imperatives. Clearly, a whole layer of commercial and regulatory imperatives would follow from these, but are beyond the scope of this chapter.

a.- Required substrate and extracellular matrix composition (*materials*);
b.- composition and rates of tissue development (*rates*);
c.- cell types present, localisation and segregation from each other (*cell types*);
d.- tissue shape and microscopic architecture (*architecture*);
e.- special local tissue functional requirements (e.g. non-thrombogenic blood vessels, tendon gliding surfaces, suppression of crystal/stone formation in urothelium).

5.3.2 Materials

In common with conventional implant design, the development of bioartificial implants is heavily dependent on the availability of suitable materials, though with different suitability criteria. There are perhaps four potential groups of material for use in soft tissues, artificial non-resorbable, artificial resorbable polymers, semi-natural, or derivatised polymer materials, and native/natural materials (i.e. grafts and transplants). Materials employed in tissue engineering will almost certainly need to be re-absorbed at least in the long term and so non-reabsorbable polymers, i.e. metals and ceramics, will not be considered further. The last group, native/natural materials includes the structures and tissues, which are the intended final product. Of the remaining groups we shall concentrate here on semi-natural, or derivatised polymer materials, i.e. biological aggregates.

Basic starting materials available

The materials, which are used in soft tissue engineering, are critical to the applications we can attempt and the outcomes we can expect. There are however relatively limited numbers of available basic structural support materials. This is simply a consequence of the type specification, which is forced upon us. They must be very weakly or non-immunogenic, stable and yet re-absorbable by biological action (this can either be through slow chemical dissolution or by cellular re-absorption). They must be easily prepared, commercially viable (i.e. inexpensive source materials), free from infection and yet of relatively defined composition. At present this is one of the major limitations of all efforts in tissue engineering and bioartificial graft work. The main categories of material are:

a.- The Collagens
b.- Hyaluronan aggregates
c.- Fibrin aggregates
d.- Fibronectin aggregates
e.- Synthetic bio-reabsorbable polymers

Note. All forms of these have been extensively investigated and there are a wide range of derivatives and composite forms. The following sections deal with each group individually.

5.3.2.1 Collagens

Intact collagenous tissues.
Collagens, in their many forms, are the only materials which have effectively spanned the prosthesis/engineered-tissue interface. In the form of whole tissue, such as tanned dermis, collagen has been used for centuries in a range of applications. The simplest form of this application has been to develop treatments for appropriate whole connective tissues (normally from animals) which preserve them and reduce any damaging host responses. This approach has evolved more recently to give 'bioprostheses' using pig heart valve and bovine tendon. In all cases chemical modification, rendering the tissue non-viable, is an essential component of the process (reviewed in Nimni et al. 1988).

The replacement of heart valves with implanted devices is now common, either using entirely mechanical/synthetic devices or bioprosthetic implants (treated porcine valves). The former requires that patients are maintained on anticoagulant therapy whilst porcine heart valve bioprostheses do not (Silver 1994). It is essential that collagenous tissues from animal sources such as this are chemically crosslinked to minimise antigenicity (and so rejection), to minimise thrombogenicity (Ishihara et al. 1981) and to produce a sufficiently stable material. Clearly, though, extensive crosslinking leads to complete tissue denaturation with the result that bio-integration is poor or inappropriate. Early attempts to prepare implantable heart valve substitutes used formaldehyde, but material stability remained poor and this was replaced by glutaraldehyde treatment (Nimni et al. 1988; Buch et al. 1970). The success of this technique led to studies on the detailed mechanisms by which glutaraldehyde alters collagen (Cheung and Nimni 1982 and 1984). Glutaraldehyde crosslinked materials were developed to the extent that there was minimal disintegration and loss of collagenous material after 30 days of incubation in culture or 48 hour digestion with the protease, papain. Additional techniques based on the carbodiimide reaction have also been described (Nimni et al. 1988). Crosslinked materials have been extensively tested in patients, with considerable clinical success (5 year survival 70-80%: ten year survival 55-70%: bioprosthesis failure rate 1%/year for years 1 to 5 and 2%/year thereafter) (Oyer et al. 1984; Cohn 1984). Problems, which arise, have related to calcification, toxicity, thrombosis, often after longer periods, many of which seem to be related to the presence of glutaraldehyde or reactive groups remaining on the material surface. The effects of long term implantation on such structures are reviewed in Ferrans et al. (1988). Failures can be ascribed to mechanical insufficiencies, particularly associated with material properties following crosslinking (Ferrans et al. 1988; Broom 1978; Ishihara et al. 1981), such as loss of compliance, or with matrix calcification. Calcification of the collagen is the most frequent and serious cause of failure (Ferrans et al. 1988) and a range of anti-calcification pre-treatments (incorporation of diphosphonates or GAGs: ref. Nimni et al. 1988) are now used to minimise the problem.

Over periods of months and years following implantation of collagenous heart valve bioprostheses, their surfaces become covered by a layer of host endothelial cells. These cells go on to deposit a layer of fibrous tissue (also host origin), known as a fibrous sheath (Spray and Roberts 1977). Such coatings can comprise elastic and collagenous deposits with smooth muscle cells, though in extreme cases they may resemble cartilage and even bone, sometimes doubling the thickness of the implant. These commonly add to the functions of the implant though thick sheaths may also be damaging (Magilligan et al. 1984). The problem of calcification of such glutaraldehyde treated substrates is significant in bioprostheses implanted for 3 years or more (Cipriano et al. 1982; Arbustini et al. 1984) and can represent a serious impediment to long term function in vivo. It is thought to be a result of changes in surface chemistry following reaction with the glutaraldehyde itself (Nimni et al. 1988; Ferrans et al. 1988). Unfortunately, the very stability produced by crosslinking of these materials limits their utilisation by suitable local repair cells as biologically compatible substrates. In effect, the substrate remains a foreign prosthesis despite its organic origins and can be regarded as similar to the many synthetic polymers now available as support materials.

Purified collagen substrates

This class of material or substrate is characterised by the use of collagen, which has been extracted from its parent tissues (normally non-human). They are free of cells and most other connective tissue components. Collagenous substrates have been prepared to support cell growth in three main forms, sponges, gels (or lattices) and films (previously reviewed in Pachence 1996). Collagen films are prepared by drying soluble collagen (including denatured collagen: -gelatin) onto surfaces to give a thin protein layer which may be further stabilised later. Since such films are 2-dimensional and non-porous in nature they will not be considered further here, being unsuitable as materials in themselves, though they can have supplementary (short-term) uses as coatings.

Sponges are dense 3-dimensional collagenous aggregates, highly porous in nature and normally prepared from insoluble collagen aggregates. Gels are natural aggregates formed by in vitro fibrillogenesis, from soluble collagen monomers. During gel formation, collagen monomers, at neutral pH and 37°C, aggregate to form a fibrillar mesh, also known as a collagen lattice. After seeding with cells (principally fibroblasts) these have been used extensively as *first stage tissues* since fibroblast seeded lattices contract to form dense cellular collagenous matrices (Elsdale and Bard 1972; Bell et al. 1979). These are amongst the most natural models of tissue substrates, which are so far in widespread use. Collagen gels and sponges are formed from interstitial collagen species, mainly type I though in some cases a proportion of type III collagen has been added. At least two specialised collagen substrates have also been described which contain, or are based on type IV collagen. These are Matrigel and Type IV/Type IV_{ox} (Madri and Williams 1983; Laquerriere et al. 1993; reviewed in Brown and McFarland 1993). Type IV collagen is the main component of basement membranes and is thought to be important in the attachment and subsequent behaviour of epithelial and endothelial cells, normally found on a basement membrane.

Collagen sponges

These materials are prepared by a number of techniques which aggregate and crosslink dispersible but essentially insoluble collagen aggregates. These insoluble aggregates can be prepared from animal tissues (commonly bovine, pig or sheep skin) to give 3-dimensional highly porous, sheet structures. It is important to make the distinction, that collagen sponges are based on aggregates of *polymerised insoluble* (as opposed to *soluble)* collagen.

Preparation of collagen sponges takes advantage of the property of insoluble polymeric collagen to swell extensively in dilute organic acid. This property was characterised and studied extensively in the late 1960s and 70s by Steven (1967) and Veis et al. (1970). In these cases insoluble polymeric collagen fibrils were isolated from other connective tissue components and shown to swell into viscous or gel-like suspensions (not solutions) at low pH. On neutralisation such acid suspensions of polymeric collagen re-precipitate and can be recovered in purified form.

Chvapil (1977) and Yannas and Burke (1980) worked extensively on the mechanisms of formation, stabilisation and pore size control. Yannas found that collagen fibrils in the cowhide suspension retained their characteristic banding pattern down to a pH of 4.25 by which time fibrils underwent gross swelling (reviewed in Yannas 1990). Addition of the GAG chondroitin-6-sulphate to such acid-swollen collagen suspensions produced a co-precipitate of collagen and GAG and this was crosslinked by a process of drastic dehydration (Yannas and Tobolsky 1967). This has proved to be a stable form of crosslinking, avoiding the use of toxic chemical crosslinking agents which frequently leave damaging residues. By careful manipulation of the physicochemical conditions during preparation (GAG content from 2-8%, temperature of freezing prior to drying etc.) it proved possible to produce materials with pore sizes of between 20 and 120 μM and rates of degradation in vivo which gave effective characteristics for repair tissue substrates (Yannas 1990 and 1988; Yannas et al. 1989). In vivo studies on this material initially concentrated on skin and peripheral nerve repair (Yannas 1988). In repair of full depth skin wounds, implantation of the collagen-GAG sponge was claimed to produce excellent repair properties characterised by good collagen architecture and minimal contracture. For nerve repair, collagen-GAG sponges were implanted inside silicone tubes and supported improved axonal regeneration across 15mm gaps over a 6-week period, compared to silicone tube-only controls. Clinical studies on collagen-GAG sponges in skin wounds have largely used the commercially produced version, known as *Integra.* In 109 burns patients the collagen-GAG sponge was as effective in *take* level as conventional allografts and formed a good base for subsequent epidermal grafting (Heimbach et al. 1988). Granulation tissue formed at 10-15 days post-implantation, new collagen filled the sponge by 18-25 days and fibres of the sponge disappeared after 30 days to leave a stable multilayered repair tissue. However, rete pegs were not re-formed at the dermal-epidermal junction and accessory structures such as hair and sweat glands did not reappear (Stern et al. 1990).

Numerous forms of collagen sponges have been prepared since their initial development. These have included sponges incorporating novel forms of chemical crosslinking, added protein and polysaccharide components, growth factors, antibiotics and metal ions. This range of materials has been tested in implants in a wide variety of tissues and surgical procedures. Most of these applications have been developed both for use as skin grafts or in some cases, for in vitro skin models for use in toxicity testing. As in the *whole tissue* bioprostheses described above, the means of collagen crosslinking has proved to be critical to the nature and success of collagen sponges. A number of forms of sponge have been prepared using stabilisation by drastic dehydration, or dehydrothermal crosslinking (Yannas 1988; Wang et al. 1994; Matsuda et al. 1992 and 1993; Koide et al. 1993). Chemical crosslinking has included techniques using diphenylphosphorylazide (DPPA) (Rault et al. 1996; Frei et al. 1994), carbodiimide reagents (CDI) (Wachem et al. 1994; Olde Damink et al. 1996), tannic acid (Heijmen et al. 1997) and thiol oxidative crosslinking (Nicolas and Gagnieu 1997). They have been used in conjunction with other macromolecular components (Vries et al. 1994), charged polysaccharides such as chitosan (Taravel and Damard 1993; Berthod et al. 1993), chondroitin sulphate and hyaluronan (Yannas 1990; Berthod et al. 1993; Murashita et al. 1996; Matsuda et al. 1990; Doillon et al. 1987), with fibrin and type III collagen (Berthod et al. 1993) and as depots for the release of growth factors (Cascone et al. 1995; Fujisato et al. 1996), drugs (Herschler 1992) and antibiotics (Matsuda et al. 1992). In addition, collagen sponges have been used as supports for the culture of fibroblasts (Maruguchi et al. 1994; Berthod et al. 1993), keratinocytes (Maruguchi et al. 1994; Hanthamrongwit et al. 1996), myoblasts (Wachem et al. 1996), chondrocytes (Fujisato et al. 1996; Nehrer et al. 1997) and many other cell types.

Collagen gels

Collagen gels are distinct from sponges in that they are invariably prepared by fibrillogenesis of soluble collagen, leading to formation of native fibrils with a typical quarter staggered molecular configuration. Use of collagen gels was developed initially as a model for interaction of fibroblasts with a 3-dimensional matrix (Elsdale and Bard 1972). When such gels (also referred to as collagen lattices) are seeded with fibroblasts and cultured, free floating over a course of days, contraction of the structure occurs (Bell et al. 1979; Bell 1995). This process is most probably a result of tractional forces exerted by resident fibroblasts on collagen fibrils as they move through and reorganise the lattice (Ehrich and Rajaratnan 1990; Grinnell 1994). Contraction produces a progressively smaller and denser matrix, which has been regarded as a tissue-like material (Bell 1995). Substantial forces can be generated within such matrices (Eastwood et al. 1994), producing collagen reorganisation (Porter et al. 1998) and reduction in thickness in tethered gels (Grinnell 1994). In addition, collagen gels have been seeded with a range of cell types including keratinocytes (Hanthamrongwit et al. 1996). A number of model tissues have been attempted, based on such contracted collagen gels but most interest has been attracted by grafting of skin replacements (Bell et al. 1984; Hull et al. 1990). The most recent of these is a bilayered commercially produced allograft (trade name *Apligraf*) based on a fibroblast-seeded collagen lattice contracted under tethered conditions (Falanga et al. 1998).

A novel and promising new development of collagen lattices as cell substrates has been the introduction of techniques that produce a defined fibrillar orientation. Indeed, some degree of fibrillar orientation was described as a secondary observation in the early studies of Elsdale and Bard (1972). Collagen fibrils in a newly formed gel have a random orientation and distribution, producing an isotropic gel. As resident fibroblasts remodel this, it is compacted, bundled and reorganised but this tends to be uncontrolled, dependent on the shape of the lattice (Eastwood et al. 1998), any tethering points (Grinnell 1994), holes or defects (Baschong et al. 1997) and the distribution of contracting cells. Methods for orientating collagen fibrils were first based on techniques for shaping and pouring the initial gelling solution (Elsdale and Bard 1972). More recently though, a technique has been described by which collagen fibrils form perpendicular to an applied high density magnetic field (Guido and Tranquillo 1993). Following from this, Tranquillo and co-workers have examined the behaviour of resident fibroblasts as they align and take on the orientation of the collagen fibrils. The dominant controlling factor here was thought to be contact guidance of cells by orientated fibrils, but such control of architecture at the cellular level opens new possibilities for the use of materials in achieving a desired form of tissue repair (Dickinson et al. 1994).

*Type IV collagens***.** Matrigel is essentially a cellular product produced in vitro by tumour cells. It is a thick layer of basement membrane laid down by transformed cells (Friman et al. 1990) and subsequently harvested. It is principally comprised of Type IV collagen but is also rich in other basement membrane components such as specialised proteoglycans, attachment factors such as laminin and nidogen, and a range of growth factors. The nature and source of Matrigel together with its effects on tumour cell behaviour mean that it is likely to remain in use largely as an experimental tool and in model systems.

Type IV/Type IV_{ox} is an aggregate of type IV collagen purified from human placenta and oxidatively crosslinked to form a stable semi-natural material (Tinois et al. 1991). It was designed principally to support growth of epithelial and endothelial cell layers, normally found on a basement membrane in mature tissues. Its use has been described in animal models of repair in the skin, dura and ear (Tinois et al. 1991; Laquerriere et al. 1993; Morgon et al. 1989). This material has so far had only very limited use and its use of human placenta as a source material may represent a major regulatory problem for wider clinical applications. In addition, whilst there is a substantial literature on the promotion of some tissue repair by basement membrane components such as laminin (in nerves), the idea that they are automatically good for epithelial repair may be flawed. Although epithelial cells rest on a type IV collagen-rich basement membrane in the *mature, fully differentiated tissue,* this behaviour changes during repair. Keratinocytes, for example, alter their extracellular matrix integrin receptors to those for temporary matrix components (collagen types I & III and fibronectin) over which they must migrate during the repair of skin wounds (Prajapati et al. 1996; Adams and Watt 1991; Kim et al. 1992).

5.3.2.2 Hyaluronan. Hyaluronan is a charged polysaccharide (glycosaminoglycans) found throughout the body associated with cell surfaces and the extracellular matrix. It is highly hydrated, with a random 3-dimensional structure and appears to be important as a lubricant between gliding surfaces in soft tissues. It has also been implicated in a range of cellular functions important in angiogenesis and tissue repair (Mast et al. 1991; Noble et al. 1993; West et al. 1985). It occurs naturally in vivo (and in solution in the laboratory) as a viscous gel, a version of which has been produced as a biomaterial (Larsen et al. 1993). A process of esterification has also been developed by which hyaluronan is crosslinked into a semi-natural biomaterial membrane. Sheets of this material, known as Hyaff (Benedetti et al. 1993), have been developed and tested by implantation into muscle. Materials can be made with varying levels of substitution and these survive for progressively longer periods in vivo, eliciting only modest inflammation and local connective tissue response (Campoccia et al. 1996). Hyaff has been developed most strongly to date for use in skin grafting (commercially available as *Laserskin* films), particularly as a carrier for keratinocytes (Andreassi et al. 1991). The uses to date for crosslinked hyaluronan membranes seem to be related more to the modest biological response elicited and the release of biologically active fragments (dependent on the effects of the esterifcation). It seems to provide little organisational information in this form, though application of native or derivatised forms to the preservation of gliding interfaces in tissue repair could represent a significant function.

5.3.2.3 Fibrin. Fibrin is an obvious candidate for a *natural biopolymer support* (comparable with collagen gels) since that is just what it is in vivo. There are now a number of forms of fibrin-glue or fibrin-sealant available (depending on the designed use). These can be made from platelet-rich-plasma or prepared from fibrinogen and thrombin (human, large pool plasma) with a bovine protease inhibitor, aprotinin, as a stabiliser (reviewed in Silver et al. 1995). They are used most widely in surgery, to join or seal tissues rapidly, but some uses have been reported as supports for tissue engineering applications, both alone or in combination with other matrix components. One composite form, Neuroplast, a combination of elastin and fibrin, has been proposed as a substitute for dura mater (San-Galli et al. 1996) and tympanic membranes (Bonzon et al. 1995).

Fibrin based materials have also been used by a number of groups as implantable growth factor depots (Pandit et al. 1998), forming a simple localised slow release source of any agent trapped within the fibrin plug. Fibrin adsorbed onto a Dacron mesh base was used to retain a cocktail of angiogenic agents, including hyaluronan, fibronectin, endothelial cell growth factor and FGF, and these promoted angiogenesis for up to 28 days (Fournier and Doillon 1996). Similar studies on the effects of growth factor loaded fibrin on fibroblast proliferation indicated that FGF in particular was stabilised by incorporation into fibrin, retaining its activity over a longer period (Roy et al. 1993).

5.3.2.4 ***Fibronectin.*** Fibronectin (Fn) is a protein which has long been associated with tissue repair, since it can be identified as an active and critical component at almost all stages of skin repair (Grinnell 1984). In most cases, its role is related to cellular adhesion, normally to elements of the ECM. Indeed, it is recognised as the first major element, laid down by fibroblasts, of a new connective tissue matrix. At this point it is found as fine fibres which act as supports and appear to guide subsequent waves of repair cells as they are recruited to the injury site (Grinnell 1984; McCarthy et al. 1996). Consequently, much of the early work on the possible therapeutic uses of Fn concentrated on application of large quantities of the native protein (normally in solution) with the apparent aim of correcting local deficiencies. Falcone et al (1984) prepared an aggregated form of Fn for testing in rat dermal wounds, but this amorphous precipitate was again used primarily to deliver a therapeutic dose of Fn, rather than as a material. Although Fn is available in substantial quantities from plasma and methods for its precipitation were described at an early stage, its use as a biomaterial was almost unknown until aggregated forms were described for contact guidance substrates (Ejim et al. 1993; Brown et al. 1994).

Such Fn contact guidance substrates were prepared by the application of a directional shear force to concentrated solutions of the purified protein. This caused its aggregation into discrete fibres (Wojciak-Stothard et al. 1997; Ejim et al. 1993) which proved to be remarkably stable after drying (figure 5.9). Further stabilisation has recently been achieved by treating the Fn-materials with trace levels of copper salts (Ahmed et al. 1998). The aim of these materials is to provide a practical form of orientational cue for recruited cells (on the aligned fibres, seen in figure 5.10) through the process of contact guidance, described previously using experimental models (Clark et al. 1991; Curtis and Varde 1964). It was predicted that orientation of repair cells would provide cues by which matrix and eventually the entire tissue can be given an appropriate architecture (figure 5.7). As discussed previously, restoration of tissue architecture around implants is a limiting feature of repair tissue function.

Since the base Fn material is an excellent cell attachment protein it acts as a very effective substrate for cells including fibroblasts, Schwann cells and endothelial cells (Ejim et al. 1993; Ahmed et al. submitted; Underwood et al. in press). In addition, adherent cells, the matrix they produced and even the repair tissue formed when

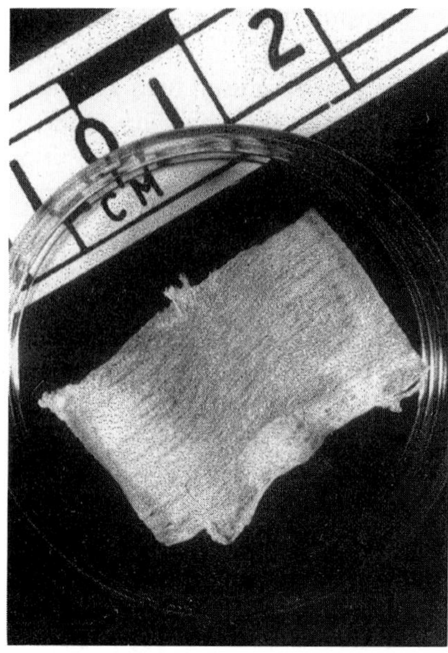

Fig. 5.9. Orientated fibre of aggregated fibronectin formed into a small mat for practical application of contact guidance of repair cells (from Ejim et al. 1993). Note the macroscopically aligned fibres parallel with the long axis of the mat.

implanted into dermal and nerve injury sites (Whitworth et al. 1995), takes on the predicted alignment. Not only do the Fn-materials bind cells effectively but also they support rapid cellular migration along the composite fibres (Ahmed 1999). Furthermore, in addition to its ability to bind a wide array of cell types, soluble fibronectin and its breakdown products are strongly chemotactic to a range of cells (Bowersox and Sorgente 1982; Talas and Brown in press). In Fn-materials, then, we have an array of active design features to act as substrate-based controls.

To understand the real importance of orientated guide materials, such as Fn-mats, it is critical to stress that a major limiting factor in biological repair in vivo, or engineering of cellular implants in vitro, is cellular recruitment. In vivo this is from surrounding host tissues. At large injury sites (e.g. full depth dermal burns) this can be many hundreds of millimetres. Fibroblasts migrate at *speeds* of less than 50 μM/h. However, without directional guidance, cell migration (during recruitment) will have no overall direction and progression into the material/injury site (i.e. their velocity, in a particular direction) will be a small fraction of their speed. By using directionally aligned Fn fibres it is possible not only to optimise adhesion and chemoattraction (properties of the protein itself) but also to bring cellular velocity, in the fibre plane, close to the speed of locomotion (Ahmed 1999). Hence, these materials optimise the major rate limiting factor in repair and engineering, namely cellular recruitment.

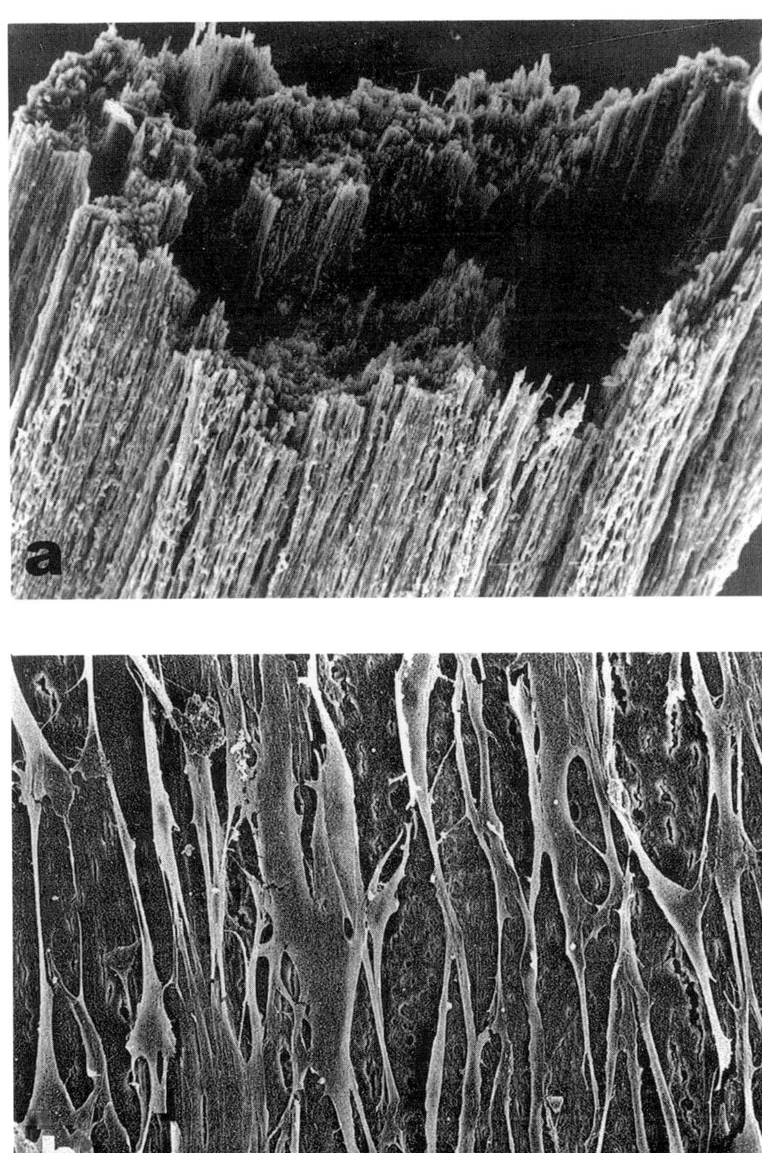

Fig. 5.10. (a) Scanning electron micrograph of a fibre form of orientated fibronectin aggregate. Note the fine fibrous surface structure of this 200μm diameter fibre, described by Underwood et al. in press. (b) Human dermal fibroblasts aligned parallel to the surface fibre topography (top to bottom orientation) of the fibronectin fibre shown in (a) (x880).

5.3.2.5 ***Resorbable synthetic polymers.*** A wide variety of resorbable synthetic polymers have been developed and used in tissue engineering to date, notably, biodegradable polymers of lactate or glycolic acid or co-polymers of both (Langer and Vacanti 1993; Putnam and Mooney 1996; Mooney et al. 1996). Complex co-polymers with biological molecules, such as that reported with crosslinked gelatin and poly L-glutamic acid are also possible, though less commonly used (Otani et al. 1996). The work of Langer and others in this area has concentrated on characterising the optimal pore size for cellular utilisation and infiltration and on polymer stability (Putnam and Mooney 1996; Ma and Langer 1999; Freed et al. 1994). In these applications the rationale has been relatively simple. A suitable gross shape and composition of the supporting polymer is seeded with cells from the tissue site(s) to be reconstructed, ideally from the patient (Langer and Vacanti 1993). After a limited period in culture, the aim is to implant such constructs to the body tissue site, with the intention that the seeded cells would reconstruct a viable natural tissue before the polymer substrate is resorbed. Tissues which have been tackled in this way, are skin, heart valve, cartilage, and urethra (Freed et al. 1994; Atala et al. 1993; Oberpenning et al. 1999; Vacanti et al. 1991; Hansbrough et al. 1992). The design and control requirements for these synthetic polymers are much the same as for semi-natural biomaterials (above) though the nature of cellular interactions is frequently governed by the adhesion proteins which coat them.

5.3.3 Control

5.3.3.1 ***Control of composition.*** The composition of a bioartificial tissue construct depends heavily on whether it is designed as a primary or secondary stage implant, figure 5.11. For example, a primary stage *tendon* repair implant may have little intrinsic tensional strength but would represent a good substrate for tenocyte ingrowth and rapid remodelling with the aim of leaving a dense aligned collagen matrix. In contrast a later stage, provisionally functional repair tissue, for tendon, would need to be composed of parallel, wide diameter collagen fibres (ideally type I) with small quantities of proteoglycan and elastin. Each *stage* represents a different set of compromises. The latter is difficult and complex to construct outside the body, at the present. The former, in contrast, normally restores very little function of the original tissue in the first instance but promotes orderly repair.

Composition of a primary stage tissue implant for articular cartilage might be comparable to that of tendon, being mainly based on growth promotion factors (proliferation and/or migration) and cell attachment protein(s) on a support material. In contrast, a secondary stage tissue implant would be quite different in composition, to actively promote specific cell phenotypic behaviour, rich in type II collagen and aggregating proteoglycans for cartilage and fibronectin and types I & III collagen for tendon. In general, composition of early stage implants are likely to be more similar between tissue sites than later stage since early stage imperatives tend to be the

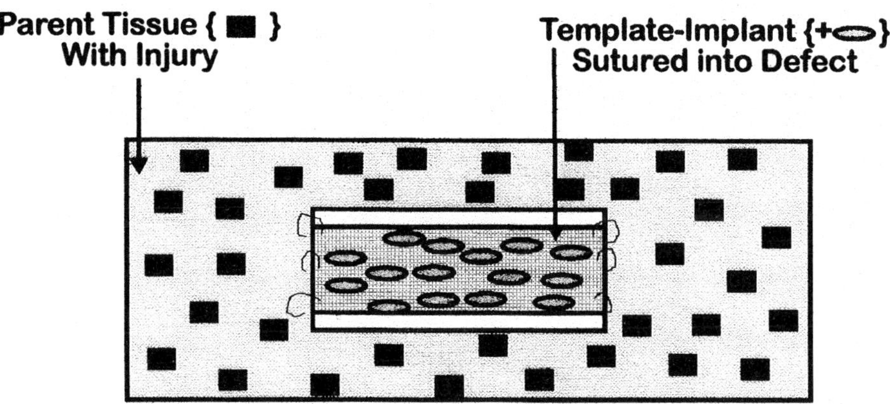

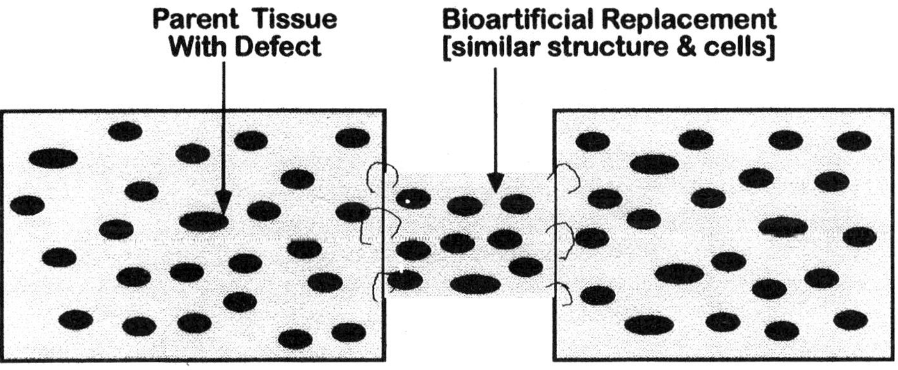

Fig. 5.11. Diagram illustrating differences between primary and secondary stage implants (for example, applied to tendon). In the primary implant the engineered tissue is designed to be a repair tissue, with a distinct matrix and cell type from the parent tissue to be replaced (upper panel). In this instance the aim is to implant a tissue which will effectively organise the progression of the natural repair process. The lower panel indicates the principle that a mature engineered tissue is implanted with the aim of providing much of the function of that tissue.

independent of tissue type (cell recruitment, attachment, segregation, proliferation and guidance). In later stages a greater level of mimic and specialisation to tissue type will be needed to provide appropriate diffusible, substrate and mechanical signals to resident cells. For example, local factors would dictate that blood vessel implants suitable to take blood flow would require an anti-coagulant polymer surface or that later stage tendon implants would require a non-adherent outer surface (perhaps based on a surface layer of hyaluronan) to promote gliding between the implant and surrounding tissues (i.e. to prevent adhesions, retaining near-uniaxial mechanical loading). Design of specific features such as this requires detailed reference to the normal and transitional (repair) tissue composition.

5.3.3.2 Control of rates of tissue formation. The rate at which the primary bioartificial tissue is remodelled and replaced is clearly going to be a balance between the rate of resorbtion of the implant and the rate of deposition of new natural matrix by resident cells. The rate of resorbtion of bioartificial polymers is largely a feature of their chemistry and this can be engineered accordingly. Hence, if long-term support is required e.g. in slowly developing tissues or where mechanical support is important, slowly resorbing polymers would be selected. Where natural or semi-natural macromolecular aggregates are used as support materials, extension of in vivo life is traditionally achieved by crosslinking and a selection of these approaches have been reviewed in the previous section. Where resorbtion of a material is due to a specific infiltrating cell type e.g. phagocytic cell types such as macrophages, it may be possible to control the rate of resorbtion by regulation of their attachment or release of extracellular matrix-degrading enzymes (chiefly matrix metalloproteinase (MMPs) and serine proteinases: reviewed in Mignatti et al. 1996). The process of cell attachment and migration over materials is regulated by different patterns of cell-matrix receptors (mainly the integrin family: see (4) below). By modifying the surface properties of any given protein material or synthetic polymer it is already possible to regulate the cell attachment and utilisation of that material (Steele et al. 1993).

The converse side of the *tissue accumulation* equation is the rate of accumulation of new native matrix replacing the fabric of the implant. Factors governing the *rate of deposition* of matrix include the type and source of cells involved. These can be stimulated by locally acting growth factors or other biochemical regulators to produce more extracellular matrix (e.g. TGF-β- and insulin-like growth factor -IGF-1). For example, promotion of cartilage deposition (Type II collagen network, rich in aggregan proteoglycan) would be first approached by seeding a bioartificial implant with active, well differentiated chondrocytes, maintaining their phenotype (i.e. production of type II collagen) and stimulating optimal production of such matrix. A major imperative, then, is to stimulate synthesis of new tissue by resident cells.

Growth factor/cytokine (e.g. TGF-β, IGF-1) delivery of this sort has been widely proposed, often using entrapment of the growth factor within the cell support material (Brown et al. 1994; Langer and Vacanti 1993) and allowing its slow release by diffusion. However, problems associated with this technology have yet to be fully tested. For example, non-localised release of potent regulators such as these could have serious penalties for other tissue functions. In nerve regeneration, stimulation of collagen production to promote strength of the implant, could lead to excessive amounts of collagen between regenerating axons resulting in fibrotic nerve repair, contraction and poor nervous function. Also, growth factors tend only to affect how much matrix is deposited. The question of its overall composition is separate and is generally a function of the phenotype of the resident cell types recruited. In our examples chondrocytes *can* produce both types I and II collagen, the proportions are altered by the environmental conditions and level of differentiation.

Overall crude accumulation of extracellular matrix is thought to be the net effect of a number of controlling factors. Crudely stated, these are: (i) cell accumulation (= proliferation rate versus cell death/apoptosis), (ii) cell movement (= cell immigration versus cell emigration and speed versus direction), (iii) accumulation of matrix (= matrix component synthesis rate versus matrix component degradation rate). Each of these can be varied, with predictable effects on matrix accumulation. Fig. 5.12 gives a highly simplified guide to the principle of balanced matrix breakdown and synthesis, representing turnover or *remodelling*. These processes are under complex biochemical control (Mignatti et al. 1996) and are primarily dependent on the number of cells participating (hence the importance of cell proliferation and migration to the tissue site).

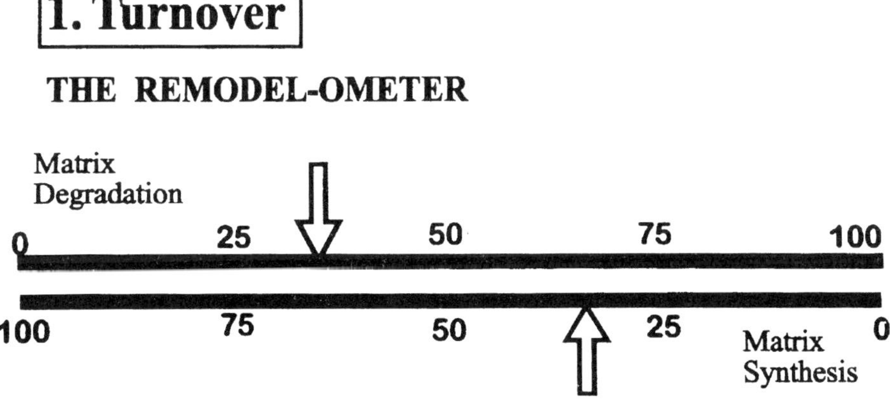

Fig. 5.12. Simplified scheme describing the overall control of matrix deposition into a tissue by cells. In this 'remodel-ometer' the net production of matrix by any group of cells will be a resultant of the rates of production and degradation. This apparently wasteful form of turnover appears to operate in all tissues throughout life, at different rates. Matrix components are produced by standard cell synthesis of proteins and polysaccharides, with all of its control levels. Degradation of extracellular matrix components is mainly achieved by protease activities (serine- and matrix metallo proteinases); themselves regulated by an intricate system of synthesis rates, proenzyme forms, activators and inhibitors.

5.3.4 Selection of cell types

The type of cell seeded into the support material can depend on the type of implant required (i.e. primary stage template or functional secondary stage implant). Seeded cells at the primary stage are commonly activated forms of the tissue cell-type or uncommitted stem cells, capable of rapid division and differentiation to an appropriate phenotype. Alternatively, the cells can act as expendable sources of growth factors, cytokines, mitogenic or chemotactic factors for the attraction and control of host cell recruitment from the implant margin. Current examples of such feeder cell populations commonly use allogeneic cells, which are progressively replaced by ingrowing host cells. In the case of tissue engineered skin replacements such as *Dermagraft*, active neonatal fibroblasts are incorporated into the implants, avoiding the cost, delay and technical problems associated with the use of the patients own (autologous) cells. The design aim here is for such cells to promote ingrowth, adhesion, migration etc. of the patients own cells into the implant and to lay down new collagen. A comparable form of approach has been described for experimental peripheral nerve implants in which Schwann cells are incorporated, releasing neurotrophic factors to promote axonal regeneration through the implant.

Seeded cells can be incorporated either over the surface of the support material or encouraged to penetrate throughout its depth. The former, coating layer of cells is ideal in the case of endothelial or epithelial cells, for example in constructs forming blood vessels or urothelial grafts. Alternatively, mesenchymal cells, required to elaborate an extracellular matrix, are normally encouraged to grow deep into the material. For good substrate utilisation pore size is important and substantial research effort in this area has now defined the ideal pore size range for given substrates such as the collagen-GAG sponge, Integra (Yannas 1990) and polyglycolic/polylactic acid sponges (Putnam and Mooney 1996).

The source of cells for seeding is critical and represents a major design feature. The simplest and possibly cheapest source is from animal tissues. Clearly, such xenogeneic implants carry serious immunological and rejection implications, requiring long term immunosuppression. The same can be said of allogeneic cells where they are used from donors or cadavers. Allograft materials also carry the possibility of infective agents and so present additional regulatory hurdles. They are attractive for commercially produced implants since large numbers of cells can be produced and stored at central production sites, far from the patients hospital. Tissue acquisition from some sites of the patient (autograft) is frequently not difficult as biopsies can be small and these patients normally expect surgery. Whilst rejection and infective agents are not a problem here, autologous cells present less obvious difficulties associated with the quality of the cells available (e.g. pancreatic island cells for insulin production, liver cells or use of cells where genetic disorders affect all of the patient's cells) and tissues which are free from malignant cells in the case of tumour surgery. Additionally, in many cases (such as in burns) there can be a dangerous lag period after the injury, whilst cells are cultured to expand the population sufficiently, prior to incorporation. Such prolonged culture periods can represent a major clinical problem.

Specific culture conditions will vary widely between cell types (details beyond the scope of this chapter). However, general strategies for cell acquisition fall under the headings of either *fine cell purification* or *minimal culture*.

Many experimental systems tend to concentrate on extraction and purification stages needed to produce homogeneous cell preparations (e.g. endothelial cells, keratinocytes, urothelial cells). In some applications these approaches may be important but they normally incur penalties in terms of the time, equipment, expertise and cost of putting cell extracts through multiple separation and testing stages.

Also, in general, the more manipulations are needed the more likely infection or cell death will be a factor. A standard technique would involve dissolution of the tissues surrounding cells, extraction of required cell species and exclusion of major contaminating types and finally testing to ensure cell purity. In conclusion, where autologous cell seeding is part of the design, protocols frequently require separate biopsy procedures. Ideally, these allow tissue samples to be taken from a range of sites and tissues, not necessarily from the site of injury. The imperative is to keep tissue culture expansion stages as short as possible, making use of added growth factors/mitogens. Indeed, the logical progression of this design is to employ *minimal culture*, direct extraction of tissue fragments, allowing seeded cells to populate the bioartificial tissue after it has been implanted.

Minimal culture cell seeding has considerable practical, cost and facility advantages, whilst in some cases being closer to the natural repair process. Tissue fragments suitable as cell donor sources are frequently available at the time of surgery, the aim being to incorporate such tissue fragments into the implant such that suitable cell populations migrate out of the fragments and colonise the implant. Examples include insertion of small pieces of nerve autograft into peripheral nerve conduits instead of seeding with isolated Schwann cells.

Also skin implants can be seeded with fragments of epithelium or clusters of keratinocytes, rather than differentiated sheets of cells (Rheinwald and Green 1975). In the former case integrin substrate receptors, which are important in migration to repair the epithelial sheet (Adams and Watt 1991; Kim et al. 1992), are comparable with those seen in the normal repair process (Prajaparti et al. 1996).

Stem cells or populations of rapidly dividing, poorly differentiated cells are currently being closely examined as sources for use particularly in bone, blood vessel and fibrous connective tissue repair. Active stromal cells from the bone marrow are now studied as potential sources of active cells for seeding into materials. These have the advantage of growing very rapidly in culture and having a relatively plastic phenotype; i.e. they can become suitable cell types in whatever site they are implanted.

Another important area of potential application is to further modify or refine the cells, which are seeded by transfecting with specified genes. This technique in principle would allow a seeded population of cells to overexpress one or more important proteins e.g. growth factors, proteases, hormones, for formation of bioartificial organs and depots.

5.3.5 Macroscopic shape and micro-architecture

5.3.5.1 Macroscopic shape and dimensions. The selection and production of the gross shape of any given implant is perhaps the easiest and obvious design feature. It is clearly subject to a wide variety of factors many of which are special, either to the tissue location or to the stage at which the implant is designed to operate. The gross shape of a bioartificial implant can be important cosmetically when it involves external or visible use, for example in replacement of external ear tissue. However, function tends to be the main imperative.

For structures requiring clear lumen such as blood vessels or urethra, most implants would start by providing such a lumen. Provision to maintain that lumen may also be necessary, either because of pressures from surrounding tissues (compressing weak implant materials, particularly when the patient moves) or from the biological process of collagen matrix contraction. Forces involved are substantial and could easily constrict or block the lumen of many biological tubes. Tubes are used as implants for peripheral nerve regeneration in order to guide axonal regeneration from the proximal to the distal stump across an injury site. However in this case the aim is that the lumen is filled with functional tissue. As a result, non-resorbable implants can constrict the central regenerated tissue, as it forms, impairing later function and making surgical removal a necessity.

Shape also has particular importance in tissues where application of mechanical loads to repair cells is critical for the formation of a functionally aligned connective tissue (i.e. with good tensile properties). The pattern of strain which is set up by uniaxial loading of a high aspect ratio (i.e. long and thin tissue substitute) is dramatically greater than the strain set up in a low aspect ratio (short and wide) tissue, given the same applied stress (Eastwood et al. 1998). It has been recently demonstrated that modest levels of uniaxial strain though a disorganised matrix can orientate resident fibroblasts. The cell behaviour identified in this and related studies (Brown et al. 1998) (bipolarity, alignment with the principal strain and deposition of fibrous matrix) will all lead to stress shielding of the cells. In effect, this is a mechanistic description of how soft tissues adapt to predominant loading patterns - the important point here being that the entire process can be profoundly influenced by initial construct shape.

5.3.5.2 Microscopic architecture. The term *tissue architecture* here is used to refer to the specific structural organisation of any tissue or construct, that is the position, thickness and polarity of cell layers, the presence of zones or layers of particular connective tissue components and the orientation of fibres. Primary stage implants would be expected to contain information to guide towards the desired final architecture whilst secondary stage bioartificial tissue implants would ideally resemble the original tissue.

One central aspect of architecture is the recruitment of appropriate cells to layers of the new tissue. This is most commonly approached at present by seeding cells into each layer. However, it is also possible to engineer the materials to favour ingrowth of only the required cell types. Such a cell selection approach can be either negative or positive, though negative selection is likely to produce more effective segregation. Such selective biomaterial surfaces can be produced which do not support attachment/migration of cells to be excluded. An example of this could use a substrate which supported poor fibroblast ingrowth but allowed neural cell attachment (including neurites and Schwann cells) to promote nerve regeneration whilst minimising fibroblast infiltration and so, potentially fibrosis.

Architecture at both the molecular and the cellular level can be regulated by combinations of contact guidance and mechanical loading (Brown et al. 1997). These are not independent factors; particularly in fibroblast populated connective tissue constructs, which are prone to contraction (endogenous loading). Ultimately, these factors may reinforce and contradict each other, depending on the design.

The main forms of experimental guidance substrates described so far use micron scale topographical features such as fibres or ridges. The three main forms are (i) resorbable polymer substrates (Curtis and Wilkinson 1997) to promote and align cellular outgrowth between cut tendon ends, the aim being to form an aligned provisional tissue, (ii) fibrous materials based on aggregated forms of fibronectin (Ejim et al. 1993; Brown et al. 1994) and (iii) aligned collagen fibrils in gel form (Dickinson et al. 1994).

Control of tissue architecture through mechanical loading can be divided simplistically, on the basis of the predominant type of loading used, into three types: tension, compression and shear. Tensional loading, particularly uni-directional, has been used to achieve orientation particularly of fibroblasts from tissues such as muscle, tendon and ligament substitutes (Eastwood et al. 1998,Vandenberg 1988). Careful analysis of the cell responses to such strains has demonstrated that fibroblasts align parallel with the principal strain, even at very modest loading levels. Compressional loading is also thought to be important in regulating the type of matrix synthesised by articular chondrocytes. Fluid flow shear has been used extensively for development of the natural orientation of vascular endothelial cells in reconstruction of blood vessels. In this case cells take on an elongate bipolar morphology, parallel with the direction of the applied shear (Levesque and Nerem 1985). In the case of tensional loads on fibroblasts and shear on endothelial cells it is possible to induce predictable cellular orientation. It has been suggested that predictions of orientation can be made using the working hypothesis that: in appropriate strain fields, *fibroblasts take on the shape and alignment which minimises the strain applied to their cytoskeleton, by the ECM to which they are attached* (Eastwood et al. 1998). That is, if there is a repetitive uniaxial tensional loading across the ECM, sufficiently great to deform the resident cells, they will minimise that deformation by assuming a long and thin morphology (i.e. bipolar-elongate), align parallel to the principal strain they experience and potentially deposit collagen in that same plane. It is becoming possible then, to design bioreactors for producing a required cell or tissue organisation, using predominantly fluid shear, tensional loading or compressional loading as directing cues. In the examples mentioned above, the cue (or combinations of cues) would be used to produce spatial and biosynthetic responses required to generate vascular, fibrous or cartilaginous tissues, respectively.

5.3.6 Special local factors: Different problems for different tissue sites

Specific examples of tissues and sites are perhaps the most effective vehicle for the discussion of theoretical aspects of bioartificial tissue design (and limitations) as well as the practical imperatives, which govern the design. The very selection of a tissue or injury site is itself governed by imperatives such as clinical, economic and social demand (frequency of occurrence, effect on life quality and employment, availability of alternative treatments, resources needed to treat by conventional means). Clearly then, examples such as chronic wounds and arthritis in the elderly, spinal and peripheral nerve injury and heart valve failure attract much research. Examples considered here are from a range of tissue types, addressing diverse clinical requirements.

5.4. EXAMPLES OF BIOARTIFICIAL TISSUES AND CONSTRUCTS

5.4.1 Organs with metabolic functions

In some respect this group represents a special category of bioartificial tissues and organs. Some are best described as *glands*. Others are the major synthetic and maintenance organs of the body, acting through the blood system, such as liver and kidney. Characteristically these have major *systemic* functions, producing hormones, growth and blood factors, removing toxic compounds etc. Consequently, there is a heavy dependency on good blood perfusion for function and this needs to be established, as an early imperative, before a bioartificial organ of this type can operate. It can be envisaged that a capillary bed may form part of the initial construction of the artificial tissue or angiogenic factors are supplied with the implant to attract a rich capillary supply as quickly as possible. In many cases the anatomical positioning of such an organ is not a primary consideration. Further, in contrast to many other examples given here its detailed structural architecture is less important.

Figure 5.13 shows a diagrammatic representation of approaches in two important examples, namely *bioartificial liver* and *pancreatic function*. Extracorporeal shunts designed to provide liver function are already under test, principally for patients awaiting transplants. Designs for implantable structures are also attracting attention. Clearly the aim here is to provide a huge exchange area with circulating recipient blood for donor cells to carry out metabolic functions (Lanza et al. 1992; Thomas and Thomas 1997). The second example involves encapsulation of pancreatic islet cells, notably within alginate, a relatively inert and stable polysaccharide shell (Tatarkiewicz 1995). These islet cells produce large amounts of insulin, the aim being to immobilise and trap such encapsulated cells in a bioartificial gland to provide diabetic patients with a steady supply of circulating insulin.

In both cases (and in most examples of this form of implant) the aim is to replace the function (either secretive or metabolic processing) of a defective host cell. Since the host, or patient's cells are defective it is almost certain that allogeneic or even xenogeneic cells must be used. Pancreatic islet cells are used from human donors whilst most bioartificial liver designs aim to use trapped porcine hepatic cells. Clearly these pose major rejection problems. The approaches used all attempt to segregate the

Organs with Metabolic Functions

Basic Imperatives - Discrete Capsular Structure
- Blood Perfusion
- Segregation of Cells & Host

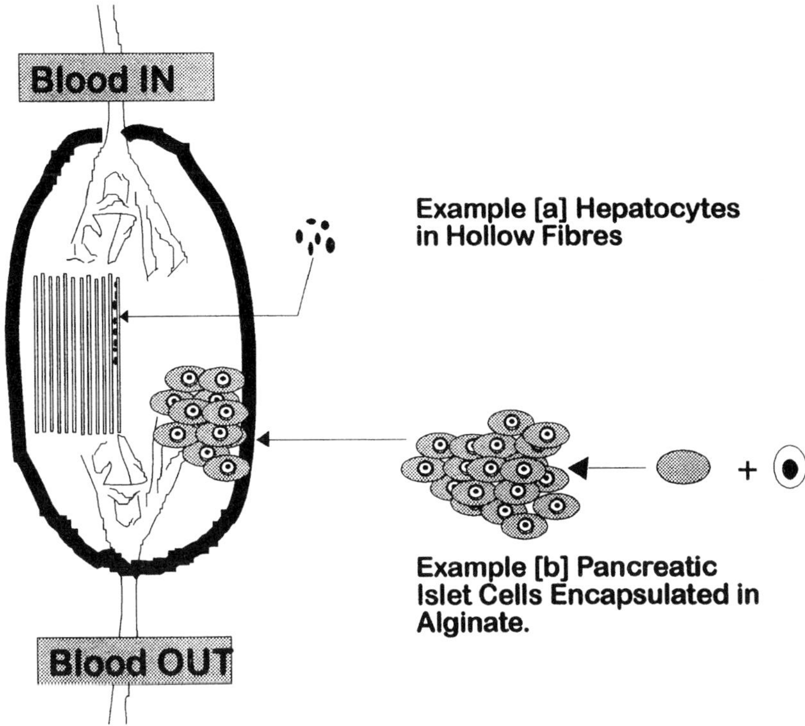

Fig. 5.13. Diagrammatic illustration of rationale for formation of bioartificial organs and glands. Example (a) shows a form of liver construct in which functional (liver) cells are segregated from the recipient circulation by entrapment in hollow fibres with semi-permeable membrane walls. Case (b) shows a cell encapsulation approach, which is being developed with the aim of forming an artificial pancreas. Though the technique is different the imperative is similar, to allow rapid and efficient exchange to occur between cells and the circulation whilst preventing direct contact which would provoke an immunological response to the foreign cells.

implanted donor cells. The idea of trapping and hiding pancreatic islet cells from immune surveillance is now well established, in which cells are encapsulated in an alginate gel. This allows insulin and other small metabolites out into the surrounding fluid, but acts as a barrier to direct contact between implanted islet cells and those of the host immune system. Similarly, the trapping of donor hepatocytes on the inner walls of hollow fibre devices (around which the host blood is allowed to flow) solves both perfusion and segregation questions simultaneously, providing excellent exchange characteristics while allowing no direct host-donor cell-cell contact (Gerlach et al. 1996). However, such liver replacements can never become integrated with the host body tissues and so are closer in nature to bioprostheses.

5.4.2 Tendons and ligaments

Attempts to replace tendon and ligament with bioartificial implants to date have relied largely on the use of fabrics, polymers and carbon fibre implants. However, these have proved far from ideal in general clinical use. These prostheses have been developed using the primary imperative (perceived surgical requirement) that the ruptured ends of the tendon/ligament lesion need to be made to carry significant tensile loads as quickly as possible after surgery. Future designs may modify this imperative, since in emphasising the need to carry early, large scale loads, stiff implants produce severe localised stress-shielding to cells of the repair tissue and the new-old tissue interface. These are wholly inappropriate organisational cues at the cellular level, which may contribute to the poor quality of repair and adhesions between gliding interfaces in conventional repair.

Natural tendon repair is regarded as a mixture of processes based on responses from 'intrinsic' (tendon-derived) cells and 'extrinsic'cells, recruited from outside the tendon (Gelberman et al. 1988). Some reports have described the guidance of intrinsic tendon repair in culture (and on grooved artificial substrates, providing a contact guidance cue, parallel with the long axis of the tendon (Curtis and Wilkinson 1997). As the arm and hand is extended and flexed, the tendons glide many centimetres relative to surrounding tissues, particularly crucial in flexor tendons which run for much of their length through tunnels, lined by synovial sheaths (specialised membranes which maintain gliding function). The preservation of gliding surfaces between tissues is particularly important in such dynamic connective tissues. In order for repaired hand tendons to regain good function it is essential that the tendon moves freely between other tissue layers. Hence, adhesions as a result of injury and repair are regarded as a common cause of poor final function and represent a major imperative in the design of implants and treatment protocols. In fact it is possible to regard reconnection of the tendon stumps and adhesion formation as conflicting imperatives since in both, stable collagenous matrices are laid down as part of an apparently common repair process. Future designs then, will aim to focus the repair and matrix integration processes at the implant-tendon interface and inhibit or block it across interfaces with surrounding tissues (summarised in figure 5.14).

Relationship of Gliding Structures in Tendon (eg. Hand Flexor Tendon)

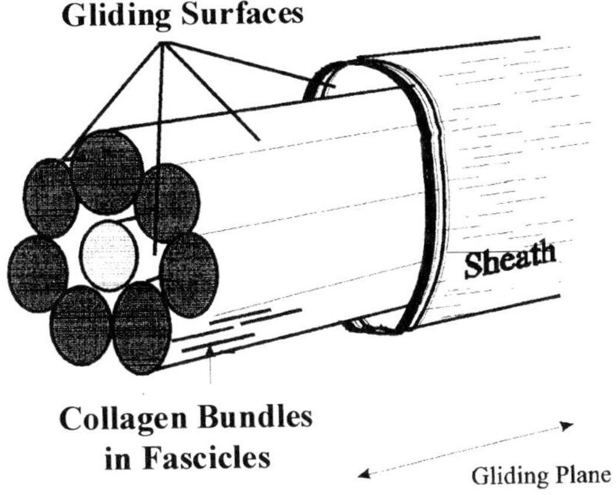

Fig. 5.14. Diagrammatic representation of the critical features needed for effective tendon repair function. Connective tissue features include dense fibre bundles arranged into independent structures, near parallel in orientation. Cell density is low and collagen fibre bundles have the appearance of moving longitudinally past each other (see figure 5.3). The epitenon, surface layer, provides a gliding surface with the surrounding tissues, often a thin tendon sheath, which is derived from synovial membrane. Tendon is fed by blood microvessels and nerves entering from the surrounding tissues. Tendon function is dominated by great tensile strength (transmitting load between muscle and bone) and a capacity for dynamic flexibility, through gliding at every level of its organisation.

5.4.3 Urothelial tissue implants and patches

Urothelium is a specialised tissue critical to normal function of the urogenital tract. Damage is common in trauma, disease and in some forms of birth defect, typically hypospadias. Hypospadia is a relatively common defect in which the urethra opens before the end of the penis. In extreme forms, conventional surgical reconstruction fails and alternative graft materials are needed.

Urothelial patches for use in this type of reconstruction have been described; based on a resorbable polyglycolic acid mesh seeded with mixed urothelial and smooth muscle cells. These produced implantable tissue structures which reorganised to give two distinct cell layers in vivo (Atala et al. 1993; Scott et al. 1991), most recently used to form urinary bladders (Oberpenning et al. 1999). Another form of urothelial construct has been reported where urothelial cells were cultured on the surface of crosslinked collagen sponges to form differentiated epithelial multilayers (Sabbagh et al. 1998).

Specific design imperatives for this tissue type relate to the need to form a continuous, differentiating urothelial cell layer, forming a functional interface with urine, as quickly as possible. At the same time, implants must have sufficient mechanical strength and elasticity until resident cells have elaborated an effective

ECM. Special problems are the tendency to become infected or to form crystals in contact with urine (Scott et al. 1991, Sabbagh et al. 1998). This point is particularly important in the early phases when the urothelial barrier function is incomplete. Even a modest tendency for a support material to act as a crystal seeding site could lead to implant failure due to the formation of 'stones' in the implanted tissue.

5.4.4 Large and medium diameter blood vessels

Completely artificial prostheses for surgical implantation and replacement of large vessels has a long and in some instances a successful history. These are based on a range of woven and knitted fabric prostheses produced from variants of Dacron, PTFE, polyurothanes etc. The pore size of these fabrics is important, with 10 to 45 μm being the most effective for surrounding tissue ingrowth. Cell and tissue ingrowth around the implant is considered to be important for success. Reformation of an endothelial-like cell lining may be provided from one of four possible routes summarised by Jerusalem et al (1987).

a.- Migration across the suture lines.
b.- Seeding by deposition from circulating cells.
c.- Immigration and transformation of cells from surrounding adventitial tissue.
d.- Migration and transformation of smooth muscle cells from the media.

Interestingly, a common feature in many successful fabric prostheses is the incorporation of a crimp into the knitting or weaving process. This crimp structure modifies the mechanical properties of the implant, producing a low modulus region in the stress-strain curve. It is possible that this mechanical feature is important in the subsequent response of connective tissue cells.

Prior to surgery the prostheses are pre-clotted with the patient's own blood such that the pores are blocked and bleeding and leakage is minimised post-surgery. A trade-off between leakage due to increased porosity and benefits of subsequent adventitial ingrowth is part of the design of these prostheses. More recently attempts have been made to seed the luminal surface of such prostheses with endothelial cells to decrease thrombogenosis and improve the long-term patency of the vessel (Shepard et al. 1986). A fully tissue engineered vessel with burst strength comparable to a natural vessel and an endothelial cell lining has recently been described by the group of Auger (L'Heureux et al. 1998). In animal studies (Noishiki et al. 1996) implants have been seeded with bone marrow stromal cells with the aim of accelerating the overgrowth of an endothelial cell lining. These authors suggested that marrow cell seeding provided angiogenic factors, which in turn improved recruitment of microvessels and cells to the implant. It is also possible that the marrow stromal cells act as a direct source of *stem* cells capable of differentiating into endothelial cells.

Tissue design imperatives (figure 5.15):

a.- Suitable for stable suturing (mechanical strength).
b.- Minimal leakage, maximal surrounding tissue infiltration.
c.- Non-thrombogenic surface (long-term patency).

Basic Features of Large Blood Vessels/Implants

Imperatives - Mechanically suitable: pressures/flow/tension
- Non-thrombogenic lumen
- Biologically stable

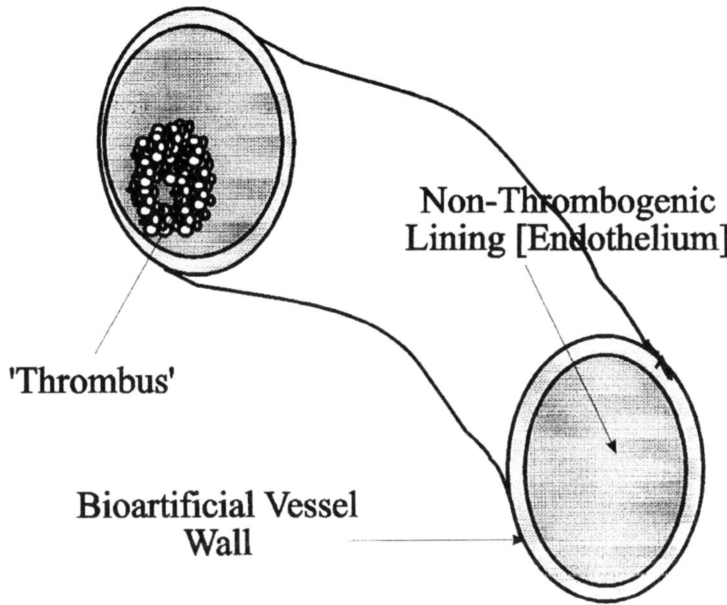

Fig. 5.15. Functional imperatives for blood vessels vary, depending on the size, type and anatomical location. In general, a structurally stable vessel wall, at the fluid pressures and shear forces required is essential. A number of forms of mechanical compliance are possible for the wall, from weak to elastic to stiff, depending on organisation and composition of the connective tissue. It is also essential that the lumen remains open despite tendencies to for thrombi on the inner surface. Hence a non-thrombogenic surface is necessary.

Conventional imperatives in this tissue are dominated by the need to form a mechanically stable, non-thrombogenic lumenal surface as soon as possible after implantation. Currently the aim is to provide this as a patent endothelial cell lining. In addition, fluid shear and pressure at many implantation sites indicates that a considerable mechanical strength is needed though some surgical options are available to temporarily divert flow whilst a mature vessel wall forms. In general the larger the vessels to be engineered, the greater the internal pressure and the more complex the nature of the native vessel wall. This seems in part to reflect more complex mechanical function, with incorporation of elastic and reactive smooth muscle layers. The biology of blood flow and vessel wall mechanical and biochemical interaction is complex and likely to present many layers if difficulty in producing functional bioartificial grafts with longterm survival.

At the opposite end of the implant spectrum, autografts of vessels (commonly the saphenous vein) are considered to be generally successful and in the case of children these grow with the child. They suffer some problems due to aneurysm formation and fibrosis due to fibroblast activity and, like all large tissue autografts, suffer complications and morbidity related to the donor site.

Microvessel formation by *guided angiogenesis* has been proposed as a mechanism for promoting optimal formation of new capillary beds in repair of bioartificial tissues (Brown et al. in press). The idea in this case is to direct the growth of new microvesels on orientated fibres of aggregated fibronectin, acting as haptotactic guides for sprouting endothelial cells. A form of this guided angiogenesis has been described in the use of fibronectin fibrous materials in nerve regeneration, where new microvascular invasion was also directed to the orientation of implanted fibronectin (Hobson et al. 1997).

5.4.5 Dermal substitutes, skin equivalents and artificial skin

Construction of bioartificial skin equivalents is arguably the most advanced area of tissue engineering. As more and more patients survive the initial trauma of massive skin loss, the dilemma of how to produce an effective *graft* to cover the wounds becomes more acute. The imperatives behind the development of skin equivalents were initially the clinical requirement to provide some form of covering for extensive full depth burns. The greater the area of burn, the less intact skin is available for grafting AND the greater is the loss of body fluids and risk of deep infection. Without early effective covering most of these patients die within days or weeks. Those who survive to receive longterm treatment often suffer severe and irreversible scarring. First imperatives then were to provide early stage, biologically effective covering. More recently, additional imperatives have been to control the scarring process, frequently by minimising contraction and even to provide grafts for coverage of chronic wounds (venous leg ulcers, pressure sores etc.)

Figure 5.16 illustrates the main features basic to most types of skin. Minimalistically, these can be divided into a barrier function epidermis separated from a vascularised, innervated mechanically strong, dermis by a dividing basement membrane. Early attempts to replace living epidermal layers can be traced back for four decades (Billingham and Reynolds 1952) though research has been increasingly

SKIN BIOARTIFICIAL IMPLANTS

[a] Natural Tissue Components/Architecture

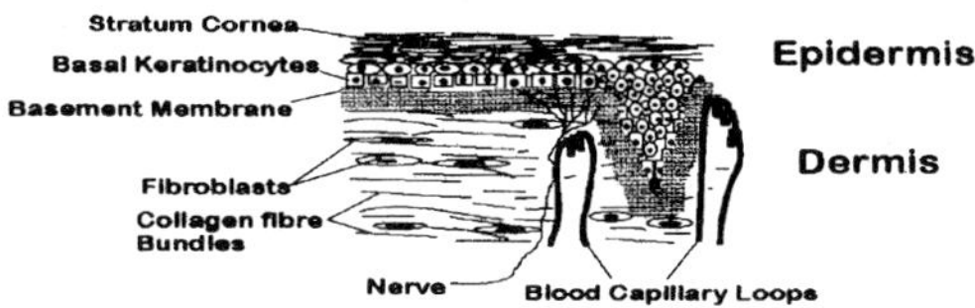

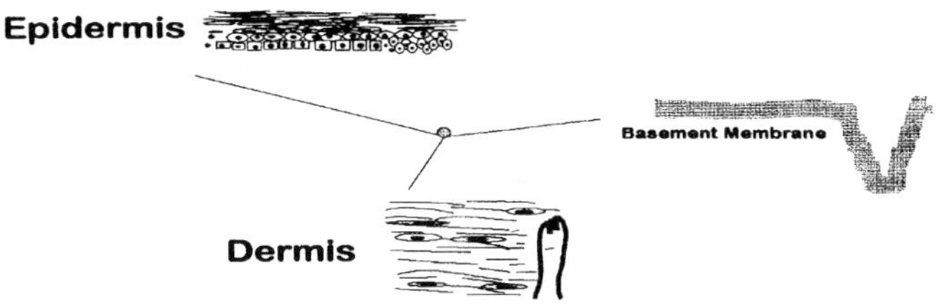

[b] Components and Assembly of Potential Bioartificial Skin

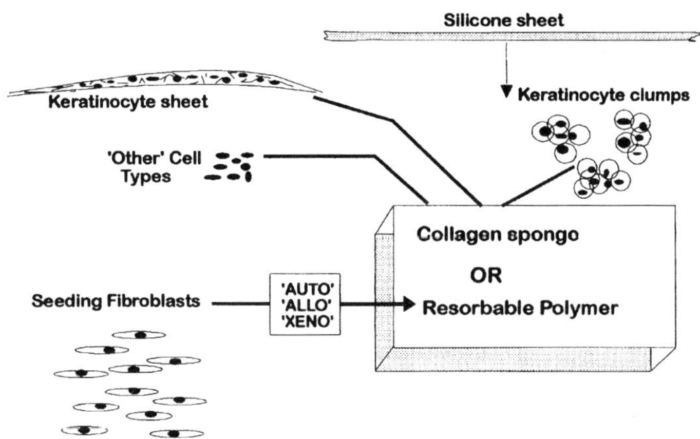

Fig. 5.16. Diagrammatic illustration of the forms taken by bioartificial skin constructs. Panel [a] shows the main tissue components of intact skin (not including specialised glands etc.). The epidermis is composed of keratinocytes and other associated cell types (e.g. melanocytes), on a basement membrane separated form the collagenous dermis. Panel [b] illustrates some forms of composite used to mimic skin structure, based on collagen or resorbable synthetic polymer, seeded with fibroblasts (auto, -allo- or xenogeneic). This is covered by a keratinocyte layer (either as a sheet of or clumps which grow to form a sheet) sometimes mixed with associated cells such as melanocytes, or covered by a silicone sheet.

active in the last 20 years with the availability of expanded sheets of keratinocytes for grafting (Rheinwald and Green 1975). Two key components have developed in parallel, but separately in the first instance. These components will be distinguished here, for convenience as *dermal substitutes* and *skin equivalents*.

Dermal substitutes are materials produced to replace or temporarily substitute for the dermis in full depth wounds. Ideally, such materials would become infiltrated by the recipient's cells and eventually remodelled and replaced by repair tissue and act somewhere between a removable dressing and a living graft.

Amongst the best examples of simple dermal substitutes are the collagen-GAG sponges, notably the form developed by Yannas et al (1980) (Dagalakis et al. 1980) containing chondroitin-6-sulphate (collagen-GAG sponges). These have been developed extensively as bilayer implants. The basal layer comprises the collagen-GAG sponge, designed to recruit and support the growth of granulation tissue (fibroblasts and blood capillaries) from the surrounding dermis and eventually full dermal repair. The second layer is a silicone sheet bonded to the surface, to reduce fluid losses until a full epithelial layer forms over the surface of the collagen-GAG sponge.

These implants have now been clinically tested and support good dermal repair with limited scar contraction (Heimbach et al. 1988). Developments and alternative forms of such collagen-based dermal substitutes have been described by Herbage et al (Rault et al. 1996), Middlekoop et al (Heijmen et al. 1997), Chvapil (1982), van Luyn et al (1992) and Matsuda et al (1993). Versions of collagen sponges containing elastin (Lefebvre et al. 1996), hyaluronan, heparan sulphate (Lefebvre et al. 1996) and chitosan (Taravel and Damard 1993 and 1996), growth factors (Cascone et al. 1995; Fujisato et al. 1996) and antibiotics (Matsuda et al. 1992) have been developed. In addition, their use has been extended beyond burns, to a range of chronic non-healing wounds (Silver 1994). Meanwhile, non-collagen synthetic resorbable polymers have been developed towards similar applications (reviewed in Langer and Vacanti 1993; Putnam and Mooney 1996; Pulapura and Kohn 1992).

Development of living artificial skin grafts was based initially on sheets of cultured human keratinocytes, designed to rapidly replace the covering epithelial layer. This structure is indeed critical to early stage patient survival through limiting infection and loss of body fluids. In the early 1970s techniques for the expansion of keratinocyte cultures were developed, leading to a technique for production of useful sheets of cells by Green and co-workers (Rheinwald and Green 1975). The current view holds that such a simple epithelial cell graft is not effective in the longterm for full thickness defects due to the fragility of resulting tissue (especially over joints) and its failure to form a basement membrane. Current work, therefore, has aimed to incorporate some form of living dermal component to meet this deficiency. As in other examples, different designs come mainly from the range of support materials chosen.

Some forms of implant have used caderveric, acellular dermis as a base material; termed de-epidermalised dermis (DED). In this case cultured keratinocyte sheets have been layered directly onto DED prior to implantation into dermal wounds, producing effective living skin grafts (Navsaria et al. 1998). Similarly, bioartificial (semi-natural) materials have been used as substrates or carriers for grafted skin cells. Integra (without its silicone layer) has been used experimentally after seeding with autologous keratinocytes (Grant et al. 1998) and crosslinked hyaluronan films have similarly been used as semi-natural keratinocyte carrier layers (Andreassi et al. 1991).

Examples of artificial skin are perhaps the most advanced practical forms of any tissue engineered grafts presently under test. Two forms are known by trade names as *Apligraf* and *Dermagraft.* Dermagraft consists of allogeneic fibroblasts (from human foreskin) within a resorbable synthetic polyglycolic acid mesh and has been reported to function effectively in clinical trials so far (Noughton et al. 1997). Apligraf consists of a bilayer of allogeneic cells, human neonatal foreskin fibroblasts and keratinocytes (Wilkins et al. 1994). The fibroblasts are seeded into a bovine type I collagen gel which is allowed to contract under tension. The surface of this gel is then seeded with keratinocytes and cultured until a cornified multilayer is formed, resembling the structure of normal epidermis.

A recent clinical study involving 275 patients with venous leg ulcers showed clear statistical benefit from the application of this material in terms of rate of wound closure (Falanga et al. 1998). Perhaps more importantly for the longterm design of implants such as this, no adverse responses were attributed to the bioartificial tissue. Firstly, there were no signs of immunological response to the bovine collagen or rejection of the allogeneic cells. The finding that there was no significant generation of antibodies to the bovine collagen is an important confirmation of the safety of native collagen-based materials (Falanga et al. 1998). The investigators found that the implant was slowly removed (remodelled) rather than being rejected (at least using this cell source). This is a critical point, indicating that for skin implants at least, bioartificial tissues may not need to use the patient's own cells. Whilst in many ways ideal, the use of allogeneic cells causes serious complications, delaying surgical procedures, introducing the complexities and costs (facilities and expertise) of local cell culture, and limiting the possibilities for commercial exploitation. The present supply of Apligraf, for immediate use (as a living product) with a 5-day shelf life, clearly would not be possible if the patient's own cells were used.

5.4.6 Peripheral nerve repair conduits

Peripheral nerve repair represents an attractive problem for the application of soft tissue engineering. Injuries to peripheral nerves are relatively common following trauma (road traffic, occupational or glass related) and surgery. They can vary from a clean cut of the hand nerve to massive loss of nerve tissue. Prospects of repair are moderate and operative reconstructions are common, though recovery of lost function is very variable, i.e. there is much that could be improved. Primary repair, where the two cut ends of a nerve can be sutured together without significant tissue tension, is the ideal option (Lundborg 1988). However, where this is not possible due to loss of tissue, it is normal to graft a nerve from another location (secondary repair with autograft). This form of grafting carries particular consequences for the donor site, which is left denervated and insensate. Even with autografting secondary repair outcomes are frequently poor. It must be stressed that following nerve injury *all* of the neural tissue downstream (distal) of the damage dies. Consequently, axons must regrow from the proximal stump of the injury site all the way to the target organ (Lundborg 1988) through whatever material is present in the injury gap.

Use of artificial or tissue engineered grafts is clearly attractive to avoid donor site morbidity. Figure 5.17 shows some of the numerous forms of implant materials used (aside from natural grafts of muscle and vein) including collagen (Doolabh et al. 1996) hyaluronan aggregate (Favaro et al. 1990) copolymers of lactide and caprolactone (Hoppen et al. 1990) and fibronectin (Whitworth et al. 1995).

Design imperatives for nerve grafts and conduits (in addition to the standard requirements of suitable substrates etc.) are as follows.

a.- Support of Schwann cell outgrowth
b.- Provision of neurotrophic factors to promote rapid regeneration
c.- Directional guidance along the axis of the repair to the distal stump
d.- Resorption of the support material after a stable regenerate has formed.

Rate of regeneration across a defect is critical to the degree of function that can be restored. Prolonged denervation of many target organs, motor or sensory, leads to irreversible degeneration and so permanent loss of function. In this application, then, a primary imperative is to achieve the most rapid regrowth possible. This can be facilitated through provision of either Schwann cells (or one or more of the growth promoting factors they produce). Schwann cells are critical support cells for regenerating axons, partly by virtue of neurotrophic factors which they produce (Lundborg 1988; Ansselin et al. 1997). For longer implants the outgrowth of Schwann cells is slow and appears to be a limiting feature. Outgrowth can be improved by provision of suitable matrix substrates or chemotactic factors or donor cells can be seeded into the implant at suitable places. Examples of this are the seeding of Schwann cells into collagen sponge (Ansselin et al. 1997) and resorbable polylactone tubes (Brown et al. 1996)

An alternative or additional approach is to supply the implant with its own neurotrophic factor depot. The simplest form of depot is that used for Fn-material conduits, where dried porous materials are allowed to swell in a solution of the factor. Nerve growth factor (NGF) and neurotrophin-3 (NT-3) used in this manner, are slowly released from the material (over up to 7 day periods, (Whitworth et al. 1996; Sterne et al. 1998).

Without suitable alignment of the regeneration, particularly over longer gaps, repair is impossible. This has been achieved in the past through use of small open tubes or conduits, which trap a fluid exudate through which nerve growth cones progress. Directional guidance is provided by the lumen. More recently, direct contact guidance has been proposed, using fibronectin materials with a fibre orientation, parallel with the axis of regeneration (Whitworth et al. 1995 and 1996). Neurites are known to align to and migrate more rapidly along fibronectin fibres in vitro. (Wojciak-Stothard et al. 1997). Aligned collagen fibrils have also been proposed as contact guidance substrates (Tranquillo RT., personal communication).

Nerve Guides & Bioartificial Guides

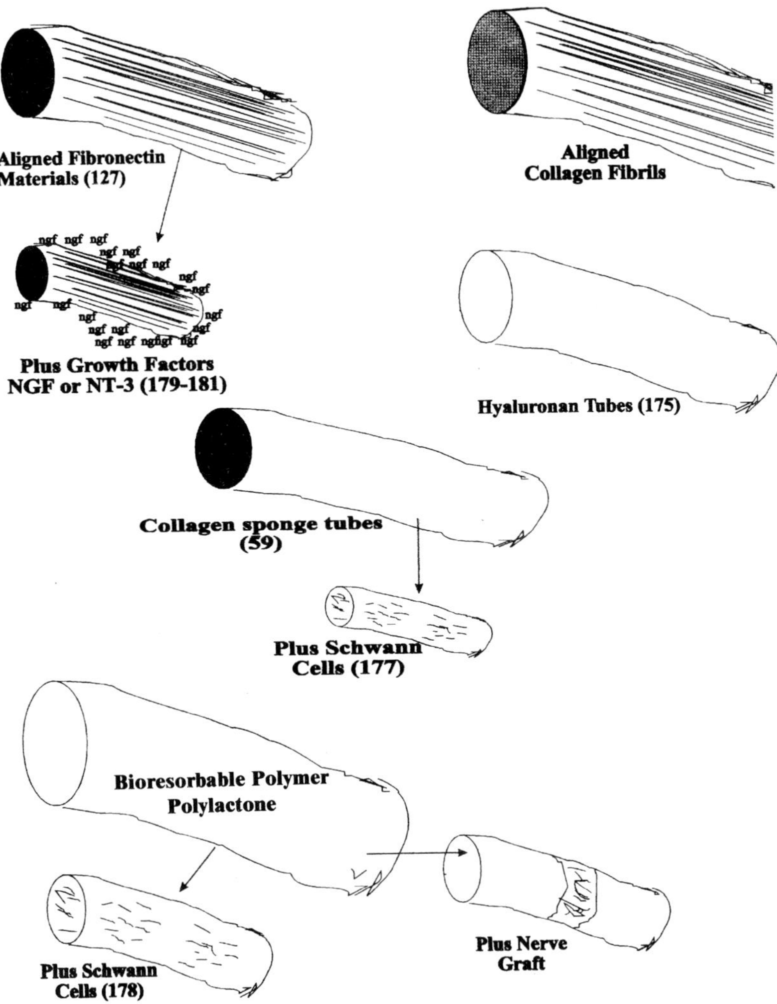

Fig. 5.17. Imperatives for peripheral nerve repair are a uniaxial structural reconstruction and a rapid rate of regeneration of axons to across the implant. Nerve guides or conduits, for promotion of repair; come in numerous forms, using two basic approaches. The first generation (evolving directly from implantable silicone tubes) are the collagen, hyaluronan and synthetic polymer (polylactone) tubes. These provide guidance and contain the repair tissue simply by virtue of their tubular structure. The second type typically has aligned fibres (in the first instance fibronectin and more recently, magnetically aligned collagen fibrils) in the form of a 'conduit' (i.e. porous but with no large lumen). The aim here is to provide contact guidance for the neural repair elements. To either tube-guides or contact guidance implants it is possible to add growth promoters, such as NGF or NT-3 neurotrophic factors, or to incorporate Schwann cells in order to speed up neurite extension.

In these cases the provision of directional guidance cues in the substrate will also increase the migration velocity of axon sprouts (even at the same speed of progress) by limiting the degree of path deflection (Ahmed 1999). It is important to distinguish between porous fibrillar guides, which potentially provide contact guidance and tubular guides where orientation is provided only by the limiting walls of the conduit. Fn-mat guides (Whitworth et al. 1995; Sterne et al. 1997) and orientated collagen fibrillar guides both provide guidance at the cellular level whilst tubes from collagen sponge (Doolabh et al. 1996), synthetic polymer and hyaluronan (Favaro et al. 1990) provide only a lumen.

Resorption of the conduit or guide material is important for nerve applications since persistence can lead to constriction of the new nerve tissue in the months following repair, producing compression injury and pain. Non-resorbable materials require a separate operation for their removal. In this respect, silicone tubes can cause constriction and clearly do not resorb and this has lead to the use of polylactone resorbable materials, as alternative conduits.

Using combinations of these approaches, then, it is now possible to achieve regeneration in rat and primate (Ahmed et al. submitted) animal models of nerve injury. The repair quality produced approaches that of nerve autografting, in terms of their structure (Whitworth et al. 1996; Sterne et al. 1997) and function (Sterne et al. 1997 and 1998), including diabetic rat nerves, where repair is slow (Whitworth et al. 1995). Clearly, this is an application where further tissue and material engineering developments in the near future are likely to significantly alter surgical practice.

5.5. CONCLUSIONS

Tissue engineering is a new and evolving field. Its interdependence on a range of other highly developed disciplines such as cell biology, biomaterials, bioengineering and surgery has allowed its rapid growth. However, this has also generated confusing approaches and aims since novel tissue engineering inevitably sits at interfaces between these disciplines.

The attempt here has been to rationalise these approaches within concepts of *design imperatives*, operating within the biological repair process and the control requirements of mammalian cells. Central to this is the need to have logical design strategies for engineering of *repair tissues* (primary TE) or *mature tissues* (secondary TE). The first depends heavily on repair biology whilst the second will be limited by advances in bioreactor design.

Examples are elaborated for both of these extremes, from nerve repair to major blood vessels, indicating how the problems of spatial control of repair may be achieved on one hand, whilst examining the problems of tissue density/asymmetry on the other. In reality, most applications can use combinations of the two and in the future will depend heavily on surgical initiative in finding new ways to use bioatificial spare parts for reconstructive surgery.

REFERENCES

Adams J.C. and Watt F.M. (1991) *J. Cell Biol.* **115**, 829.

Ahmed Z. (1999) PhD Thesis, University of London.

Ahmed Z., Brown R.A., Ljungberg C., Wiberg M. and Terenghi G. (1999) *Scand. J. Plast. Reconstr. Surg.* **33**, 1.

Ahmed Z., Idowu B.D. and Brown R.A. (1999) *Biomaterials* **20**, 201.

Andreassi L., Casini L., Trabucchi E., et al. (1991) *Wounds* **3**, 116.

Ansselin A.D., Fink T. and Davies D.F. (1997) *Neuropath. Appl. Neurobiol.* **23**, 387.

Arbustini E., Jones J.M., Moses R.D., Eidbo E.E., Carroll R.J. and Ferrans V.J. (1984) *Am.J.Cardiol.* **53**, 1388.

Arnoczky S., Adams M., DeHaven K., Eyre D., Mow V., Kelly (1988) In *Injury and Repair of the Musculoskeletal Soft Tissues*, eds. Woo, S.L.-Y. and Buckwalter J.A. (AAOS., Park Ridge, Illinois) p. 487.

Atala A., Freeman M.R., Vacanti J.P., Shepard J. and Retik A.B. (1993) *J. Urol.* **150**, 608.

Ayad S., Boot-Handforth R., Humphries M., Kadler K., Shuttleworth A. (1994) *The Extracellular Matrix Facts Book* (Academic Press, London) p. 88.

Baschong W., Sutterlin R. and Aebi U. (1997) *Eur. J. Cell Biol.* **72**, 189.

Bateman J.F., Lamande S.R., Ramshaw J.A.M. (1996) in *Extracellular Matrix* vol 2. ed. Comper W.D. (Harwood Academic, Amsterdam) p. 122.

Bell E. (1995) *J. Cell Eng.* **1**, 28.

Bell E., Iverson B. and Merill C. (1979) *Proc. Natl. Acad. Sci* **76**, 1274.

Bell E., Sher S., Hull B. (1984) *Scanning Elect. Microsc.* **4**, 1957.

Benedetti L., Cortivo R., Berti T., Berti A., Pea F., Mazzo M. and Abatangelo G. (1993) *Biomaterials* **14**, 1154.

Berthod F., Hayek D., Damour O. and Collombel C. (1993) *Biomaterials* **14**, 749.

Billingham R.E. and Reynolds J. (1952) *Br. J. Plast. Surg.* **5**, 25.

Birk C.E. and Trelstad R.L. (1980) *J. Cell Biol. J. Anat.* **131**, 81.

Birk D.E. Silver F.S, Trelstad R.L. (1991) in *Cell Biology of Extracellular Matrix* ed. Hay E.D., 2nd edition. (Plenum Press, New York) p. 221.

Bonzon N., Carrat X., Deminiere C., Daculsi G., Lefebvre F. and Rabaud M. (1995) *Biomaterials* **16**, 881.

Bowersox J.C. and Sorgente N. (1982) *Canc. Res.* **42**, 2547.

Broom N.D. (1978) *J. Thorac. Cardiovasc. Surg.* **76**, 202.

Brown R.A. and McFarland C.D. (1993) *Curr. Opinion Therap. Patents.* **3**, 1117.

Brown R.A., Blunn G.W. and Ejim O.S. (1994) *Biomaterials* **15**, 475.

Brown R.A., Pajapati R., McGrouther D.A. and Eastwood M. (1998) *J. Cell Physiol.* **175**, 323.

Brown R.A., Smith K.D. and McGrouther D.A. (1997) *Wound Repair Regen.* **5**, 212.

Brown R.A., Terenghi G. and McFarland C.D. (1999) in *The New Angiotherapy* eds Fan T.-P.D. and Auerbach R. (Humana Press Inc., Totwa New Jersey).

Brown R.E., Erdmann D., Lyons S.F. and Suchy H. (1996) *J. Reconstr. Microsurg.* **12**, 149.

Buch W.S., Kosek J.C. and Angell W.W. (1970) *J. Thorac .Cardiovasc. Surg.* **60**, 673.

Burkitt H.G., Young B., Heath J.W. (1993) *Weater's Functional Histology 3rd edition.* (Churchill-Livingstone).

Byers, P.D., Brown, R.A. (1990) in *Methods in Cartilage Research* eds. Maroudas, A. and Kuettner, K. (Academic Press, London) p. 319.

Campoccia D., Hunt J.A., Dohetery P.J., Zhong S.P., O'Regan M., Benedetti L. and Williams D.F. (1996) *Biomaterials.* **17**, 963.

Cascone M.G., Sim B. and Downes S. (1995) *Biomaterials* **16**, 569.

Cipriano P.R., Billingham M.E., Oyer P.E., Kutsche L.M. and Stinsin E.B. (1982) *Circulation* **66**, 1100.
Clark P; Connolly P; Curtis A.S; Dow J.A; Wilkinson C.D. (1991) *J. Cell Sci.* **99**, 73.
Cleary E.G., Gibson M.A. (1996) in *Extracellular Matrix* vol 2 ed. Comper W.D. (Harwood Academic, Amsterdam) p. 95.
Cohn L.H. (1984) *Chest.* **85**, 387.
Comper W.D. (1996). in *Extracellular Matrix* vol 2 ed. Comper W.D. (Harwood Academic, Amsterdam) p. 1.
Curtis A.S.G. and Varde M. (1964) *J. Nat. Can. Inst.* **33**, 15.
Curtis A.S.G. and Wilkinson C.D. (1997) *Biomaterials* **18**, 1573.
Cheung D.T. and Nimini M.E. (1982) *Connect. Tiss. Res.* **10**, 187.
Cheung D.T. and Nimini M.E. (1982) *Connect. Tiss. Res.* **10**, 201.
Cheung D.T. and Nimini M.E. (1984) *Connect. Tiss. Res.* **13**, 109.
Chvapil M. (1977) *J. Biomed. Mater. Res.* **11**, 721.
Chvapil M. (1982) *J. Biomed. Mat. Res.* **16**, 245.
Dagalakis N., Flink J., Stasikelis P., Burke J.F. and Yannas I.V. (1980) *J. Biomed. Mater. Res.* **14**, 511.
Dickinson R.B; Guido S; Tranquillo R.T. (1994) *Ann. Biomed. Eng.* **22**, 342.
Doillon C.J., Silver F.H. and Berg R.A. (1987) *Biomaterials* **8**, 195.
Doolabh V.B., Hertl M.C. and Mackinnon S.E. (1996) *Rev. Neurol.* **7**, 47.
Eastwood M., McGrouther D.A. and Brown R.A. (1994) *Biochim. Biophys. Acta* **1201**, 186.
Eastwood M., Mudera V.C. McGrouther D.A., Brown R.A. (1998) *Cell Motility. Cytoskel.* **49**, 13.
Ehrich H.P. and Rajaratnan J.B. (1990) *Tissue Cell* **22**, 407.
Ejim O.S., Blunn G.W. and Brown R.A. (1993) *Biomaterials* **14**, 743.
Elsdale T. and Bard J. (1972) *J. Cell Biol.* **54**, 626.
Falanga V., Margolis D., Alvarez O., et al. (1998) *Arch. Dermatol.* **134**, 293.
Falcone P.A., Bonaventura M., Turner D.C. and Fromm D. (1984) *Plastic Reconstruct. Surg.* **74**, 809.
Favaro G., Bortolami M.C., Cereser S., Pastorello D.A., Callegrao L. and Fioi M.G. (1990) *Trans. Am. Soc. Artif. Intern. Organs* **36**, 291.
Ferrans V.J.,Hilbert S.L., Tomita Y., Jones M. and Roberts W. (1988) in *Collagen*, vol III, ed. Nimni M.E. (CRC Press Boca Raton) p. 1.
Fosang A.J., Hardingham T.E. (1996) in *Extracellular Matrix* vol 2, ed. Comper W.D. (Harwood Academic, Amsterdam) p. 200.
Fournier N. and Doillon C.J. (1996) *Biomaterials* **17**, 1659.
Frank C., Amiel D., Woo S.L.-Y. and Akeson W. (1985) *Clin. Orth. Rel. Res.* **196**, 15.
Freed L.E., Vunjak-Novakovic G., Biron R.J., et al. (1994) *Bio. Tech.* **12**, 689.
Frei V., Huc A. and Herbage D. (1994) *J. Biomed. Mater. Res.* **28**, 159.
Friman R., Giaccone G., Kanemoto T., Martin G.R., Gazdar A.F. and Mulshine J.L. (1990) *Proc. Natl. Acad. Sci. USA.* **87**, 6698.
Fujisato T., Sajiki T., Liu Q. and Ikada Y. (1996) *Biomaterials* **17**, 155.
Gelberman R., Goldberg V., An K.N. and Banes A. (1988) in *Injury and Repair of the Musculoskeletal Soft Tissues*, eds. Woo S.L.-Y. and Buckwalter J.A. (AAOS, Illinois) p. 5.
Gerlach L.C., Schnoy N., Vienken J., Smith M. and Neuhaus P. (1996) *Int. J. Artif. Organs* **19**, 610.
Grant I., O'Byrne A., Green C., Martin R. (1998) *Proc. Eur. Tissue Repair Soc.* p. 41.

Grinnell F. (1984) *J. Cell Biochem.* **26**, 107.
Grinnell F. (1994) *J. Cell Biol.* **124**, 401.
Guido S. and Tranquillo R.T. (1993) *J. Cell. Sci.* **105**, 317.
Hansbrough J.F., Cooper M.L., Cohen R. et al. (1992) *Surg.* **111**, 438.
Hanthamrongwit M., Reid W.H. and Grant M.H. (1996) *Biomaterials.* **17**, 775.
Hanthamrongwit M., Wilkinson R., Osborne C., Reid W.H. and Grant M.H. (1996) *J. Biomed. Mater. Res.* **30**, 331.
Hardingham T.E., Fosang A.J. (1992) *FASEB J.* **6**, 861.
Heijmen F.H., Pont J.S. du, Middlekoop E., Kreis R.W. and Hoekstra M.J. (1997) *Biomaterials* **18**, 749.
Heimbach D., Luterman A., Burke J., et al. (1988) *Ann. Surg.* **208**, 313.
Heldin C.H. and Westermark B. (1996) in *The Molecular and Cellular Biology of Wound Repair*, 2nd ed. ed. Clark R.A.F (Plenum Press, New York) p. 249.
Herschler J. (1992) *Ophthalmology* **99**, 666.
Hickey D.S. and Hukins D.W.L. (1980) *J. Anat.* **131**, 81.
Hobson M.I., Brown R.A., Green C.J. and Terenghi G. (1997) *Br. J. Hand Surg.* **50**, 125.
Hoppen H.J., Leenslag J.W., Penning A.J., Lei B. van der and Robinson P.H. (1990) *Biomaterials* **11**, 285.
Hukins D.W.L. (1982) in *Collagen in Health and Disease* eds. Weiss J.B. and Jayson M. (Churchill-Livingstone, Edinburgh) p. 49.
Hull B.E., Finley R.K. and Miller S.F. (1990) *Surg.* **107**, 496.
Ishihara T., Ferrans V.J., Jones M., Boyce S.W. and Roberts W.C. (1981) *Am. J. Cardiol.* **48**, 443.
Ishihara T., Ferrans V.J., Jones M., Boyce S.W. and Roberts W.C. (1981) *Am. J. Cardiol.* **48**, 665.
Jackson D.A. (1982) in *Collagen in Health and Disease* eds. Weiss J.B.and Jayson M. (Churchill-Livingstone, Edinburgh) p. 466.
Jerusalem C., Hess F. and Werner H. (1987) *Cell Tiss. Res.* **248**, 505.
Kim J.P, Zhang K, Chen J.D, Wynn K.C, Krammer R.H. and Woodley D.T. (1992) *J. Cell Physiol.* **151**, 443.
Koide M., Osaki K., Konishi J., et al. (1993) *J. Biomed. Mater. Res.* **27**, 79.
Kuettner K.E., Pauli B.U., Gali G., Memoli V.A., Schenk R.K. (1993) *J. Cell Biol.,* 743.
L'Heureux N., Paquet S., Labbe R., Germaine L. and Auger F.A. (1998) *FASEB J.* **12**, 47.
Langer R. and Vacanti J.P. (1993) *Science* **260**, 920.
Lanza R.P., Sullivan S.J. and Chick W.L. (1992) *Diabetes* **41**, 1503.
Laquerriere A., Yun J., Toillier I., Hemet J. and Tardie M. (1993) *J. Neurosurg.* **78**, 487.
Larsen N.E., Pollak C.T., Reiner K., Leshiner E. and Balazs E.A. (1993) *J. Biomed. Mater. Res.* **27**, 1129.
Laurent T.C, Fraser J.R.E. (1992) *FASEB J.* **6**, 2397.
Lefebvre F., Pilet P., Bonzon N., Daculsi G. and Rabaud M. (1996) *Biomaterials* **17**, 1813.
Levesque M.J. and Nerem R.M. (1985) *J. Biomech Eng.* **107**, 341.
Lundborg G. (1988) in *Nerve Injury and Repair* (Churchill Livingstone, Edinburgh) p. 149.
Luyn M.J. van, Wachem P.B. van et al. (1992) *J. Biomed. Mater. Res.* **26**, 1091.
Ma P.X. and Langer R. (1999) in *Tissue Engineering Methods and Protocols* eds. Margan J.R. and Yarmush M.L. (Humana Press, Totowa, NJ) p. 47.
Madri J.A. and Williams S.K. (1983) *J. Cell Biol.* **97**, 153.
Magilligan D.J., Oyama C., Klein S., Riddle J.M. and Smith D. (1984) *Am. J. Cardiol.* **53**, 945.

Maruguchi T., Maruguchi Y., Suzuki S., Matsuda K., Toda K. and Isshika N. (1994) *Plast. Reconstr. Surg.* **93**, 537.

Mast B.A., Flood L.C., Haynes J.H., et al. (1991) *Matrix* **11**, 63.

Matsuda K., Suzuki S., Isshika N. and Ikada Y. (1993) *Biomaterials* **14**, 1030.

Matsuda K., Suzuki S., Isshika N., Yoshioka K., Okada T. and Ikada Y. (1990) *Biomaterials* **11**, 351.

Matsuda K., Suzuki S., Isshika N., Yoshioka K., Wada R., Hyon S.R. and Ikada Y. (1992) *Biomaterials* **13**, 119.

McCarthy J.B., Iida J. and Furcht L.T. (1996) *in The Molecular and Cellular Biology of Wound Repair* 2nd ed., ed. Clark R.A.F. (Plenum Press, New York) p. 373..

Mignatti P., Rifkin D.B., Welgus H.G. and Parks W.C. (1996) in *The Molecular and Cell Biology of Wound Repair*, 2nd edition ed Clark R.A.F. (Plenum Press New York) p. 427.

Mooney D.J., Mazzoni C.L., Breuer C., et al. (1996) *Biomaterials* **17**, 115.

Morgon A., Disant F. and Truy E. (1989) *Acta Otolaryngol.* **107**, 450.

Murashita T. Nakayama Y., Hirano T. and Ohashi S. (1996) *Br. J. Plast. Surg.* **49**, 58.

Navsaria H.A.,Harris P.A., Philp B., Linge C., Sanders R., Green C. and Leigh I.M. (1998) *Wound Repair Regen.* **6**, A507.

Nehrer S., Breinan H.A., Ramappa A., et al. (1997) *Biomaterials* **18**, 769.

Nicolas F.L. and Gagnieu C.H. (1997) *Biomaterials* **18**, 815.

Nimni M.E. (1988) in *Collagen* vol. I ed. Nimni M.E. (CRC Press, Florida), p.1.

Nimni M.E., Cheung D.T., Strates B., Kodama M. and Sheikh K. (1988) in *Collagen*, vol III, ed. Nimni M.E. (CRC Press Boca Ratan) p. 1.

Noble P.M., Lake F.R., Henson P.M. and Riches D.W. (1993) *J. Clin. Invest.* **91**, 2368.

Noishiki Y., Yasuko T., Yamane Y. and Matsumoto A. (1996) *Nature Medicine* **2**, 90.

Noughton G., Mansbridge J. and Gentzkow G. (1997) *Artif. Organ.* **12**, 1203.

Oberpenning F., Meng J., Yoo J.J. and Atala A. (1999) *Nature Biotech.* **17**, 149.

Olde Damink L.H., Dijkstra P.J., Luyen M.J. van, Wachem P.B. van, Nieuwenhis P. and Feijen J. (1996) *Biomaterials* **17**, 765.

Otani Y., Tabata Y. and Ikada Y. (1996) *Biomaterials* **17**, 1387.

Oyer P.E., Stinson E.B., Miller D.C., Jamieson S.W., Mitchell R.S. and Shumway N.E. (1984) *Eur. Heart J.* **5**, 81.

Pachence J.M. (1996) *J. Biomed. Mater. Res.* **33**, 35.

Pandit A.S., Feldman D.S., Caulfield J. and Thompson A. (1998) *Growth Factor.* **15**, 113.

Porter R.A., Brown R.A., Eastwood M., Occleston N. and Khaw P. (1998) *Wound Repair Regen.* **6**, 157.

Prajapati R.T., Al-Ani S., Smith P.J. and Brown R.A. (1996) *Cell Eng.* **1**, 143.

Pulapura S. and Kohn J. (1992) *J. Biomater. Appl.* **6**, 216.

Putnam A.J. and Mooney D.J. (1996) *Nature Medicine* **2**, 824.

Rault I., Frei V., Herbage D., Abdul-Malak N. and Huc A. (1996) *J. Mater. Sci. Mater. Med.* **7**, 215.

Rheinwald J.G. and Green H. (1975) *Cell* **6**, 331.

Roy F., DeBlois C. and Doillon C.J. (1993) *J. Biomed. Mater. Res.* **27**, 389.

Sabbagh W., Masters J.R.W., Duffy P.G., Herbage D. and Brown R.A. (1998) *Br. J. Urol.* **82** (in press).

San-Galli F., Deminiere C., Guerin J. and Rabaud M. (1996) *Biomaterials* **17**, 1081.

Scott R., Gorham S.D., Aitcheson M., Bramwell P., Speakman J. and Meddings R.N. (1991) *Br. J. Urol.* **68**, 421.

Schor S.L., Schor A.M. (1987) *Bioessays*, **7**, 200.

Shepard A.D., Eldrup-Jorgensen J., Keough E.M. et al. (1986) *Surgery* **90**, 318.

Silver F.H. (1994) in *Biomaterials, Medical Devices and Tissue Engineering* (Chapman & Hall, London) p. 153.

Silver F.H. (1994) in *Biomaterials, Medical Devices and Tissue Engineering*. (Chapman Hall, London) p. 46.

Silver F.H., Wang M.C. and Pins G.D. (1995) *Biomaterials* **16**, 891.

Spray T.L. and Roberts W.C. (1977) *Am. J. Cardiol.* **44**, 319.

Steele J., Johnson G., McFarland C., et al. (1993) *J. Biomat. Sci.*

Stern R., McPherson M. Pharm D. and Longaker M.T. (1990) *J. Burn Care Rehabil.* **11**, 7.

Sterne G.D., Coulton G.R., Brown R.A., Green C.J. and Terenghi G. (1997) *J. Cell Biol.* **139**, 709.

Sterne G.D.,Brown R.A., Green C.J. and Terenghi G. (1997) *Eur. J. Neurosci.* **9**, 1388.

Sterne G.D.,Brown R.A., Green C.J. and Terenghi G. (1998) *J. Anat.* **193**, 273.

Steven F.S. (1967) *Biochim. Biophys. Acta.* **140**, 522.

Talas G. Brown R.A. and McCrontter D.A. (1999) *Biochem. Pharmacol.* **57**, 1085.

Taravel M.N. and Damard A. (1993) *Biomaterials* **14**, 930.

Taravel M.N. and Domard A. (1996) *Biomaterials* **17**, 451.

Tatarkiewicz K. (1995) *J. Cell Eng.* **1**, 39.

Thomas F.T. and Thomas J.M. (1997) in *Principles of Tissue Engineering* eds. Lanza R., Langer R. and Chick W. (R.G..Landes, Austin, Texas) p. 309.

Tinois E., Toillier J., Gaucherand M., et al. (1991) *Exp. Cell Res.* **193**, 310.

Toole B.P. (1991) in *Cell Biology of Extracellular Matrix* ed. Hay E.D., 2nd edition (Plenum Press, New York) p. 221.

Underwood S., Afoke A., Brown R.A., McLeod A.J. and Dunnill P. (1999) *Bioprocess Eng.* **20**, 239.

Urban J.P. (1994) *Br. J. Rheum.* **33**, 901.

Ushiki T., Chizuka I. (1990) *Cell Tiss. Res.* **260**, 175.

Vacanti C.A., Langer R., Schloo B. and Vacanti J.P. (1991) *J. Plast. Reconstr. Surg.* **88**, 753.

Vandenberg H.H. (1988) *In Vitro Cell. Devel. Biol.* **24**, 609.

Veis A., Bhatnagar R.S., Shuttleworth C.A. and Mussell S. (1970) *Biochim. Biophys. Acta.* **200**, 97.

Vries H.J.C. de, Middlekoop E., Mekkes J.R., Dutrieux R.P., Wildevuur C.H.R. and Westerhof W. (1994) *Wound Rep. Reg.* **2**, 37.

Wachem P.B. van, Luyen M.J. van and Costa M.L. da (1996) *J. Biomed. Mater. Res.* **30**, 353.

Wachem P.B. van, Luyen M.J. van, Olde Damink L.H., Dijkstra P.J., Feijen J. and Nieuwenhis P. (1994) *Int. J. Artif. Organs* **17**, 230.

Walbeehm E.T. and McGrouther D.A. (1995) *J. Hand Surg.* **20B**, 270.

Wang M.C., Pins G.D. and Silver F.H. (1994) *Biomaterials* **15**, 507.

West D.C., Hampson I.N., Arnold F., et al. (1985) *Science* **228**, 1324.

Whitworth I.H., Brown R.A., Dore C., Green C.J. and Terenghi G. (1995) *J. Hand Surg.* **20B**, 429.

Whitworth I.H., Brown R.A., Dore C., Green C.J. and Terenghi G. (1996) *J. Hand Surg.* **21B**, 514.

Whitworth I.H., Terenghi G., Green C.J., Brown R.A., Stevens E. and Tomlinson D.R. (1995) *Eur. J. Neurosci.* **7**, 2220.

Wilkins L.M., Watson S.R., Prosky S.J., Meunier S.F. and Parenteau N.L. (1994) *Biotechnol. Bioeng.* **43**, 747.

Woessner F. (1982) in *Collagen in Health and Disease* eds. Weiss J.B. and Jayson M. (Churchill Livingstone, Edinburgh). P. 506.

Wojciak-Stothard B, Denyer M, Mishra M, Brown R.A. (1997) *In Vitro Cell Devel. Biol.* **33**, 110.

Woo S.L.-Y. Maynard J., Butler D. et al. (1988) in *Injury and Repair of the Musculoskeletal Soft Tissues* eds. Woo S.L.-Y. and Buckwalter J.A. (AAOS., Park Ridge, Illinois) p. 133.

Woodhead-Galloway J. (1982) in *Collagen in Health and Disease* eds. Weiss J.B. and Jayson M (Churchill-Livingstone, Edinburgh) p. 28.

Yannas I.V. (1988) in *Collagen, Vol III, Biotechnology*, ed. Nimni M.E. (CRC Press, Boca Raton) p. 87.

Yannas I.V. (1990) *Angew. Chem. Int. Ed. Engl.* **29**, 20.

Yannas I.V. and Burke J.F. (1980) *J. Biomed. Mater. Res.* **14**, 65.

Yannas I.V. and Tobolsky A.V. (1967) *Nature* **215**, 509.

Yannas I.V., Burke J.F., Gordon P.L., Huang C. and Rubenstein R.H. (1980) *J. Biomed. Mater. Res.* **14**, 107.

Yannas I.V., Lee E., Orgill D.P., Skrabut E.M. and Murphy G.F. (1989) *Proc. Natl. Acad. Sci. USA* **86**, 933.

Chapter 6

Mechanical Characterisation of Tendons *in Vitro*

Chapter 6

Mechanical Characterisation of Tendons *in Vitro*

DAN BADER and HELIO SCHECHTMAN

6.1. GENERAL FEATURES OF TENDONS

Tendons are highly fibrous regular connective tissues, glistening white in appearance, in which the fibres are regularly orientated with respect to one another to form thicker bundles. Tendons connect muscles to structural elements such as bone. The form taken by a specific tendon depends on the contraction of the associated muscle, its orientation with respect to the relevant joint and often on the availability of the bony surface into which the tendon must insert. Thus, the proximal tendon of the human semimembranous muscle is a flat band-like structure, reflecting the shape of the short angle fibres of the muscle as it connects with the tendon (Herzog and Loitz 1994). Other tendons adopt the form of cords, for example the proximal tendon of the human biceps brachii muscle, and may be round, oval or elongated in cross-section. Tendons act as linking elements transmitting muscular pulls and external loads. They are highly resistant to extension but are relatively flexible, and can therefore be angulated around bone surfaces or deflected beneath retinacula to alter the direction of the muscular pull. In the situations, in which tendons pass over a bony prominence or turn through a digital sheath, they can be subjected to compressive loading. Thus local areas of tendon could contain fibrocartilage tissue.

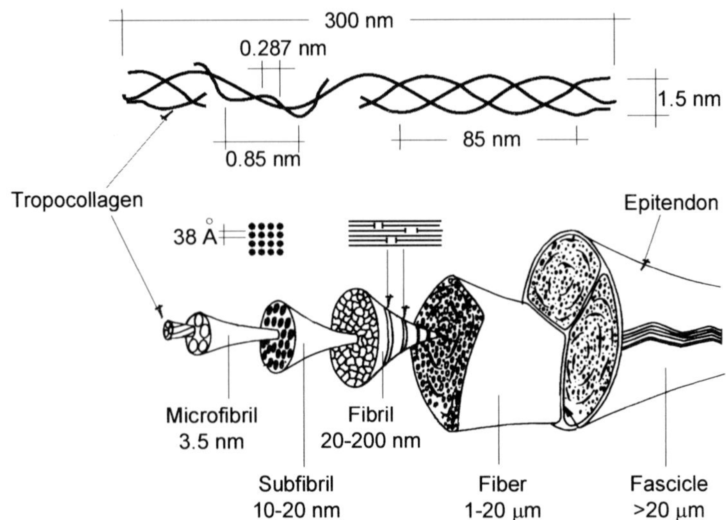

Fig. 6.1. Structural features of the collagen fibres in tendons (based on Kastelic and Baer 1980).

Tendons consist of fascicles of *collagen fibres* (see chapter 8) largely running parallel to the long axis of their structure, as indicated in Figure 6.1. Their surface is generally smooth, although longitudinal ridging due to the arrangement of coarse fasciculi is quite common in larger tendons. Bundles of collagen *fibrils* each 0.02 to 0.20 μm in diameter, assemble together into *fibres* with a diameter of between 1 and 20 μm. These fibres bundle together into the *fascicles*, within which the fibres are more or less longitudinally orientated and are bound by a small amount of an amorphous mucoprotein cement.

It is well established that the fibres demonstrate a planar crimping, of wavelength of between 100 to 300 μm. The areolar connective tissue which permeates the tendon between its fascicles provides a route for vessels and nerves. The blood supply of tendons is provided by a relatively sparse array of small arterioles, which run longitudinally from the adjacent muscular tissues. These arterioles ramify in the interfascicular spaces, where they intercommunicate freely and are accompanied by veins. The longitudinal network in the tendon is augmented by small vessels from the surrounding areolar connective tissue or, where present, the synovial sheets. The vascular networks are of low density, reflecting the minimal metabolic requirements of tendons.

The nerve supply of the larger tendons, such as the Achilles tendon, appears to be mainly afferent in nature, with no clear evidence of vasomotor control. Specialised afferent receptors, neurotendinous endings known as Golgi tendon organs, exist particularly near the myotendinous junction. Each is about 500μm long and 100 μm in diameter and consists of small bundles of tendon fibres enclosed in a delicate capsule. When tendons are stretched, these neurotendinous endings activate and initiate myotactic reflexes, which inhibit the development of excessive tension during muscular contraction.

6.2. STRUCTURE AND COMPOSITION

Tendons may be considered to be unidirectional fibre-reinforced composites. The building block of the fibrous phase consists of *tropocollagen molecules*, which reinforce a matrix made up of a *hydrated proteoglycan gel*. Tendon also contains the large glycoprotein, *fibronectin*. The presence of this molecule is important in the interaction between the tendon cells and the extracellular matrix, cell-to-cell adhesion and cell migration.

The tropocollagen molecule, 300 nm long and 1.5 nm wide, has a molecular weight of approximately 300,000 daltons. Its molecular form is ideally designed to support tensile loads, to which the structural composites are subjected. The mechanical integrity of the collagen is considerable due to the presence of both inter- and intra-molecular cross-links. Collagen, predominantly in the form of type 1, constitutes approximately 30 % of the wet weight of tendons and 80% of its dry weight. The collagen fibres may be considered to be largely independent, although stress can be transferred from one fibre to its neighbour by shear in the matrix or by more specific cross-links.

Single fascicles and groups of fascicles are surrounded by sheaths, termed the endotenon and peritenon respectively. The tendons are surrounded by some loose connective tissues, termed the epitendon (Figure 6.1) or paratendon, which comprises small collagen fibrils widely separated by cells and possibly small amounts of elastin. This structure functions as a sleeve to permit gliding of the tendon over extratendinous tissues as well as through synovial sheaths at the digits.

Four distinct zones have been identified at the insertion between tendon and bone. The fibrous tendon itself gradually changes to fibrocartilage, which is characterised by a higher concentration of proteoglycans and cartilage-like cells. It has been suggested that this region is important in ensuring that the tendon fibres do not bend, splay out or become compressed at a hard tissue interface and are therefore offered some protection (Benjamin et al. 1986). A calcified fibrocartilage layer is also present within the tendon insertion and is adjacent to the bone region.

There are at least two cell populations represented in the major anatomical compartments of tendon. The epitendon contains a large, polygonal to spherical cell, known as the *tendon epitenon synovial cell* (TSC). The TSC is embedded in a lipid and proteoglycan rich matrix containing only about 25% collagen. The internal portion of tendon contains *fibroblasts* (TIF), which are in tightly packed rows amidst linear and branching collagen fascicles and bundles (Banes et al. 1988). Both cell types will be subjected to a combination of shear stresses during gliding and tension as a result of muscle contraction. In general the cellular material occupies about 20% of the total tissue volume, with the remaining volume occupied by the extracellular matrix.

6.2.1 Clinical features and ageing

During ageing, changes occur in the composition of tendon. In particular the collagen content decreases with age, with an associated decrease in the mechanical strength, stiffness and ability to withstand deformation. Ageing of tendons is also characterised by a reduced ability to adapt to environmental stress and loss of tissue homeostasis.

The most common tissue injuries are lacerations, ruptures and tendinitis. These can result from two basic mechanisms. A single impact macro-trauma, such as a blow to a leg or a twisting injury of a joint, will injure bone, muscle, tendon, ligament, and even neurovascular elements. The other mechanism of injury is repetitive microtrauma caused by the repeated exposure of tissue to low magnitude force, which itself will not result in tissue injury (Micheli 1986). The number of overuse injuries is estimated to be about 30 to 50 % of all sports-related injuries in the U.S.A. (Jarvinen 1992). Tendon injuries are common examples of such injuries as, during physical activity, much of the force is focused on the tendon component of the muscle-tendon-bone unit. Thus rapid elongation of this unit with maximum uncoordinated muscle contraction may rupture healthy tendons.

The process of healing takes a form typical of connective tissues, involving phases of inflammation; proliferation and remodelling of newly formed extracellular matrix. Maintaining the blood supply to the tendon is critical to prevent necrosis of collagen. Another factor that affects the long-term success of healing, particularly in tendons of the hand, is the avoidance of adhesion between the repair site and the tendon sheath (Herzog and Loitz 1984). In addition, suturing the ends of the damaged tendon and controlled passive motion will facilitate tendon gliding during joint motion. However, adult tendons have a low metabolic rate and vascularity. Increasing intratendinous tension causes a decrease in blood perfusion. Due to persistent hypoxia, sections of the tendon may undergo fibrocartilaginous metaplasia (Uhthoff et al. 1976). In these cases, chondrocytes may mediate calcium deposition, which may proceed to the formation of discrete nodules within the tendons. This will inevitably alter the biomechanical properties of the whole tendon.

6.3. BIOMECHANICS OF TENDONS

6.3.1 Load Carriage

Tendons act as linking elements connecting muscles to bones, thus transmitting muscular pulls and external loads. In slow concentric activities, where the inertial effects may be neglected, the maximal load to which the tendon may be subjected is the muscle isometric tetanic contraction, approximately equal to 0.35N per square millimetre of muscle belly (Guyton 1986). As an example, the isometric stress in the patellar tendon can be estimated at 29 MPa, based on the cross-sectional areas of 125 mm^2 and 10,300 mm^2 for the tendon and the Quadriceps femoris muscle respectively. However, most daily activities consist of quick eccentric movements, where inertial effects play an important role. Experimental studies have indicated that these dynamic activities are associated with tendon stresses in the range of 42 to 110 MPa, the latter exceeding the established values of the ultimate tensile strength (Wahrenberg et al. 1978; Komi et al. 1992). However, in most cases human tendons are so thick that there is no possibility of rupture through one single application at the maximum load.

Normal healthy individuals are estimated to walk approximately 1 to 1.5 million strides per year (Wallbridge and Dowson 1982). During locomotion, the musculoskeletal system is subjected to a continuous and constant external load, the body weight. Movement is achieved by muscular contraction and the consequent production of torque around the joints of the lower limbs. Evidently, any specific muscle-tendon unit produces a cyclic force with a constant maximal value, which is proportional to the external load. Due to muscle tone, a small amount of tension is always present ensuring that the muscle-tendon units are taut even when the muscle is relaxed. Moreover, any possible slackening due to creep of the tendon would be eliminated by a reduction in the length of the muscle. Therefore, the *in vivo* repetitive loading pattern of tendons in the lower limbs may be broadly classified as a tension-tension square wave, as observed in the *in vivo* tensile load pattern in the Achilles tendon during various form of locomotion (Komi et al. 1992).

Tendon forces can be determined either directly or indirectly. The latter uses mathematical models based on kinetic and kinematic measurements (Crowsninshield and Brandt 1981; Morrison 1970). However optimisation schemes are necessary to solve these indeterminate problems and validation of the methods remains a question. Direct measurement of tendon forces involves the use of force sensors, often in the form of buckle transducers (An et al. 1990; Barry and Ahmed 1986; Komi 1990). The frame and crossbar arrangement of the buckle transducer is woven through the tissue structures. However due to its positioning on the tendon surface, it is vulnerable to impingement from surrounding soft tissues and bone. More recently an implantable force transducer has been described (Xu et al. 1992; Korvick et al. 1996). This device consists of a curved beam strain-gauged on both sides, which is implanted into the mid-substance of a tendon. The maximum force recorded when the device was positioned in the patellar tendon of a goat was equivalent to one-third of its ultimate failure load, corresponding to a period of trotting. The shape of the tendon force was very similar to that recorded for the ground reaction force. The results suggested that the patellar tendon functions in both the toe-in and initial linear regions of its stress-strain curve (Korvick et al. 1996).

6.3.2 *In vitro studies – Experimental problems*

The load bearing function of tendons has prompted a plethora of biomechanical studies. In particular, uniaxial tensile testing of animal and human tendons has been performed over many decades. Examples of seminal studies and review papers include (Rigby et al. 1959; Abrahams 1967; Benedict et al. 1968; Kastelic and Baer 1980; Haut 1983; Butler et al. 1984; Stouffer et al. 1985; Baer et al. 1988).

The model most commonly employed is that of the *rat-tail tendon* (RTT). The overall mechanism of deformation of the RTT involves the gradual straightening of the initially crimped collagen fibrils followed by fibril extension in the elastic region and then shear-slip and ultimate rupture. The stress-strain curves of RTT as a function of age (Kastelic and Baer 1980), capture the overall deformation process; a small toe-in region followed by a linear region, up to 2% depending on age, and then permanent yield. In mature tendon, two distinct yield regions are found representing possibly two damage processes. In young animals, only a single yield region is seen which can extend to a strain of 17% (Kastelic and Baer 1980). The presence of water affects dramatically the shape of the stress-strain curve and four distinct hydration regimes have been identified (Baer et al. 1988).

However, the mechanical testing of human soft tissues, such as tendons and muscles is fraught with practical difficulties involving gripping the specimen, the measurement of cross-sectional area and the degree of hydration during both specimen preparation and testing. These issues have been examined in a comprehensive thesis involving a large number of human tendons from a variety of sources (Schechtman 1995). All the specimens were obtained from routine post-mortem examinations, with preparation and storage detailed in a previous publication (Schechtman and Bader 1994). This storage procedure, involving freezing the specimens in self-sealing plastic bags, has been shown to have minimal effects on the mechanical properties of biological tissues (Viidik and Lewin 1966).

6.3.2.1 Clamping the specimens. Ensuring a firm grip is certainly one of the major issues in testing specific soft tissues which, unlike ligaments, are devoid of bony attachments. A firm grip is a function of an optimum matching of the clamping device and the specimen. Freezing the ends of some animal tendons, with a large aspect ratio and relatively uniform cross-sectional area, has proved a successful gripping arrangement. For other tendons, several designs of clamping devices have been reported in the literature ranging from the use of serrated jaws to drill-chucks (Pradas and Calleja 1990; Schwerdt et al. 1980; Minns et al. 1973; Haut and Little 1972; Partington and Wood 1963). It follows that no definitive clamping device exists, and the precise details of the experiment will determine the optimum matching conditions.

The design incorporating clamps, which tighten during a tensile test, has been reported by several authors (Butler et al. 1984; Woo 1982; Schechtman and Bader 1994). The latter authors designed a set of special self-tightening clamps, which employed pairs of wedges with sandblasted, ridged, flat gripping surfaces. They conducted a preliminary investigation to assess the optimum arrangement, which ensured that specimens were gripped without subsequent damage during any tensile testing procedure. This required a minimum specimen length of 20mm to be inserted into each clamp and a torque of 10 Nm applied to the locking screws.

Tendon specimens were tested in a Universal screw-driven testing machine (Instron Ltd., UK, model 6025), equipped with a load cell (2518-204 / 1 kN). The length of the specimen between the clamps, defined as the *free-length* region, was measured at the first non-zero load registered by the load cell. The crosshead speed was chosen to provide a strain rate of 0.01 s^{-1}. The tests were conducted until the specimens, which were constantly kept moist by spraying with buffered Ringer's solution at room temperature, exhibited gross macroscopic failure. The maximum load and extension to failure, as measured from the grip-to grip separation, were recorded and values of ultimate tensile strength (UTS) and its corresponding strain were calculated.

Tests were performed on a series of human tendon specimens. The influence of the free-length of the specimen was examined with respect to the failure strain (Figure 6.2). A threshold value of 35 mm could be defined for the free-length region of the specimen. Specimens with a value above the threshold demonstrated a mean strain of 10.6 $\pm$ 3.0 %, while below the threshold values of 17.8 $\pm$ 9.2 % were recorded, the difference was statistically significant at the 5 per cent level. In addition, the variability associated with the shorter specimens was considerably greater. These results suggest

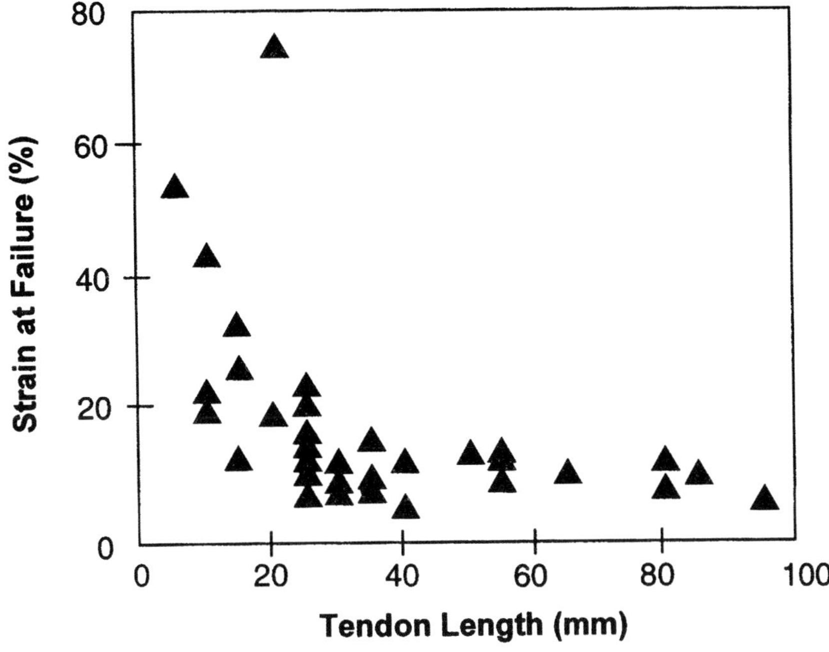

Fig. 6.2. The failure strain of human tendons as a function of their free length

that with short specimens, the effects of stress concentrations arising at the clamps and possible specimen slippage can not be ignored. Similar findings have been reported (Haut 1986). In a similar manner data indicated that there was a maximum limit for cross-sectional area, typically 10 mm^2. The grips could not provide efficient load transfer for large area specimens, thereby producing abnormally high failure strains. This precluded the use of whole human tendons with relatively large cross-sectional areas such as the Achilles, Patellar and Quadriceps Femoris tendons.

6.3.2.2 Effects of hydration. Thawing and testing of tendons is usually conducted in a moist environment that simulates the physiological conditions, such as osmotic pressure and pH. However, it has been reported that the tensile strength decreases reversibly by 5%/0.1pH unit on either side of pH 7.5 (Elden 1968). Moreover, the environmental conditions may also affect the physical dimensions, such as has been observed with respect to water absorption by tendons.

The issue of hydration was investigated by the authors (Schechtman 1995). Intact tendons from the Extensor Digitorum Longus of the human foot were either *immersed* in a beaker containing buffered Ringer's solution or kept *moist* by wrapping in paper towels soaked in the same solution. The change of weight was monitored over a period

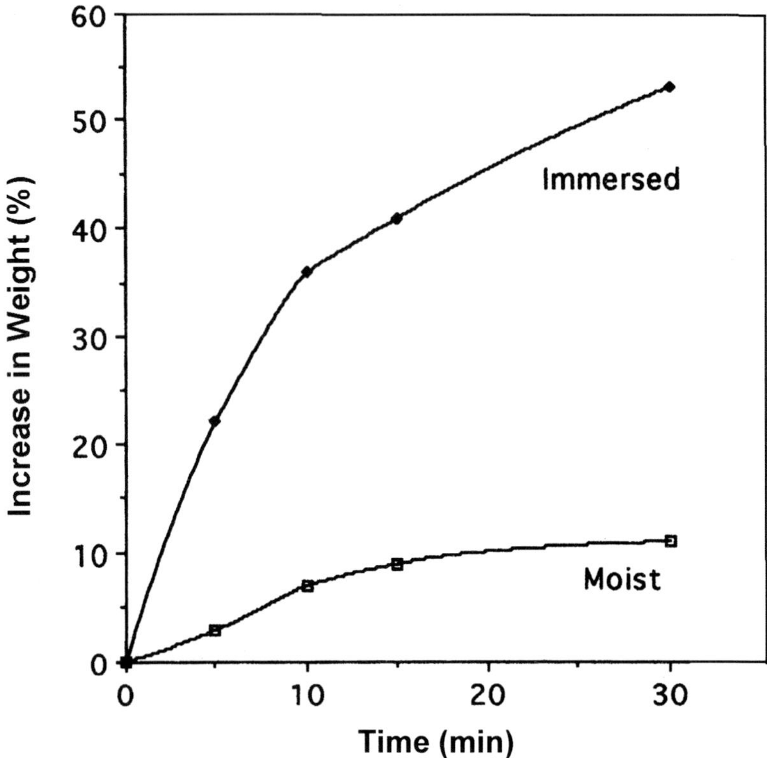

Fig. 6.3. Increase in weight due to absorption of Ringer's solution as a function of time

of 30 minutes. The results, as illustrated in Figure 6.3, revealed a large difference in fluid uptake between the two environments. There was a total increase in weight of over 50% when specimens were immersed in solution, compared to a value of approximately 12% for the moist specimens.

In separate study using thick irregular-shaped thick tendons, such as the human Achilles tendon, longitudinal sections were obtained by cutting in between tendon fascicles with a knife with parallel blades separated by a gap of 1.5 mm. This produced specimens with a cross-sectional area small enough to be adequately gripped during a tensile test. However results were even more dramatic with these *cut* specimens than was observed with *intact* specimens. For example, weight increases of over 60% were achieved within 10 minutes of full immersion in solution. The cut tendons also exhibited a considerably reduced tensile strength compared to the equivalent intact tendon specimens. Thus it was concluded that only *intact tendon specimens* should be used and kept moist by wrapping in paper towels soaked in buffered Ringer's solution, to ensure minimal dimensional swelling.

6.3.2.3 Cross-sectional area measurements. A firm grip assures that the tensile load is transferred to all the potential load bearing components within the specimen. The calculation of the tensile stress, however, is also a function of the cross-sectional area of this load bearing collagenous components. Correct measurement of the load-bearing elements is, thus, critical. The literature reveals several measurement techniques for cross-sectional area, the most popular of which involves wet gravimetric methodology (Bennett et al. 1986; Mathews and Ellis 1968; Ellis 1969; Abrahams 1967). However, these authors have alluded to the problems associated with this technique. Ellis (1969) compared the performance of several techniques on the area of cat tendon specimens. Results indicated that a local measurement, using an area micrometer, produced repeatable values, which were approximately 40% lower than the values using gravimetric procedures.

A similar design to that described by Ellis (1969) was used by the authors. The area micrometer consisted of interchangeable slots of known dimensions and a plunger connected to a micrometer head. The cross-sectional area was calculated from the product of the width of the slot and the distance of the plunger from the slot base. In a separate investigation, the cross-sectional area of the specimens was measured locally, using a slot 3 mm wide and 5 mm thick. The pressure applied by the plunger on the specimen was in the range of 97 kPa to 133 kPa. The accuracy and reproducibility of this method was estimated to be approximately ± 2% (Schechtman and Bader 1994).

Human tendons were measured both globally using a standard gravimetric protocol and locally, every 5 mm along its length, using the area micrometer. A further examination involved dehydration of the specimen and measuring the cross-sectional area using the area micrometer. The results of the three methods are presented in Figure 6.4. The cross-sectional area value was 4.7 mm^2 for the moist gravimetry procedure and the average value by the area micrometer was 2.79 ± 0.62 mm^2 for the moist tendon, with a minimum value of 1.74 mm^2. These values are equivalent to 60% and 37% of the average value estimated by the wet gravimetric technique. These significant differences will inevitably affect the estimated values of the ultimate tensile strength, as the specimen would be expected to fail at its minimum cross-section area. In addition, the dehydrated tendon yielded a mean area of 1.03 ± 0.28 mm^2 and a minimum value of 0.55 mm^2. Comparison of the area profiles of the moist and the dehydrated tendon clearly indicate similar trends (Figure 6.4). Thus the minimum cross-sectional area occurred in both cases at a position approximately 50 mm from one end of the specimen. Therefore, it could be argued that the local variation in cross-sectional area of the intact tendon specimen was due to the load bearing elements with no obvious local variation in liquid uptake.

6.3.2.4 Strain measurements. Strain measurements in tendons are clearly important in estimating their material properties in healthy and repairing states. However, the physical nature of the specimens generally precludes the use of contacting measurement sensors, which will influence the loading response of the tendons. In the simplest case, a gross estimate of specimen strain may be determined from the displacement of the crosshead of the loading system, termed the *grip-to-grip displacement*. In order to measure local strains, previous studies have proposed optical

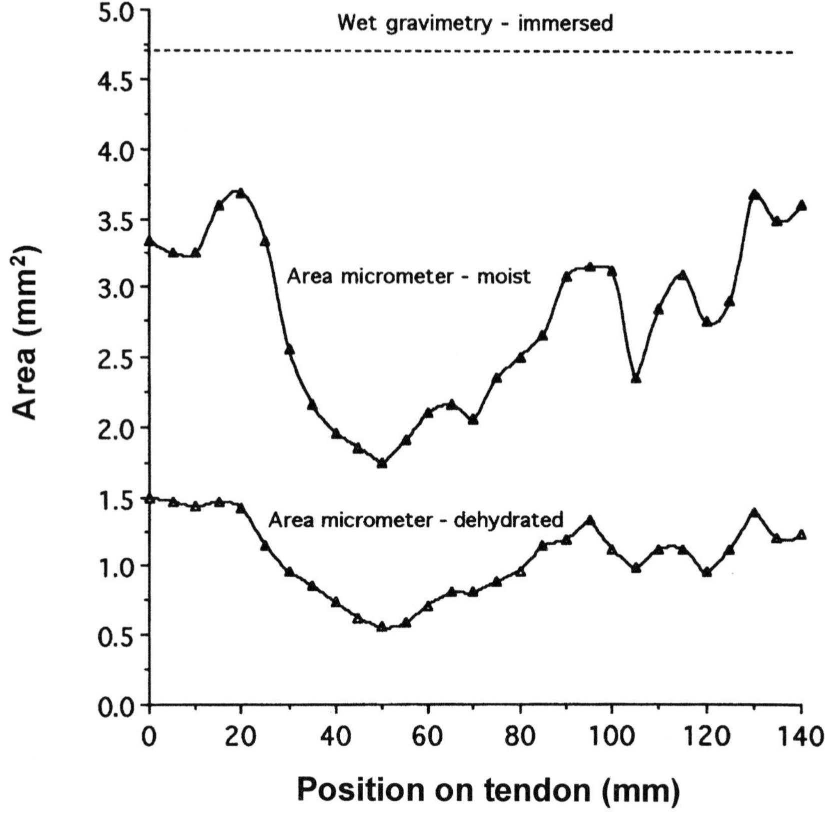

Fig. 6.4. Estimation of cross-sectional area for tendon specimen in various states of hydration.

techniques to track markers on the surface of the tendon, during the loading regimens. This has involved the use of high-speed cameras (Butler et al. 1984), a video dimensional analyser (Woo et al. 1976) and a video-based analysis system (Smutz et al. 1996). The latter report determined the accuracy of the system, which has the potential for measuring strain in three dimensions and the ability to estimate the strain field on the surfaces of the soft tissue specimens. None of these techniques, however, provide any information at the microstructural level of tendon and certainly do not provide information on the local molecular changes in tendons subjected to applied loading.

When using intact human tendons, which can not be cut and shaped into dumbell specimens, it is very difficult to monitor local strains about the point of fracture. Therefore, many authors still employ the grip-to-grip displacement to estimate global strains within the specimens up to fracture.

6.3.2.5 Establishing test conditions. Considering the problems associated with aforementioned factors, specific recommendations have been defined for the testing of human tendons, as detailed in Table 6.1. These were employed by the authors in all subsequent tests.

Table 6.1. Recommended specimen dimensions and conditions for the static and dynamic mechanical testing of human tendons (based on Schechtman 1995).

Intact tendon specimens
Tendon specimens with a relatively uniform cross-sectional area smaller than 10 mm^2 and a minimum grip-to-grip length of 35 mm. The foot tendons, extensor hallucis longus (EHL) and extensor digitorum longus (EDL) were suitable.
Specimens need to be kept moist by wrapping them in paper towels soaked in buffered Ringer's solution, prior to testing
Cross-sectional area measurements using the area micrometer. The thinnest section of the free-length region was used in subsequent stress calculations.
Applied clamping torque of 10 Nm.
Strain estimated from the grip-to-grip displacement

6.3.3 Static testing

The authors tested to failure a range of human tendons, namely 12 EDL and 12 EHL from the foot, at an equivalent strain rate of 0.01 s^{-1} using the conditions and methods cited in Table 6.1. From the resulting relationship between force and grip-to-grip displacement, values of the ultimate tensile strength (UTS) and failure strain were calculated, based on the original minimum area of the free length region and its length, respectively.

A typical stress-strain curve for the EDL, as presented in Figure 6.5, demonstrates non-linear behaviour. The initial region of the curve, the toe-in region, is characterised by a small increase in stress with increasing strain, up to a value of approximately 20 MPa. A linear region, with an approximately constant modulus of elasticity follows the toe-in region. A third region, the failure region, is typified by a well-defined maximum value followed by a sharp decrease in stress. A tangent modulus was estimated from the linear region of the stress-strain relationship.

The results indicated mean ultimate tensile strengths (UTS) of 99.9 ± 12.2 MPa and 87.1 ± 12.5 MPa, for the EDL and EHL tendons respectively. The corresponding failure strains were 15.3 ± 2.6 % and 17.6 ± 4.2 %. The mean tangent modulus values (E) were 1135 ± 222 MPa and 932 ± 197 MPa respectively. The statistical analysis indicated that both the UTS and the tangent modulus for two tendon types were significantly different at the 5 per cent level, while their failure strains were not significantly different ($p=0.13$).

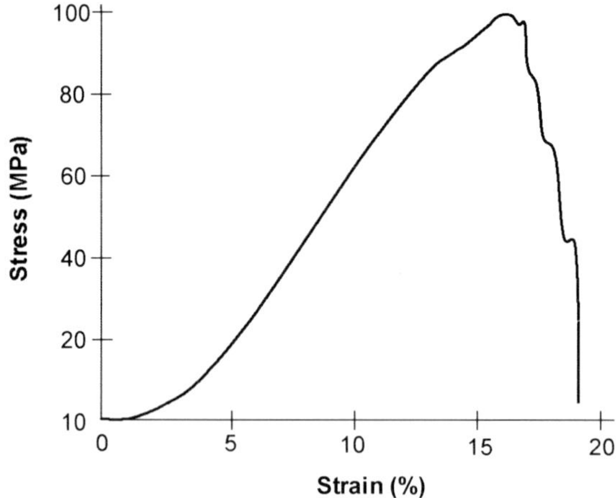

Fig. 6.5. Typical stress-strain behaviour of an EDL tendon when subjected to uniaxial tension at a rate of 0.01% s^{-1} (based on Schechtman and Bader 1997).

6.3.4 Dynamic testing

Cyclic loads can induce resonance in a system if the frequency of the load is similar to its natural frequency. Resonance is characterised by a dramatic increase in the amplitude of the induced displacement which is, however, absent if the system possesses hysteresis energy losses. Consequently, tendons must present hysteresis energy losses, although they must not be too large or the metabolic cost of any activity would be prohibitive.

The viscoelastic behaviour of the whole musculoskeletal system has been studied via its various components. The myotendinous complex has been investigated, generally, in terms of the compliance and stiffness and the response of the neural receptors (Baratta and Solomonow 1991; Proseke and Morgan 1987; Rack et al. 1983). The viscoelastic behaviour of tendons greatly influences the mechanical response of the musculoskeletal system to applied loads. Therefore, its characterisation in terms of the dynamic modulus and its components is of physiological importance.

Several studies have investigated the viscoelastic behaviour of tendons using a variety of techniques. For example, Mason (1965) investigated the viscoelastic behaviour of rat tail tendon by the wave attenuation method with strain, in the range of 1% to 3%, as the independent variable at a frequency of 20 kHz. H.Schwerdt et al (1980) studied the response of the human flexor digitorum tendons of the hands to sinusoidal cyclic loads at frequencies up to 9.5 Hz, with strains in the range of 0.5% to 5% as the independent variable. Bennett and colleagues (1986) measured the elastic modulus of several mammalian tendons by calculating the slope of a tangent to hysteresis loops at frequencies in the range of 0.2 Hz to 11 Hz. The mechanical properties of human palmaris longus tendons of the hands and the extensor hallucis longus tendons of the feet were also investigated (Hubbard and Soutas-Little 1984). Their results showed that the elastic modulus, as measured by the tangent to a hysteresis loop, was strain rate dependent but independent of the age of the specimens. More recently, the elastic modulus of both wallaby and tiger tail tendons have been examined

(Wang et al. 1991). The measured modulus, as obtained from the slope of the tangent to hysteresis loops at a frequency of 1.1 Hz, was found to be independent of temperature over the range 20 °C to 41 °C.

In a separate study, the present authors examined the dynamic characterisation of seven human EDL and EHL tendons using the method of force oscillations and dedicated software on a hydraulic testing machine (MTS Systems Co., USA, model Elastomer 830). Specimens were subjected to cyclic tension-tension loads at frequencies in the physiological range of 1 to 4 Hz. The static load was set at equivalent values corresponding to prescribed levels between 10% and 80% of the calculated UTS, approximately 100 MPa. For all test conditions, the dynamic amplitude load was set at an equivalence of 5% of the UTS.

Figure 6.6 illustrates the effects of static stress on the mean values of the dynamic tensile modulus, K*, at a frequency of 1 Hz. It can be seen that modulus increased monotonically in the range of 10 % to 60 % of the UTS, reaching a peak value of approximately 1.8 GPa. There was a small increase in the dynamic modulus with frequency, although it was insignificant when compared to the increase due to mean static stress. At each frequency a second order polynomial expression was fitted through the estimated values for K*. The polynomial model in Figure 6.6 produced a high correlation coefficient.

A similar trend was also observed for the storage modulus, K', the real component of K*, with peak values of 1.8 GPa occurring at a stress level of 60 % the UTS. By contrast, the loss modulus, K'', the imaginary component of K*, was less than 8 % of the value of the storage modulus. There was little obvious trend in loss modulus values with respect to mean static stress. However, close examination of the frequency data revealed a small increase in loss modulus, from 37 MPa at 1 Hz to 50 MPa at 2-4 Hz.

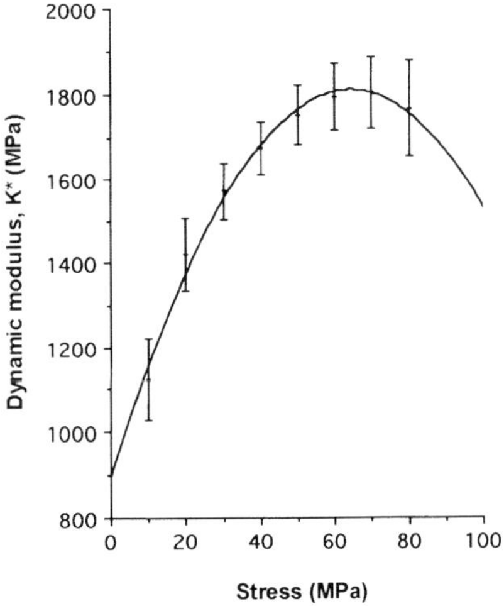

Fig. 6.6. The response of dynamic tensile modulus versus mean static stress for a human tendon at 1 Hz.
$y = 897.5 + 28.47\,x - 0.22\,x^2$; r= 0.99

A statistical analysis indicated no differences between the major viscoelastic parameters estimated for any of the seven human tendon specimens. Indeed, the variability between specimens was significantly less than that due to static stress levels.

The influence of various input factors on the dynamic viscoelastic properties of tendons can be summarised in association with related studies in Table 6.2. In all cases, there was an increase in modulus values with imposed stress or strain. The values of dynamic tensile and storage tensile modulii were largely independent of frequency. The apparent small increase in these parameters with frequency, could be explained in terms of the strain rate dependence of viscoelastic tendons (Hubbard and Soutas-Little 1984; Van-Brocklin and Ellis 1965; Abrahams 1967).

Table 6.2. Comparative results of the dynamic behaviour of tendons

Source	Procedure	Control variable	Frequency	D. Modulus
Mason (1965)*	Wave attenuation	Strain 1%-3%	20kHz	1-3 GPa
Schwerdt et al. (1980)**	Forced oscillations	train 0.5%-5%	0.5–9.5 Hz	0.3–4 GPa
Bennett et al. (1986)***	Hysteresis loops	Stress 30-70 MPa	0.2–11 Hz	1.5 GPa
Schechtman and Bader (1994)****	Forced oscillations	Stress 10-80% UTS	1–4 Hz	1–2GPa

* Rat tail tendon
** Flexor Digitorum in the human hand
*** Average for several mammalian tendons
**** Extensor Digitorum Longus and Extensor Hallucis Longus in the human foot

In any viscoelastic system, the energy loss is a function of the loss modulus, the frequency and the strain. In the particular case of tendons, the hysteresis energy losses would be independent of the mean static stress, but dependent on the dynamic amplitude. The effect of frequency is, however, complex due to the interdependence of strain rate and frequency in the methodology employing a sinusoidal form of loading. In the physiological situation the reported small increase in the loss modulus from 1 Hz to 2 Hz, may be important in optimising the performance of tendons. At low frequencies associated with normal walking, the energy losses should be small to ensure a low metabolic cost. At higher frequencies, associated with vigorous activities or impact loading, the energy loss must be relatively high in order to protect the musculoskeletal system regardless of the metabolic cost.

A comparison of the estimated mechanical parameters for tendon must take into account the loading history. The tangent modulus estimated from the static tensile test is solely a function of loading the tendon specimens. The dynamic modulus, however, is derived from both loading and unloading the tendon specimens by small amplitudes at different stress levels. The loading phase presents a behaviour similar to that observed in the static test. The unloading phase, however, represents a limited elastic recovery of the fibres from a stressed state. In view of energy considerations for the viscoelastic tendon, the gradient of the unloading phase will necessarily be greater than that from the loading phase. Thus the absolute value of the dynamic modulus, K*, will always be greater than the corresponding static tangent modulus. The changes in dynamic modulus as a function of the static stress (Figure 6.6) can be explained in terms of the relative contributions of the gradients of both the loading and unloading phases. Up to 20 % UTS, both gradients will increase resulting in a net increase in dynamic modulus. Between 20 % and 60 % UTS, the gradient of the loading phase remains constant, as evidenced by the linear region in Figure 6.5, while the gradient of the unloading phase will increase resulting in a net increase in dynamic modulus. Beyond this region, the reduction in gradient of the loading phase produces a small net decrease in dynamic modulus.

The polynomial model (Figure 6.6) extrapolates below the minimum tested level of 10 % UTS, to predict a finite value of tangent modulus, approximately 0.9 MPa, at infinitesimally small stress levels. This model, however, is based on the properties of the collagen fibres alone and does not take into account their structural organisation. Thus the model would need to be modified to take into account the crimped nature of the collagen fibres in their unloaded state, as well as the influence of the associated ground substance.

The adopted procedures for dynamic characterisation provide a non-invasive measure of both the mechanical integrity of human tendons and some important viscoelastic parameters.

6.3.4.1 Fatigue testing. The practical problems associated with soft tissue testing, which are particularly critical in long term cyclic testing, has limited the number of fatigue studies (Wang et al. 1995; Weightman et al. 1978). The former study investigated the fatigue behaviour of wallaby tail tendons under sinusoidal loading. Such tendons are ideal specimens for investigation as they present a large aspect ratio, with a length often exceeding 400 mm and a relatively uniform cross-sectional area. Results indicated a series of linear relationships between the logarithm of fatigue life and the peak tensile stress, at loading frequencies ranging from 1.1 Hz to 50 Hz (Wang et al. 1995). This dependence on loading frequency may be a direct result of the use of sinusoidal loading, which will introduce a change in the loading rate of the specimen with frequency. In the fatigue tests, rupture occurred at shorter times than would be predicted from creep failure alone as demonstrated by the same researchers (Wang and Ker 1995).

A recent study by the authors has addressed the *in vitro* fatigue behaviour of human tendons (Schechtman and Bader 1997). Specimens prepared from EDL tendons from a variety of donors were subjected to a cyclic square tension-tension stress waveform at physiological frequencies. Ten specimens were tested at each of the nine prescribed maximum stress levels of between 10% and 90% of the UTS. The minimum stress level was set at 1% UTS. This protocol allowed the use of statistical models for the distribution of fatigue life.

All specimens failed in the free-length region between the grips. Examination of the fatigued tendon specimens revealed some disruption of the fibres and clear evidence of fraying, caused by inter- and intra-fibrillar friction as the fibres slid past one another during failure (Schechtman and Bader 1997). The mean values for the failure strain of the 90 specimens was 14.2 $\pm$ 5.6 %. There was no statistical difference between the failure strains at each of the nine different stress levels.

There was considerable variation in fatigue life at each stress level. For example, at 40% of the UTS the fatigue life ranged from 1,137 to 39,547 cycles. As a consequence, a linear model based on the median value, equivalent to a 50 % probability of failure, or survival, was employed as illustrated in Figure 6.7. The relationship between stress and the median fatigue life produced a statistically significant linear model of the following form:

$$S = 101.25 - 14.83 \log (N) \qquad (6.1)$$

where S is the stress normalised to the percentage of the UTS and N is the number of cycles to failure. This model predicted a static strength of 101.3 MPa, which was clearly within one standard deviation of the experimental data obtained in the quasi-static tensile tests. The linear model also suggested the absence of an endurance limit.

The probability of failure at each stress level was found to be adequately described by both the log-normal and the Weibull statistical distributions. However, these distributions differ substantially in their hazard functions, i.e. the probability of failure as a function of time (Lawless 1982). The log-normal predicts zero probability of

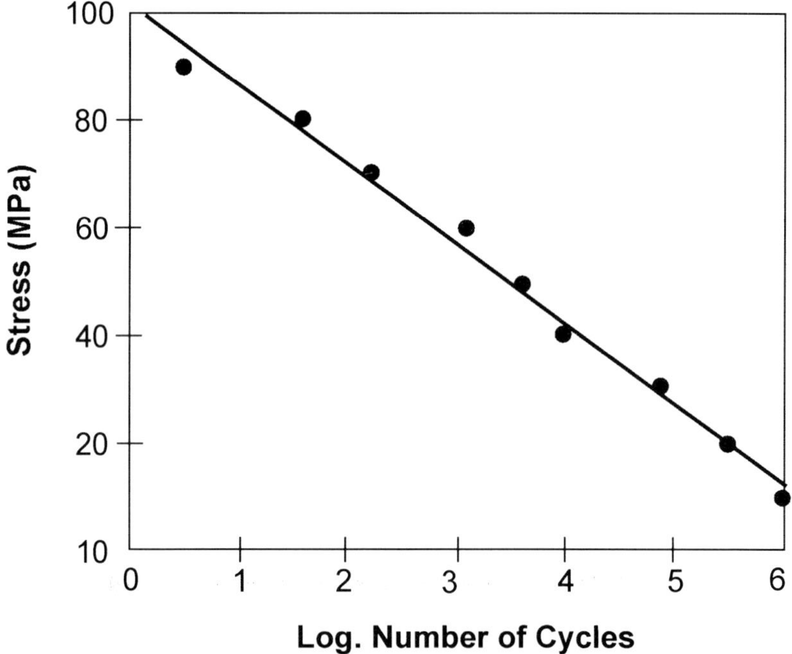

Fig. 6.7. Normalised stress versus logarithm of number of cycles to macroscopic failure. Each value represents the median of 10 human tendon specimens.

failure at extremes of time, with the maximum probability occurring at some intermediate value of time. However, the Weibull distribution generally presents a hazard function, which increases monotonically with time. Therefore, the log-normal would predict an endurance limit, whilst the Weibull distribution implies the absence of such a limit. Although the model did not predict an endurance limit, no fatigue experiment was performed below a stress level of 10% of the UTS.

The fatigue life of tendons *in vivo* will depend upon the stresses to which they are subjected. At a stress level of 20 % of the UTS, the fatigue life based on the *in vitro* linear model for the 50 % probability of failure was of the order of 300,000 cycles. This value is equivalent to a period of about three months of normal walking activity. However, such an *in vitro* assessment could not take into account the *in vivo* processes of healing and remodelling. Consequently, a modified approach was required to predict these combined processes *in vivo* to explain the presence of intact tendons throughout the majority of the population.

A cumulative damage model for metallic structures was first proposed by J. Palmgren (1924) and validated experimentally by M. Miner (1945). The cumulative damage model was extended to self-healing living structures and presented by C. Nash (1966), in the following form:

$$D(t) = D_S(t) + D_A(t) + D_D(t) - H(t) \tag{6.2}$$

where $D_s(t)$ is the damage associated with mechanical stressing, which in fatigue is described by the Miner-Palmgren model. $D_A(t)$ is the damage associated with ageing, $D_D(t)$ is the damage associated with disease and $H(t)$ is the damage repaired by healing. These factors are inter-related. Damage associated with ageing would depend upon the prior *in vivo* loading history. This term was not accounted for in the present experiment, which, for practical reasons, largely employed tendons specimens derived from relatively aged donors (Schechtman and Bader 1997). In addition, both ageing and disease will inevitably produce structural changes, which will affect the mechanical behaviour of tendon specimens and their repair potential. The terms associated with ageing and disease can be neglected if the mechanical stressing upon a healthy structure spans over a short period of time, as was simulated in the study.

The self-healing model was simplified to:

$$D(t) = \sum \left\{ \frac{n_i}{N_i} \right\} - H(t) \tag{6.3}$$

where $D(t)$ is the cumulative damage index. This parameter ranges from a value of *0*, representing the undamaged state prior to mechanical fatigue, to *1*, the state of failure due to fatigue. Such a model was adapted to describe the behaviour of compact bone (Carter and Caler 1985). The term $\sum\{n_i/N_i\}$ is the stress related damage, where n_i and N_i are the number of cycles at a stress level of S_i and the number of cycles to failure at that same stress level respectively.

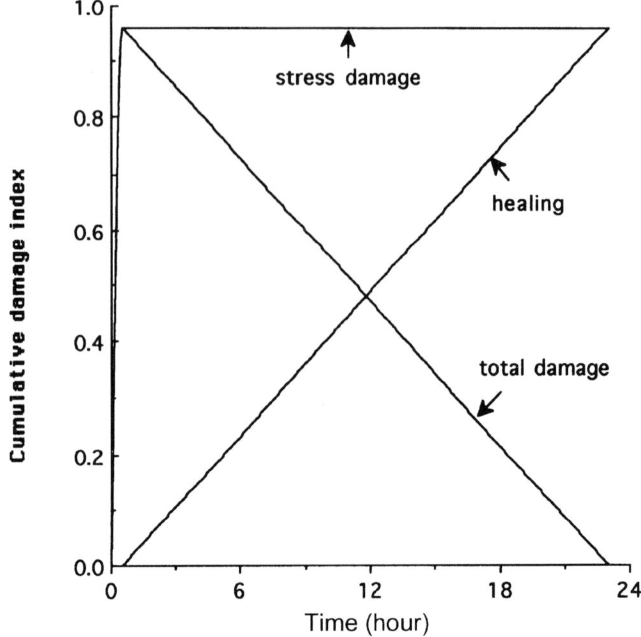

Fig. 6.8. *In vivo* model of stress related damage and associated healing for human tendons (based on Schechtman and Bader 1997).

A graphical depiction of this model, illustrated in Figure 6.8, involving stress related damage and healing, was proposed by H.Schechtman and D. Bader (1997). They employed a healing rate of 1 % per day based on previous experimental data (Noyes 1977; Hayashi 1996; Woo et al. 1987). This rate was found to be sufficient to eliminate, in less than 24 hours, any fatigue damage on a tendon subjected to a stress of 20 MPa during daily normal locomotion. Therefore the self-healing, or *in vivo*, model would predict that accumulated damage might occur if either the number of load cycles were increased at the same stress level or the stress level was increased. It is clear that the healing mechanism could be responsible for reducing the damage rate at high stress levels and establishing an endurance limit at low stress levels.

The practical implications of the data could be illustrated using an example of an athlete, who might be required to double their normal daily mileage prior to an event. In this case, after a month the accumulated damage would amount to 30 % and overuse injuries might occur. Alternatively, this accumulated damage can be considered to be equal to 30 % of the fatigue life, estimated at approximately 94,000 cycles at 20 % of the UTS. This value lies only above the lowest individual value recorded for the fatigue life at this stress level (Schechtman and Bader 1997). Therefore, a conservative estimate of probability of failure (Johnson 1964), would lead to approximately 7 % of the population presenting with fatigue failure of tendons after this number of cycles.

6.3.4.2 ***Partial fatigue testing.*** The authors extended their investigation on human tendons *in vitro*, by examining the effects of partial fatigue on specific mechanical parameters, which have been detailed in the previous sections. Specimens prepared from 12 intact EDL tendons of the foot were subjected to partial fatigue, equivalent to 25% of the median fatigue life, namely 78, 513 cycles (Figure 6.7). A cyclic square tension-tension stress waveform was employed at a physiological frequency of 4 Hz. The maximum stress was set at 20 MPa, which is equivalent to 20% of the UTS. This value was based on estimated values in the literature (Carlstedt and Nordin 1980; Ker et al. 1988). The minimum stress was set at 1 % UTS. Dynamic characterisation was performed at stress levels of 10% and 20% of the UTS prior to and following partial mechanical fatigue, in a similar manner to that described in section 6.3.4 of this chapter. Subsequent quasi-static tests were performed on a selection of tendons.

Damage was expressed as the ratio of a specific mechanical parameter measured after the partial fatigue process divided by the corresponding value prior to it. Hence, in the case of dynamic parameters this was simply the ratio of the values estimated from characterisation experiments. By contrast, the damage ratios of the static tensile parameters were the ratios of the values estimated from the tensile test to failure after partial fatigue divided by the group values of the EDL tendon, as quoted in section 6.3.3.

After partial fatigue, the value of the dynamic modulus, K*, was largely determined by the value of the storage modulus, K'. Values ranged from 516 MPa to 1187 MPa and 782 MPa and 1549 MPa at stress levels of 10% and 20% of the UTS, respectively. The individual damage ratios and mean values for K* are presented in Table 6.3.

Table 6.3. Damage ratios of selected mechanical parameters

	K* (10% UTS)	K* (20% UTS)	UTS	TM
1	0.87	0.91	–	–
2	0.84	0.93	–	–
3	0.48	0.58	0.29	0.49
4	0.87	0.91	0.59	1.04
5	0.85	0.89	–	–
6	0.92	0.96	–	–
7	0.93	0.94	0.64	1.01
8	0.61	0.78	0.39	0.61
9	0.79	0.90	–	–
10	0.64	0.79	0.39	0.62
11	0.98	0.98	0.54	0.92
12	0.97	0.97	0.61	1.05
Mean	0.81	0.88	0.49	0.82
SD	0.16	0.11	0.14	0.24

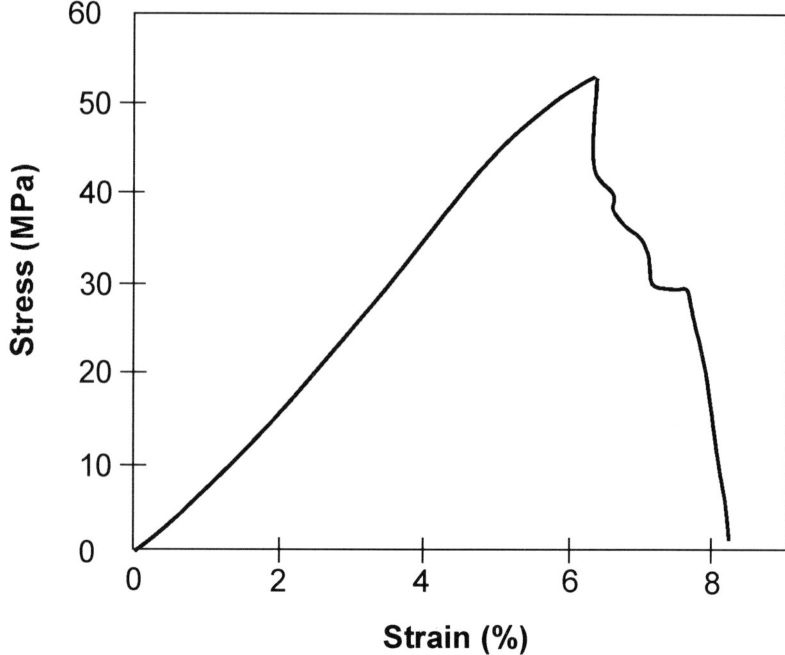

Fig. 6.9. Typical stress-strain behaviour of an EDL tendon, which has been previously subjected to partial fatigue in a cyclic tension-tension stress waveform at a frequency of 4 Hz.

Although the damage ratios were generally greater at the higher stress level, the differences were not statistically significant at the 5 per cent level. A similar finding was observed with the damage ratios for both the storage and loss modulii.

A typical stress-strain curve obtained in the quasi-static tensile testing of one partially fatigued tendon is presented in Figure 6.9. The stress-strain relationship appears to be non-linear in form, similar to that obtained for non-fatigued specimens (Figure 6.5), with a short toe-in region followed by an approximately linear region demonstrating a constant tangent modulus and finally a failure region.

The associated damage ratios for UTS and tangent modulus (TM) are also presented in Table 6.3. It is clear that the range of damage ratios of the UTS was lower than the corresponding range of the other static and dynamic parameters, the differences being statistically significant at the 5 per cent level. No statistically significant differences were observed when comparing results for the dynamic, storage, loss or tangent modulii.The relationship between the damage ratios for the dynamic modulus at 10% UTS and for both the tangent modulus and the UTS are presented in Figure 6.10. Linear models are demonstrated for both graphs, each resulting in a statistically significant correlation coefficients at the 1 per cent level.

Microscopic examination of the partially fatigued tendons, which were not tested to failure, revealed well aligned fibres forming, in general, an organised microstructure. This contrasts with the previous observations of fully fatigued specimens.

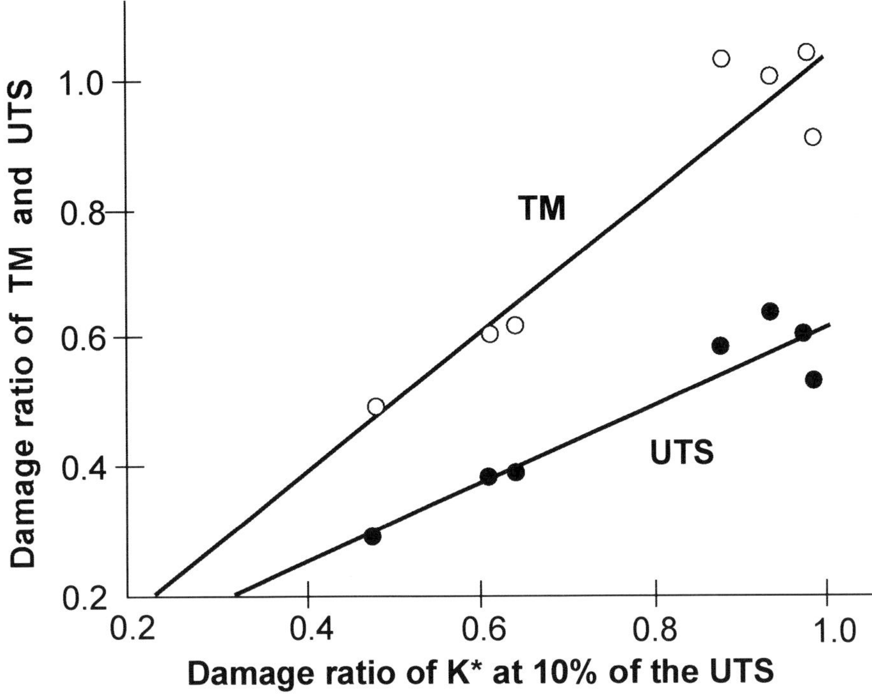

Fig. 6.10. Influence of partial fatigue on the relationship between the damage ratios of the dynamic modulus at a stress level of 10% of the UTS and the tangent modulus (TM) and the ultimate tensile strength (UTS)

For TM, $y = -0.057 + 1.121x$; $r=0.96$, $p<0.01$

For UTS, $y = -0.003 + 0.633x$; $r= 0.95$, $p< 0.01$

The damage ratio, by definition, ranges from 0 to 1 in a linear relationship to the cumulative damage index. From the test protocol, with a cumulative damage index of 0.25, the corresponding damage ratios would be expected to be of the order of 0.75. Indeed, for all the mechanical parameters, with the exception of the UTS, the mean damage ratios were close to this value, ranging from 0.81 to 0.93 (Table 6.3). By comparison, the mean damage ratio of the UTS was 0.49, suggesting damage in excess of that which would be produced by fatigue alone.

Comparative analysis of the damage ratios of static and dynamic mechanical parameters suggested the use of the damage ratio for dynamic tensile modulus as a good indicator of damage inflicted by mechanical fatigue. Such a measurement, using wave attenuation methodology, could be used to assess the integrity of tendons, particularly in those subjects presenting with symptoms at the clinic.

6.4. TENDON REPAIR STRATEGIES

Tendons, like ligaments, will remodel in response to the mechanical demands placed upon them (Hayashi 1996). This manifests itself as an increase in strength and stiffness when subjected to enhanced activity levels such as during physical training. By contrast, reducing the stress below normal levels, such as by stress shielding or immobilisation would produce a decrease in strength and stiffness of the tendons.

As has previously been discussed tendons are not well vascularised nor well innervated, therefore, the healing response is limited. Much effort has been directed in understanding the mechanisms associated with the stimulation of tendon healing. One such study has investigated the potential for mechanical stimulation in conjunction with growth factors to stimulate tendon cell activity in vitro (Banes et al. 1995). They reported the application of load using a commercial strain unit (Flexercell, Flexcell Intl. Corp., Mckeesport, USA), in which cells were attached to a collagen substrate at the base of culture plates. Negative pressure was applied in a cyclic manner, to provide deflection of the base of the plate. Results highlighted the complex mechanisms involved in the mechanical control of cell division and maintenance of matrix in tissue required to resist high tensile strains.

In a recent study, mesenchymal stem cells have been used within a biomaterial implant inserted into partial and full-thickness gap defects of rabbit tendons (Butler et al. 1998). This procedure produced accelerated tendon repair, as measured both in biomechanical and histological terms. Such a tissue engineering approach needs further development if a tendon is to repair sufficiently to exhibit a normal structure-function relationship.

6.5. FINAL COMMENTS

This chapter highlights the problems associated with the biomechanical testing of human tendons, particularly involving dynamic properties measured over a prolonged testing period. Specific test conditions have been established to examine the *in vitro* behaviour of selected tendons, such as those found in the human foot, with appropriate physical dimensions. A series of *in vitro* tests have been described and have resulted in the estimation of both static and dynamic parameters which could be used in a design template. In addition, models also needed to be developed to account for the predicted healing behaviour *in vivo*. However biomechanical studies are still required to examine other tendons, such as the human Achilles tendon and tendons of the elbow and shoulder, which are of great interest to the clinician due to their susceptibility to damage during a range of physical activities.

Acknowledgements

The authors gratefully acknowledge the support of the Brazilian Government (CAPES/MEC) and of the Department of Morbid Anatomy of the Royal London Hospital.

REFERENCES

Abrahams M. (1967) *Med. Biol. Eng.*, **5**, 433.

An K-N., Berglund L., Cooney W.P., Cho E.Y.S. and Kovacevic N. (1990) *J. Biomechanics*, **23**, 1269-1271.

Baer E., Cassidy J.J. and Hiltner A. (1988) in *Collagen: Biotechnology* Vol. 2, ed. Nimni M (CRC Press, Florida) p. 177.

Banes A.J., et al. (1988) *J. Orthopaedic Res.*, **6**, 83.

Banes A.J., Tsuzaki M., Hu P., Brigman B., Brown T., Almekinders L., Lawrence W.T., Fischer T. (1995) *J. Biomechanics*, **28**, 1505.

Baratta R. and Solomonow M. (1991) *J. Biomechanics*, **24**, 109.

Barry D. and Ahmed M.A. (1986) *J. Biomech. Eng.*, **108**, 149.

Benedict J.V., Walker L.B. and Harris E.H. (1968) *J. Biomechanics*, **1**, 53.

Benjamin M., Evans E.J. and Copp L. (1986) *J. Anatomy*, **49**, 89.

Bennett M.B., Ker R.F., Dimery N.J. and McNeil-Alexander R. (1986) *J. Zool London (A)*, **209**, 537.

Butler D.L., Grood E.S., Noyes F.R., Zernicke R.F.and Brackett K. (1984) *J. Biomechanics*, **17**, 579.

Butler D.L., Awad H., Young R., Boivin G.P., Smith F., Fink D. and Caplan A. (1998) in *Proceedings of the Third World Congress of Biomechanics* (Sapporo, Japan) p. 126.

Carlstedt C. A. and Nordin M. (1980) in *Biomechanics of Tissues and Structures of Musculoskeletal System* ed. Nordin M. and Frankel V.H (Lea and Febiger, London) p. 59.

Carter, D.R. and Caler, W.E. (1985) *Journal of Orthopaedic Research*, **3**, 84.

Crowsninshield R.D. and Brandt R.A. (1981) *J. Biomechanics*, **145**, 793.

Elden, H.R. (1964) *Biochimica et Biophysica Acta*, **79**, 592.

Elden, H.R. (1968) *Int. Rev. Connect. Tissue Res.*, **4**, 283.

Ellis D.G. (1969) *J. Biomechanics*, 2, 175.

Guyton A.C. (1986) *Textbook of Medical Physiology*, 7th Ed. WB Saunders Co. Philadelphia.

Haut R.C. (1983) *Journal of Biomechanical Engineering*, **105**, 296.

Haut R.C. (1986) *J. Biomechanics*, **19**, 951.

Haut R.C. and Little R.W. (1972) *J. Biomechanics*, **5** , 423.

Hayashi K. (1996) *J. Biomechanics*, 29, 707.

Herzog W. and Loitz B. (1984) in *Biomechanics of the Musculoskeletal System* ed. Nigg B.M. and Herzog W. (Wiley. Chichester) p. 133.

Hubbard R.P. and Soutas-Little R.W. (1984) *J. Biomech. Eng.*, **106**, 144.

Järvinen M. (1992) *Sports Med.*, **11**, 493.

Johnson L.G. (1964) *The Statistical Treatment of Fatigue Experiments*, Elsevier. London.

Kastelic, J. and Baer, E. (1980) in Soc. Exp. Biol., Symp. XXXIV, p. 397.

Ker R.F., McNeil-Alexander R. and Bennett M.B. (1988) *J. Zool. Lond.*, **216**, 309.

Komi P.V., Fukashiro S.and Järvinen M. (1992) *Clin. Sports Med.*, **11**, 521.

Komi, P.V. (1990) *J. Biomechanics*, **23** Suppl. 1, 23.

Korvick D.L., Cummings J.F., Grood E.S., Holden J.P., Feder S.M. and Butler D.L. (1996) *J. Biomechanics*, **29**, 557.

Lawless J.F. (1982) *Statistical Models and Methods for Lifetime Data*, John Wiley and Sons. New York.

Mason P. (1965) *Kolloid Z. Z. Polymere*, **202**, 139.

Matthews L.S. and Ellis D. (1968) *J. Biomechanics*, **1** , 65.

Micheli L.J. (1986) *Acta Med. Scand.*, suppl. **711**, 171.

Miner M.A. (1945) *J. Applied Mech. (ASME Trans.)*, **67**, A159.
Minns R.J., Soden P.D.and Jackson, D.S. (1973) *J. Biomechanics*, **6**, 153.
Morrison J.B. (1970) *J. Biomechanics*, **3**,51.
Nash C.D. (1966) ASME Publication 66-WA/BHF-3, *Fatigue of Self-healing Structure: A Generalized Theory of Fatigue Failure*, ASME - American Society of Mechanical Engineers, New York.
Noyes F.R. (1977) *Clin. Orthop. Rel. Res.*, **123**, 210.
Palmgren A. (1924) *Z. Ver. Dt. Ing.* **68**, 339.
Partington F.R. and Wood G.C. (1963) *Biochimica et Biophysica Acta*, **69**, 485.
Pradas, M.M. and Calleja, R.D. (1990) *J. Biomechanics*, **23**, 773.
Proske U. and Morgan D.L. (1987) *J. Biomechanics*, **20**, 75.
Rack P.M.H., Ross H.F., Thilmann A.F. and Walters D.K.W. (1983) *J. Physiol.*, **344**, 503.
Rigby, B., Hirai, N., Spikes, J. and Eryring, H. (1959) *Journal of General Physiology*, **43**, 265.
Schechtman H. and Bader D.L. (1994) *Eng in Medicine*, **208**, 241.
Schechtman H. and Bader D.L. (1997) *J. Biomechanics*, **30**, 829.
Schechtman H. (1995) Ph.D. Thesis, University of London, London.
Schwerdt H., Constantinesco A. and Chambron J. (1980) *J. Biomechanics*, **13**, 913.
Smutz W.P., Drexler M., Berglund L.J., Growney E. and An K. (1996) *J. Biomechanics*, **29**, 813.
Stouffer D.C., Butler D.L. and Hosny D. (1985) *J. Biomech. Eng.*, **107**, 158.
Uhthoff H.K., Sarkar K. and Maynard J.A. (1976) *Clin.Orthop. Relat.Res.*, **118**, 164.
Van Brocklin J.D. and Ellis D.G. (1965) *Arch. Phys. Med. Rehab.*, **46**, 369.
Viidik, A. and Lewin, T. (1966) *Acta Orthop. Scand.*, **37**, 141.
Wahrenberg H., Lindbeck L. and Ekholm J. (1978) *Scand. J. Rehab. Med.*, **10**, 99.
Wallbridge N. and Dowson D. (1982) *Eng. in Medicine*, **11**, 95.
Wang, X.T. and Ker, R.F. (1995) *Journal of Experimental Biology*, **198**, 831.
Wang X.T., Ker R.F. and McNeil-Alexander R. (1995) *Journal of Experimental Biology*, **198**, 847.
Wang X.T., De Ruijter M.R., McNeil-Alexander R. and Ker R.F. (1991) *J. Zool.*, **223**, 491.
Weightman B., Chappell D.J. and Jenkins E.A. (1978) *Ann. Rheum. Dis.*, **37**, 58.
Woo S.L-Y., Gomez M.A., Sites T.J., Newton P.O., Orlando C.A. and Akeson W.H. (1987) *J. Bone Joint Surg.*, **69**(A), 1200.
Woo S.L-Y. (1982) *Biorheology*, **19**, 385.
Woo, S. L-Y., Akeson, W.H. and Jemmott, G.F. (1976) *Journal of Biomechanics*, **9**, 785.
Woo S.L-Y., Orlando C.A., Camp J.F. and Akeson W.H. (1986) *J. Biomechanics*, **19**, 399.
Xu W.S., Butler D.L., Stouffer D.C., Grood E.S.. and Glos, D.L.(1992) *J. Biomech. Eng.*, **114**, 170.

Chapter 7

Biomimicking Materials with Smart Polymers

Chapter 7

Biomimicking Materials with Smart Polymers

TORIBIO FERNANDEZ-OTERO

7.1. INTRODUCTION

Organs in living creatures are structured on the basis of assembling organic and inorganic materials embedded in aqueous solutions of salts and organic compounds. The availability to nature of pristine chemical compounds to build, through a multistepped evolution, the necessary structural components was very limited: inorganic salts, small organic compounds, CO_2 and energy (light or heat). The way chosen by nature to overcome the problem was to develop a multitude of catalyzed reactions: *enzymatic processes*. A great number of these occur simultaneously in different parts of every small living cell of any multicellular being. The great chemical effort of synthesis from strictly limited number of original chemicals was balanced by a property (unavailable from industrial materials) of the final materials: *multifunctionality*. The resulting components are, at the same time, structural materials, sensors, actuators; they are able to accommodate to new conditions (physical or chemical) and are able to self-repair (Jeronimidis and Atkins 1995). Figure 7.1 summarizes these facts, indicating that the same biological molecule can generate, by changing structures or shapes, materials having different functions.

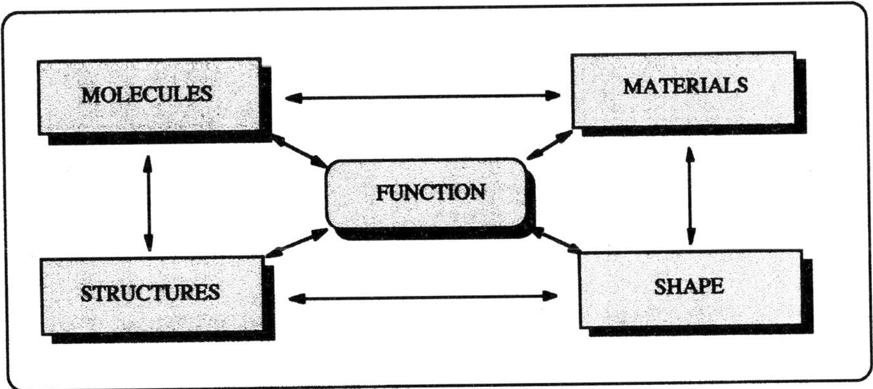

Fig. 7.1. In biology, a defined molecule yields material where different shape or different structure determine different functions, e.g. collagen in tendons, muscles or corneal tissues.

Table 7.1. Some important differences between biological materials and industrial materials

BIOLOGICAL MATERIALS	INDUSTRIAL MATERIALS
Non-homogeneous	Homogeneous
Variable composition	Constant composition
Non-isotropic	Isotropic
Non-linear properties	Linear properties (prevail)
Soft and wet	Hard and dry
Multifunctional	Monofunctional
Self-repairing	Protected against degradation
Intelligent (smart)	Passive functions

In spite of the great effort developed by chemists, biochemists and engineers to develop stereosynthesis of organic compounds and new catalysts, human technology nowadays is only able to reproduce (bioduplicate) a few of the living processes of synthesis (Viney 1993). Some differences between biological materials and industrial materials, related to the topics of this chapter, are collected in Table 7.1.

7.1.1 Biomimicking

By tradition, biomimetic materials are considered as those artificial materials (at least the processing step) the microstructure of which copies that of the natural materials. This leads to the concept of biomaterials as those materials that are used to repair bones, tendons, arteries, valves, ball-and-sockets joints, etc. Hard, pure and dry traditional materials such as metals and metallic alloys, ceramics and polymers are being used once their biocompatibility has been demonstrated.

A crucial fact attracts our attention: only those biological materials with passive functions and low water content are being mimicked. Nevertheless if we consider biomimicking as taking inspiration from nature to obtain ideas and transfer them into different technological or scientific fields, we become much more attracted by active organs, devices and functions. Natural devices like muscles, brain, nerves, electric organs, eyes, glands, etc, excite our imagination, challenging our knowledge about materials and materials properties and applications. These organs and devices are constituted by soft, wet and complex components: water, biological polymers, small organic components and inorganic salts: a long way from the traditional industrial materials (Scheme 7.1).

BIOLOGICAL MATERIALS
ARE

SOFT WET

COMPLEX INTELLIGENT

CONDUCTING POLYMERS ARE NON-STOICHIOMETRIC COMPOUNDS

WHICH COMPOSITION OF COUNTERIONS

CAN CHANGE FROM 0% TO 50%

ELECTROCHEMICAL METHODS
ALLOW

SMALL, CONTINUOUS AND REVERSIBLE

CONTROL OF THE COMPOSITION

Scheme 7.1. Most important differences between biological and industrial materials. Conducting polymers, non-stoiquiometry and electrochemical control of either, composition and any related property.

Materials containing water are particularly avoided by engineers and materials scientists when developing new devices and new technologies. This chapter is focused on those aspects and related questions: Is it possible to develop, use and control soft wet and complex materials bearing such a multifunctionality that they can biomimic active biological functions?

Those aspects will be considered and studied in relation to intrinsically conducting polyconjugated polymers. A short introduction about such soft and complex materials, their synthesis and properties when in aqueous solutions is required.

7.2. CONDUCTING POLYMERS

Intrinsically conducting polymers are materials able to allow an electron flow along the polymeric chain: they are monodimensional conductors at a molecular level. This name is applied to different kind of polymeric materials: polyconjujated, metal-polymers, some charge-transfer complexes having at least a polymeric component, etc. In this chapter we will focus on polyconjugated base materials, which are constituted by families of different basic components: polyacetylene, polyaniline, polypyrrole, polythiophene, polyphenylvynilene, etc (figure 7.2).

7.2.1 Electrosynthesis

The flow of an anodic current through a solution containing the monomer, an electrolyte and a solvent promotes the formation of a polymeric film on the metallic electrode. The film can be peeled from the electrode for suitable applications and studies. The materials can be also generated in homogeneous media using a redox couple. The material is then collected as a powder.

Both chemical and electrochemical synthesis are fast ways, through complex mechanisms, to obtain mixed materials (Otero 1999 and references therein). Different simultaneous reactions were detected and studied during electrosynthesis:

1. Electrochemical polymerization

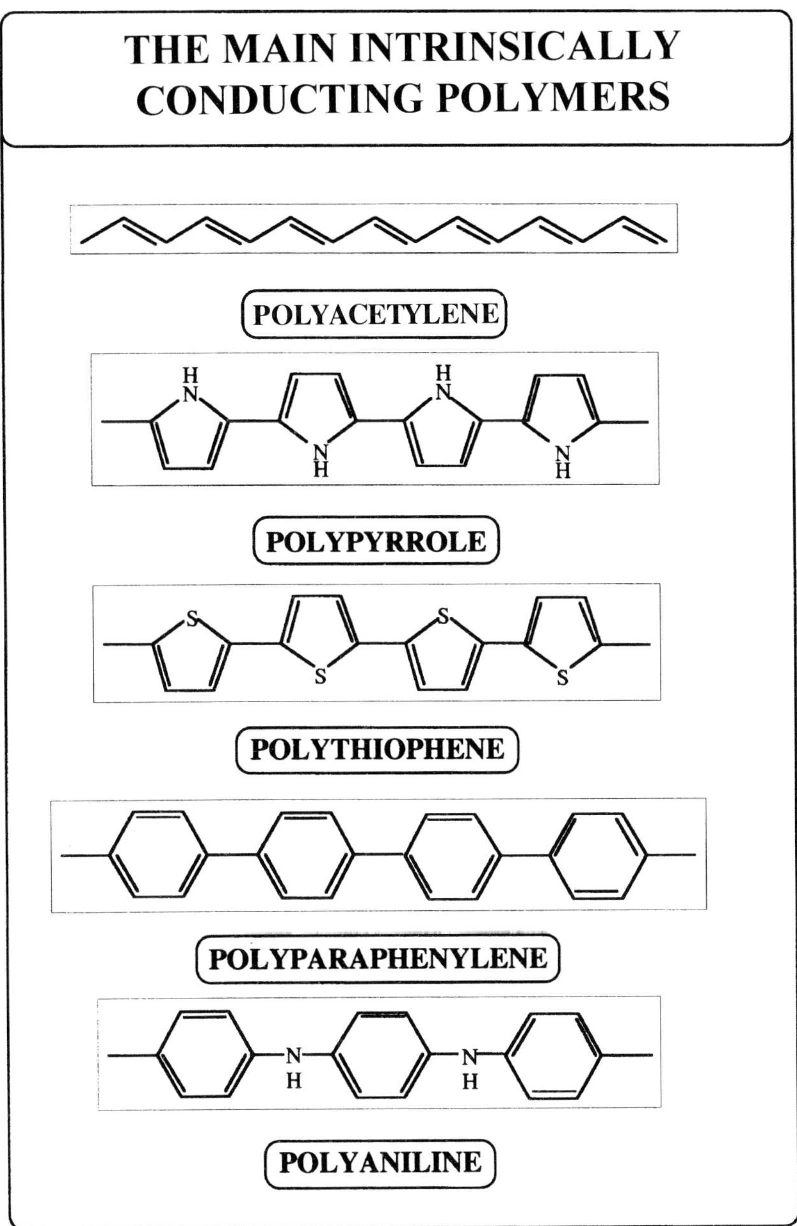

Fig. 7.2. Some of the most usual chains of conducting polymers (monodimensional, non-crosslinked and non-degraded, that means theoretical)

1. Polymeric oxidation

$$(pPy)_s + (n\,ClO_4^-)_{aq} + mH_2O \leftarrow\rightarrow [\,pPy^{n+}(ClO_4^-)_n(H_2O)_m\,]_{gel} + (\,ne^-\,)_{metal}$$

1. Chemical polymerization

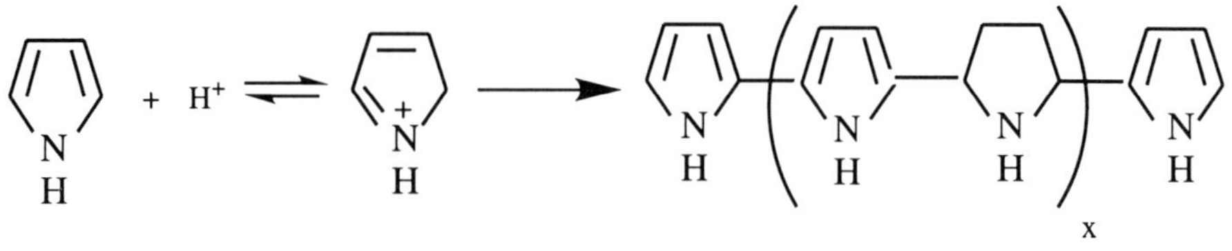

+ H^+

x

1. Polymeric degradation

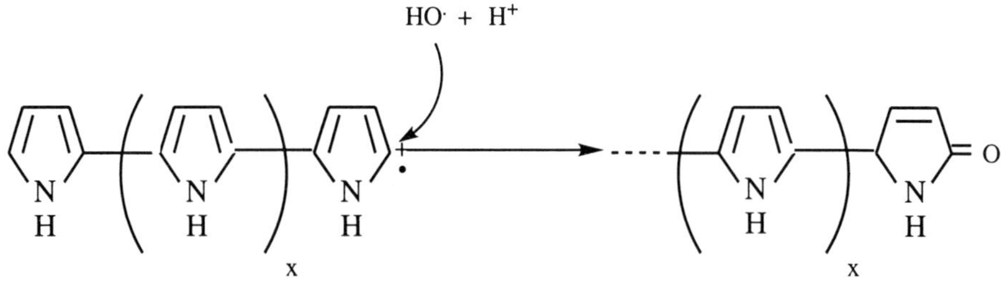

$HO^{\cdot}$ + H^+

x

x

O

5. Cross-linking of the polymeric network

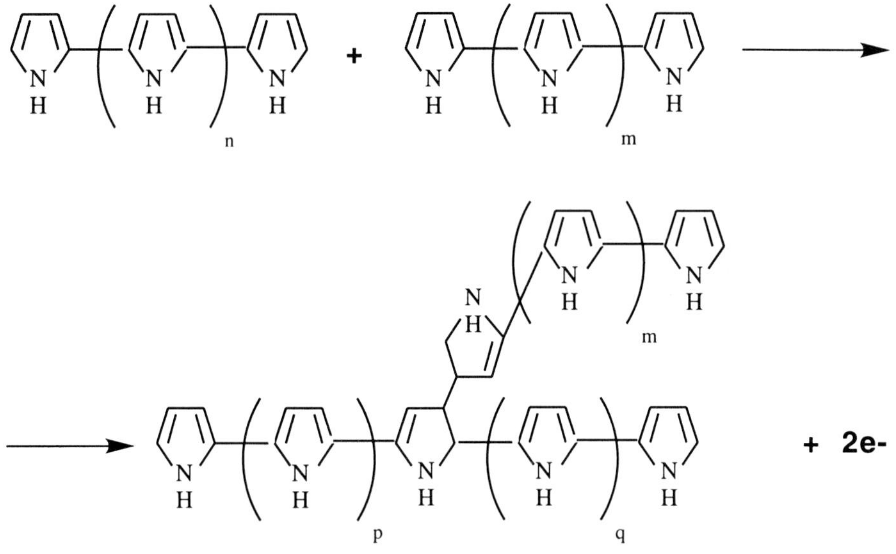

+

n

m

m

p

q

+ 2e-

p+q+1=n

6. Adsorption of the polyelectrolyte

$$(Polyelectrolyte)_{sol} \rightarrow (Polyelectrolyte)_{ad}$$

The final material is a mixed material determined by the relative rates of these parallel processes. All these kinetics are influenced in a different way by every variable of synthesis, and so both composition and properties of each material are a function of the specific values for the experimental chemical and physical variables of synthesis. Every property is related to different shape, dimensions and thicknesses of the films. The optimization of every property requires specific chemical and physical conditions during the synthesis of the material.

7.2.2 Oxidation and reduction processes in conducting polymers

Most of the properties of technological interest that we are looking for, related to polyconjugated conducting polymers, are bound to the electrochemical oxidation-reduction processes taking place when a polymeric film is studied in an electrolytic medium containing a solvent and a solved salt. There we have the three components of a soft, wet and complex material: polymeric chains forming an amorphous network, water (when working in aqueous solutions) and inorganic salts.

Starting from the neutral state of the polymer, strong polymer-polymer interactions are present giving a solid and compact structure. When a neutral film is electrochemically oxidized, positive charges are generated along the polymeric chains, whatever their position at the surface or in the bulk. This promotes repulsion between chains and the opening of the polymeric structure by conformational movements with generation of free volume (Figure 7.3). Solvated counterions are forced to penetrate into the polymer from the solution in order to keep electroneutrality in the solid. Together the polymer solvent molecules penetrate inside the film due to the high interaction between positive charges along the chains and the water dipoles. Under those conditions a complex, soft and wet material (a gel) is formed.

Opposite processes occur during reduction: electrons are injected into the solid, positive charges are eliminated and counterions and solvent molecules are expelled to the solution. As result of this, two main effects occur: the polymer recovers its neutral state and the volume of the film decreases.

In general a key point related to the oxidation of a chain of an ideal α–α'–polypyrrole film is that it can be considered as a non-stoichiometric reaction. So, if we consider the oxidation in an electrolytic medium containing ClO_4^-,

$$(pPy)_s + (n\ ClO_4^-)_{aq} + mH_2O \leftarrow\ \rightarrow [\ pPy^{n+}(ClO_4^-)_n(H_2O)_m\ ]_{gel} + (\ ne^-\ )_{metal}$$

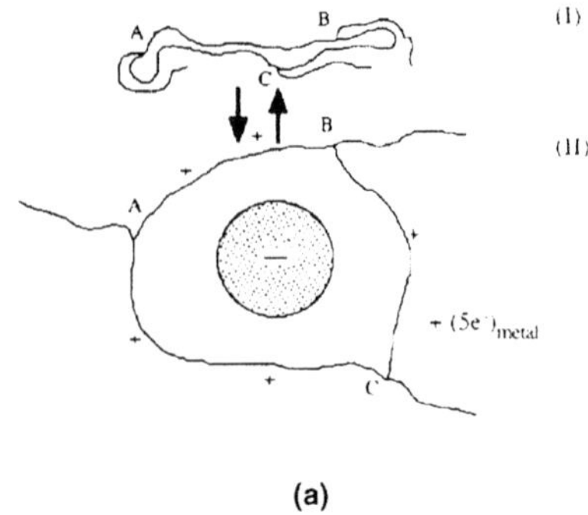

(a)

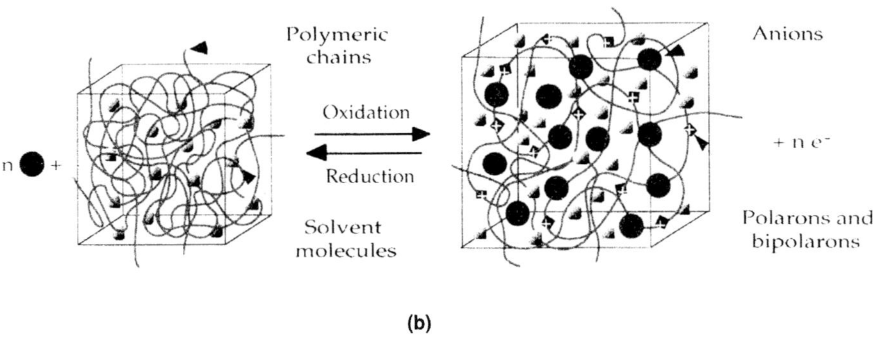

(b)

Fig. 7.3. (a) Two-dimensional representation: (I) Entangled structure after reduction at high cathodic potentials. (II) High anodic potentials are needed to inject positive charges, open the structure and allow counterions to penetrate. (b)Three-dimensional representation: A compact element of volume (having a length l) increases its length to $l + \Delta l$ during oxidation: electrons are lost from the polymer, channels are opened and hydrated counterions penetrate from the solution to maintain electroneutrality.

where pPy represents the polypyrrole chain, and the suffix indicates solid (s), solvated (aq), gel or metal. The number of positive charges (n) which can be stored by the chain moves from zero, when the chain is in the neutral state, to *i*/3, where *i* is the number of pyrrole units contained in the chain. This fraction implies that the generally accepted maximum density of charge stored in a conducting polymer before the polymer degrades (overoxidizes) is one charge for every three monomeric units.

From a theoretical point of view, increasing energies are required to extract the first, second, third, etc, electrons from a chain. From an experimental point of view we never use an independent and ideal α–α'–polypyrrole chain, but reticulated solid films having thousands of different conjugation lengths and a lot of irregularities. The consequence is that the oxidation process occurs during a large range of potential without any differentiation of successive electronic losses. Only the use of films generated by evaporation from oligomeric solutions, or some electrogenerated films where olygomers are directly formed, gives two maxima related in the literature to the formation of polarons and bipolarons.

7.2.3 ***Electrochemical control***

The electrochemical methods allow a perfect control of the oxidation and reduction processes related to conducting polymers. The conducting polymer under study can so be submitted to a triangular potential sweep (figure 7.4a′), to square potential steps (figure 7.4b′) or to square current steps (figure 7.4c′). The concomitant responses to these signals, cyclic voltammograms (figure 7.4a), chronoamperograms (figure 7.4b) and chronopotentiograms (figure 7.4d) are obtained.

As can be observed in the voltammogram during the anodic excursion of the potential, oxidation currents are present over a broad potential range. The charge consumed at every potential gives the number of electrons extracted from the polymeric chains forming the film, equal to the number of monovalent counterions penetrating from the solution to keep the electroneutrality. But the oxidation can be stopped at any point (any charge, and any composition of the material) by stopping the polarization or can be reversed from any point by reversing the sense of the potential sweep. A similar control can be performed through the current or the consumed charge.

Voltammogram and chronoamperogram shapes are a consequence of the non-stoichiometry of the electrogenerated compound. During oxidation, the counterion content moves in a continuous and controllable way from zero to around a 50% (w/w).

The groups of conducting polymers containing counterions inside the molecular structure (self-doping), or as immobile macromolecules (composites with polyelectrolytes incorporated during polymerization) or immobile hetero-macro-ions (like hybrid polymers) interchange cations during oxidation and reduction processes (figure 7.5).

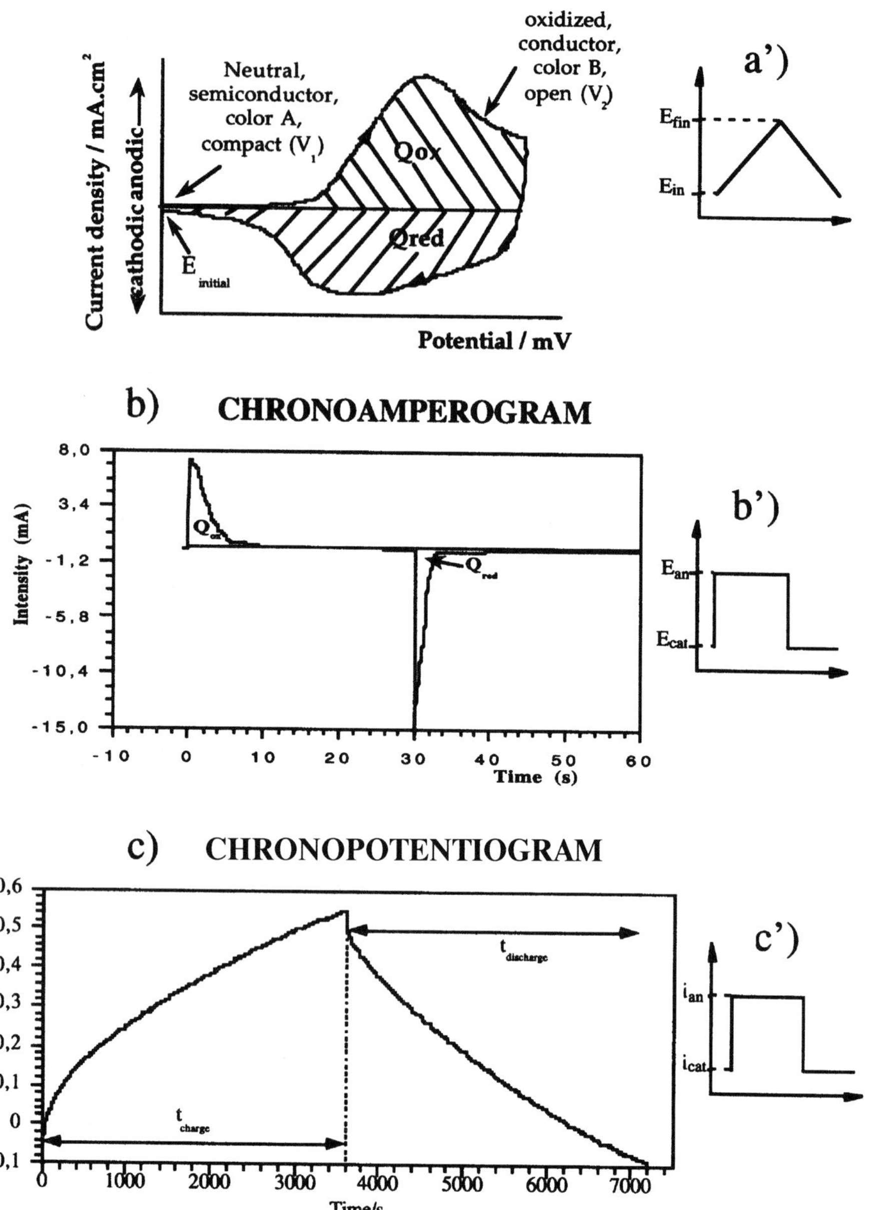

Fig. 7.4. Electrochemical system: two active electrodes (anode and cathode), a reference electrode, two interfaces (two simultaneous reactions: oxidation and reduction), one solution (ionic conductor), a power generator and two wires (electronic conductor).

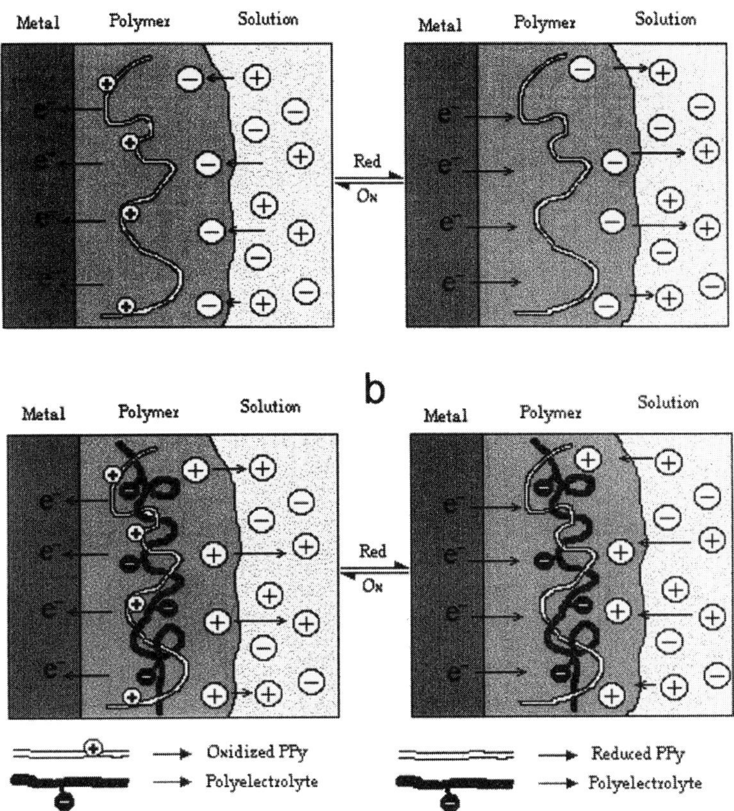

Fig. 7.5. Reduction/oxidation of (a) a material formed by a basic conducting polymer promoting expulsion/inclusion, respectively, of anions; (b) of a composite conducting polymer - polyelectrolyte promoting inclusion / expulsion, respectively, of cations.

7.2.4 Related properties: multifunctionality

Changes in the composition, as stated above, means that any property related to composition must also change in a continuous way, in a similar proportion thus, the electronic conductivity which shifts under electrochemical control across a range of several orders of magnitude (10^{-6} to 103 $S.cm^{-1}$ in polypyrrole). In a similar proportion change properties like: volume, color, charge storage, porosity, solubility (when we work with oligomeric films in specific solvents or electrolytes), or transduction properties as electron-anion, electron-cation or electron-chemical. All those properties are bounded, simultaneously, to the oxidation state of the polymer (Table 7.2): the

Table 7.2. Physical transitions and properties linked to the electrochemical transition in a conducting polymer and concomitant biological functions mimicked by the electrochemically induced property.

TRANSITIONS	CONTROLLED PROPERTY	BIOLOGICAL FUNCTION
Neutral/oxidized	Composition	
Discharged/charged	Charge storage	Electric organ
Shrinked/expanded	Electro-chemo-mechanical	Muscle
Transparent/opaque	Electrochromic	Skin mimicking
Compacted/expanded	Electroporosity	Membranes
Free ion/free electron	Ion/electron transduction	Nervous interfaces
Free ion/compound	Ion modulation	Medical dosage (glandes)

material is multifunctional. This state being under electrochemical control, any intermediate stationary state can be attained applying an appropriate potential. If the oxidation state can be changed in a continuous and reversible way (Scheme 7.1), that means that the correlated properties can be also changed in a similar way.

7.2.5 Mimicking biological functions

The above-mentioned properties, linked and controlled by the electrochemical reactions of the soft and wet material, mimic most of the functions characteristics to, and developed by, the biological organs in mammals, as is shown in table 7.2.

7.3. ARTIFICIAL MUSCLES: ELECTROCHEMOMECHANICAL PROPERTIES

Starting from a partially oxidized polymer, oxidation correlates with a continuous increase of volume related to the inclusion of counterions and water, whereas a continuous decrease of volume occurs along with the reduction process. The new free volume is generated by conformational changes of the polymeric molecules assisted by the strong power of the electrochemical reaction. These electrochemically stimulated conformational changes promoted by electric pulses and connected to a flux of ions are the origin of the electro-chemo-mechanical properties of conducting polymers giving, at molecular level, a molecular motor (Figure 7.6).

Considering the high conductivity of the polymeric chains, the electric pulses arrive virtually simultaneously at any point in the polymer (in a similar way to the calcium release in every myofibril of muscles).

ELECTROCHEMICALLY STIMULATED MOLECULAR MOTOR

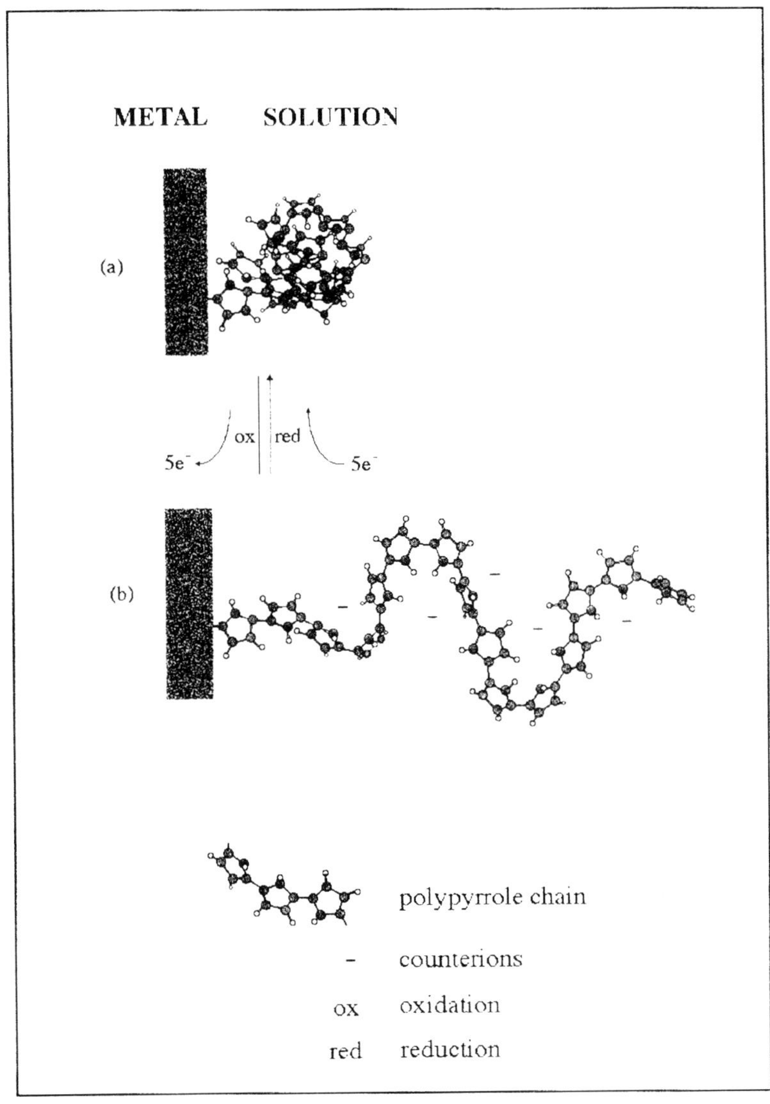

Fig. 7.6. Molecular motor: reversible conformational changes (mechanical energy) stimulated by oxidation or reduction of the polymeric chain.

7.3.1 Changes of volume

Here we will focus on the reversible and controllable change of volume linked to electrochemical reactions in the film, promoted by an electric current. Murray detected this main feature of conducting polymers in 1982 (Bourgmayer and Murray 1982). Okabayashi (1987) made direct studies of polyaniline, resulting in a variation of volume during oxidation by a factor of 2. Slama and Tanguy (1989) for polypyrrole or Tourillon and Garnier (1984) for polythiophene obtained similar results. Otero et al. confirmed this result for polypyrrole from density measurements in dry films: oxidized and reduced states showed similar densities (1.51 g cm^{-3}), the weight of the oxidized film being 50% higher due to the incorporation of counterions during oxidation. Variations of volume for polyacetylene films around 6.6%, which corresponds to a length variation of 1.8%, were reported by Baughman *et al.* (1990)

The use and application of those changes of volume is the origin of electrochemomechanical devices: sensors, actuators, electrochemopositioning devices, artificial muscles, etc, as will be explained in following sections.

7.3.2 Life and movement. Eukariotic muscles

In general, movement is an intrinsic property of living creatures. This is true at different structural levels, including: ion transfer through membranes, separation of replicated chromosomes, beating of cilia and flagellae or, the most common, contraction of muscles. These contractions enables the organism to carry out organized and sophisticated movements such as walking, running, flying, swimming, breathing, to digest foods, etc, generating mechanical energy.

Muscles are elegant devices developed through thousands of years of evolution to transform chemical energy into mechanical energy and heat. This transformation is triggered by an electric pulse arriving from the brain through nerves, which promotes an increase of Ca^{+2} inside the myofibrils from 10^{-7} to 10^{-3} M. The increase of the ionic concentration promotes conformational changes in the troponim-tropomyosin system, allowing the muscle to contract. The energy required for these conformational changes is generated by ATP hydrolysis, this ATP being the bonding ion between myosin heads and actin filaments. ATP is restored from ADP through the glucose cycle. All these processes take place in aqueous media. A muscle can be considered as an electro-chemo-mechanical actuator (figure 7.7). Thus, molecular movements occurring in biological macromolecules generate the macroscopic movements developed by a muscle. Several points should be stressed:

- A muscle is a complex system where water, ions, macromolecules and small organic molecules play important roles.
- A nervous pulse promotes ionic interchanges between the myofibril and the surrounding in a few microseconds.
- The free energy of ATP hydrolysis drives conformational changes in the myosin head, resulting in the net movement of myosin along the actin filament

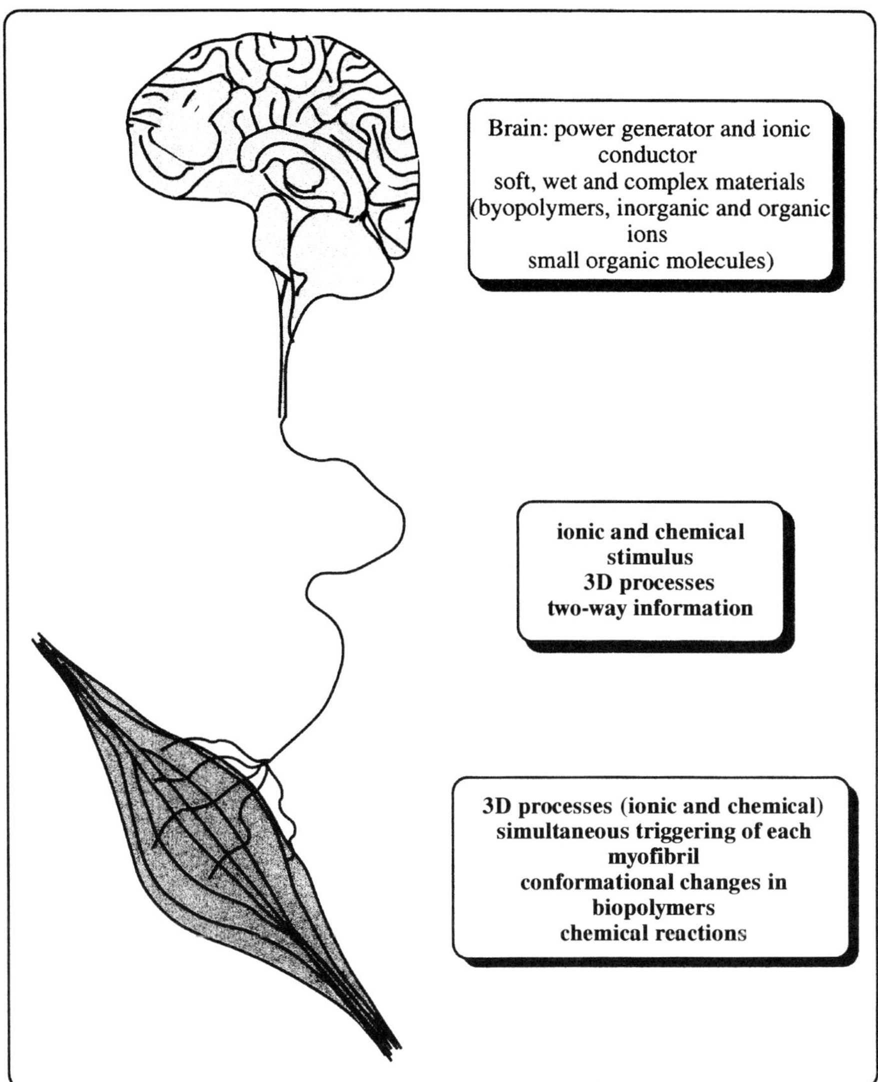

Fig. 7.7. An electric (ionic) pulse arrives from the brain through nerves to the muscle where it triggers conformational changes in proteins and chemical reactions. All the processes are three-dimensional. The generator (brain) is, at the same time an ionic conductor.

- The movement occurs through the formation of complexes between two macromolecules (myosin and actin) and an ion, ATP, and the subsequent dissociation of these complexes with formation of ADP.
- The high energy content of ATP is restored from the ADP by transferring energy through glycolysis.
- Muscles work at constant temperature and the heat generated during these transformations by entropic requirements has to be eliminated.
- The contraction of muscle is relaxed by Ca^{+2} release from the myofibril when the nervous pulse ceases.
- Interchange of water and ions other than calcium play important roles in muscle's contraction
- The final result is the generation of mechanical energy from chemical energy though conformational changes promoted by the formation and dissociation of ionic complexes bridged by ATP^{4+} ions.
- Once relaxed, a muscle recovers its initial position by the work of a complementary muscle.

This initial approach to the natural actuators evidences the interactions between electric currents (ionic), chemical reactions, mechanical work, and heat production. We can complete the picture of muscles as electro-chemo-mechanical actuators working at constant temperature, in a complex aqueous medium and able to relax to the initial state.

The similarity of nervous pulses and electric currents was shown by Galvani´s experiment: an electric current can simulate a nervous pulse. An electric pulse sent through the nerves of a dissected frog's claw was able to promote the contraction of the claw. The experiment does not work at all if the dissected frog is dehydrated: nervous pulses and chemical reactions in muscular fibers are related to ions flowing in aqueous media and through cellular membranes.

So, to develop an electrochemomechanical device mimicking natural muscles we are looking for a molecular machine based on conformational movements along macromolecules, stimulated by electric pulses linked to ionic fluxes, working in aqueous media at constant temperature and able to translate these molecular movements to macroscopic movements.

7.3.3 Approach through electrochemical systems

These hypotheses drive our attention to electrochemistry and electrochemical systems. They link electric pulses generated by an electronic equipment, sent through metal wires to an electrode-electrolyte interface where chemical reactions take place, assisted by the electric current, at constant temperature, in aqueous media and connected to an ionic flux required to maintain electroneutrality.

An electrochemical process requires, at least, two electrodes (anode and cathode). Taking into account the internal resistance of both, electrolyte and electrode-electrolyte interfaces, a fraction of the electrical energy supplied to the system is transformed to heat, which has to be eliminated in order to maintain a constant temperature.

All the previous steps have a quite close similarity to those developed by muscles. The most important difference between muscle and the usual electrochemical systems is based on its chemical nature. The central components of muscle are the molecular machines constituted by proteins: *biopolymers*. Proteins like *actin* and *myosin* are molecular engines designed by chemical evolution for the conversion of chemical energy into mechanical energy. Conversely, the most usual components of the most common electrochemical reactions are metals, metal oxides, small organic molecules and gases.

This panorama force us to include macromolecular components into the electrochemical systems in order to advance in attempting to mimic natural muscles. In the literature two main families of macromolecules can be found that are useful from an electrochemical point of view: ionic conductors (non-electroactive), or electronic and ionic conductors (electroactive). If we attempt to work in aqueous media having an open polymeric structure including water and ions, dry materials like ionic conductors (PEO, etc) are eliminated. Two families are still available: non-active gels (from an electrochemical point of view) and electroactive conducting polymers. We consider the existence of electrochemical activity when electrons are extracted from, or injected into, the macromolecular chains with the concomitant formation or rupture of covalent or ionic bonds.

7.3.4 Artificial muscles from conducting polymers

Polymer gels and proteins do not work as electronic conductors, so electro-osmotic and diffusion processes have to be used as intermediates to convert electrical energy to mechanical energy. This results in low actuation rates and high working potentials.

The availability of electronically conducting polymers, jointly with their redox properties promoting reverse changes of volume, opens new possibilities to develop molecular machines, as was postulated by Baughman, see (Otero 1997) and references therein.

On the one hand, small changes of potential (of about 0.1 - 0.5 V, that is, almost two orders of magnitude lower than previous systems) are sufficient to attain composition variations of about 30% with high reversibility. Times required to complete these variations range between 3 and 50 s, longer than in piezoelectric systems but clearly shorter than in polyelectrolyte gels.

On the other hand, conjugated polymers can generate mechanical stresses of around 100 MPa during work as electro-chemo-mechanical devices, whereas polymer gels only yield stresses of 1 MPa. The only negative aspect related to conducting polymers is that the current efficiency to produce mechanical work is rather low: 0.1-1%, depending on the kind of polymer considered.

From an overview of all these features, it can be concluded that conducting polymers offer excellent expectations for their application as electrochemomechanical actuators.

7.3.5 Artificial muscles formed by bilayer structures

Electrochemically promoted transitions from the neutral state of a conducting polymer to the oxidized state and reverse reductions to the neutral state again, are accompanied by swelling and shrinking processes. The polymer film changes from the solid state to a gel and back again. All the macroscopic movement is based on the conformational changes induced in chains by the electrochemical reaction. This molecular device gives very small macroscopic movements.

The construction of an electrochemomechanical device requires the translation of these microscopic conformational changes into macroscopic movements. This problem has been solved in nature by introducing anisotropy in such a way that the uniform swelling-shrinking processes are broken, giving unidirectional stresses. Among the different possibilities we had, a bilayer structure was chosen in the first stages of the research: a conducting polymer film (3 x 1 cm) was stuck to an adherent, flexible and non conducting polymeric film (Otero and Rodríguez 1993). The bilayer was held at the top with a metallic clamp to allow electrical contact. Once formed, the bilayer was checked in aqueous solutions of different salts. An area of 1x2 cm was introduced into the solution, keeping the clamp out of the liquid. As counterelectrode a platinum sheet was used (Figure 7.8). The construction of the bilayer is conditioned by the availability of conducting polymer films of high structural homogeneity. Such films can be obtained from electropolymerization techniques, which have been previously described. See references in (Otero 1999; Otero and Grande 1997).

When the bilayer is used as a working electrode the electric current flow and the concomitant electrochemical processes and change of volume occur only in the layer of conducting polymer. This electrochemical stimulation and generation of free volume is transformed into a stress gradient across the polymer-polymer interface, able to bend the bilayer. The system is similar to the bilayer thermometry performed by two metallic sheets having different expansion coefficients. Here the molecular movement in the conducting film, produced during oxidation and reduction (swelling and shrinking) is transferred into an angular macroscopic movement of the free end of the bilayer around the fixed one. The bending degree depends on the oxidation level, which can be controlled either through the current density flowing across the system or by the electric potential to which the conducting polymer was submitted (in this case a reference electrode is required). If both, the oxidation depth and the movement rate are stimulated by a constant anodic current, both related processes can be stopped at any point by stopping the current flow, and can be reversed by changing the sense of the current flow.

When such devices became able to describe angular movements through more than 360 degrees, dragging several hundreds times their own weight; they were named *artificial muscles*. In fact, the use of electrochemomechanical properties related to polyconjugated materials for the fabrication of artificial muscles was reported and patented in 1992 by Otero et al. Since then various researches described different devices using polypyrrole, polyaniline and poly (3-alkylthiophene). It must be remarked that they are secondary machines: no direct transformation of electric energy to mechanical work exists. Intermediate electrochemical processes, with flow

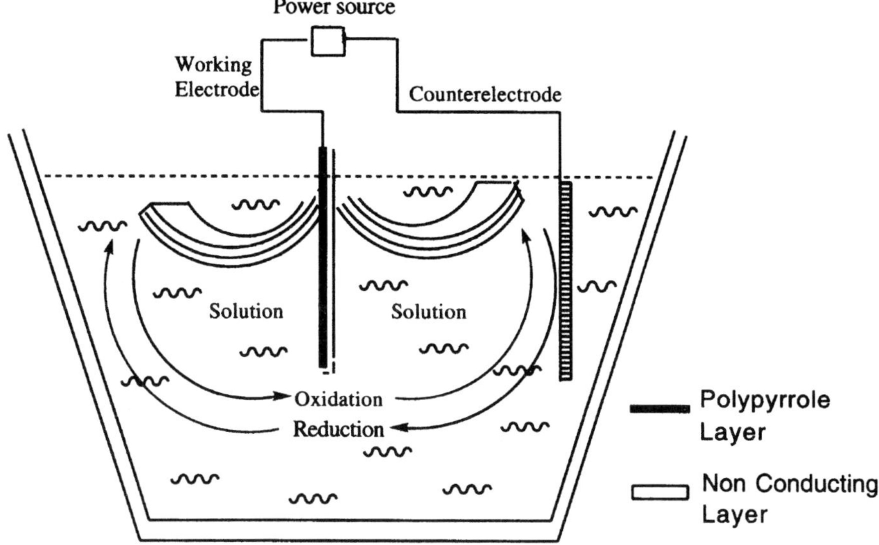

Fig. 7.8. Scheme of the movement of an artificial muscle formed by a bilayer polypyrrole film/non conducting plastic tape during current flow, starting from the vertical position. The flow of a cathodic current through the conducting film promotes its reduction with expulsion of counterions and water. Polypyrrole shrinks and the bilayer bends to the left. Opposite processes and movements occur during oxidation.

of electrons (involving changes in chemical bonds) and ions through the polymer jointly with conformational changes, along polymeric chains are required. The electrochemical nature of this process will differentiate devices constructed from conducting polymers from those based on polyelectrolyte gels.

7.3.6 Artificial muscles as electro-chemo-positioning devices

In a typical voltammetric response for a polypyrrole film a correlation between the electrical charge consumed to oxidize the polymer and the potential applied at each moment can be established. If the stress gradient at the polymer-polymer interface is linked to the relative change of volume and this is related to the stationary charge consumed at every potential of polarization, the angle described by the free end of the bilayer will be related to the electric potential. This fact was experimentally confirmed (Otero 1999; Otero and Grande 1997). The reversibility of the movement is guaranteed by the reversibility of the redox process. So each position was recovered when the bilayer was submitted to the corresponding potential.

These experimental facts are important from a structural point of view, supporting our hypothesis that the electrogenerated polypyrrole film is a polydisperse sample of conjugation lengths. This polydisperse and crosslinked sample acts like a non-stoichiometric compound having at every potential a defined oxidation depth related to a distribution of polarons and bipolarons.

The position of the free end of the bilayer depends only on the oxidation depth and this is related to a defined potential, being independent of any of the variables such as the distance to the counterelectrode. The rate of the movement is under control of the electrochemical reaction rate, so the time required to recover each position depends on the parameters acting on that electrochemical reaction, mainly concentration and electrolyte type and temperature.

7.3.7 ***The working muscle***

Both oxidation and reduction states of the conjugated polymer can be reached at constant potential, at constant current or through any other variation of potentials or currents, like linear sweeps, pulses, sinusoidal waves, trapezoidal waves, etc. In any case, along a complete oxidation cycle the free end of the bilayer describes an angular movement related to the vertical position greater than 360°. During oxidation, the expansion of the polyconjugated material pushes the flexible non-conducting layer to the concave part of the bend. During reduction, if the conjugated material was in an intermediate oxidation state when the bilayer was constructed, the free end recovers the original vertical position and goes on to describe an angle greater than 180° in the opposite direction. Now, the shrinking of the conducting polymer promotes strains of contraction at the interface giving an opposite bend: the free end of the bilayer moves towards the polypyrrole side.

This movement is able to produce mechanical work. So a bilayer containing 5 mg of polypyrrole is able to lift a steel sheet (200 mg) connected to the bottom of the bilayer. The bilayer was submitted to anodic and cathodic currents of 5 mA. This device takes around 30 s to cross over 180° from the left side to the right side and vice versa.

Movements linked to the reduction process are faster than those related to oxidation reaction, due to a different kinetics of conformational changes, as will be pointed later. Muscles able to lift a steel sheet (weighing 1000 times the conducting film weight) over more than 200 cycles have been built in our laboratory.

In spite of this magnitude, the percentage of electrical energy transformed to mechanical energy is very low (around 1%). This fact seems caused by the use of very thick films of both conducting and inactive polymer related to the distance from the polymer-polymer interface where stress gradient occurs additional polymer consumes electrical charge, does not produce work and has to be lifted. The use of thinner films, even though this poses important experimental difficulties, is one of the fields of interest in attempts to improve the energy conversion efficiency.

7.3.8 The three layers muscle

Taking into account that the bilayer requires the presence of a counter-electrode to allow current flow through the solution, a new device was developed in order to exploit the same current twice: a three-layer conducting polymer/flexible layer/conducting polymer. Its construction is easy: once a bilayer is obtained, a second conducting polymer film is made to adhere to the free side of the non-conducting tape. This inactive tape acts not only as support for stress gradients, but also as electronic insulator between the conducting films. One of the conducting films acts as anode, swelling and pushing the device. The second active film acts as cathode, shrinking by reduction and lifting the device. There is no direct electronic contact between both films owing to the presence of the non-conducting layer in the middle. Therefore the electric flow takes place by ionic conduction through the solution. The device can be improved by coating it with a film of cellophane or polyacrylamide gel containing an electrolyte, as reported by MacDiarmid et al. A "shell-type" multilayer actuator is obtained in this case, able to work in air.

7.3.9 Muscles working in air

A working muscle requires the presence of a solution, which support requirements from counterions and water. Due to the structure of the triple layer counterions requirements are minimal because they flow from one of the electroactive layer into the other. Under those conditions attempts were performed in order to find a tape bearing a high ionic conductivity without any electronic conductivity jointly with adherence and flexibility. These properties are fulfilled by the lithium perchlorate solved in poly (epichlorohydrine-co-ethylene oxide). This solid electrolyte developed by De Paoli et al. allowed us the construction of a triple layer polypyrrole / polyelectrolyte / polypyrrole (Otero 1999). Since the ions move through the tape no aqueous solution is required and the device works in air. Ionic movements, stresses and bending are represented in figure 7.9.

Nevertheless when we described similitude between muscles and artificial muscles we underline the importance to use aqueous materials and the importance of the water interchange on volumetric variations during redox processes. Now we confirm those hypotheses: the solid muscle does not work if the relative humidity in air during the experiment is lower than a 60%.

7.3.10 Control of the movement rate

The rate of the movement depends on every one of the variables acting on the electrochemical reaction taking place in the solid film. Both anodic and cathodic overpotentials have a strong influence on the redox kinetics. At constant overpotential, any increase on the electrolyte concentration (which is one of the chemical components acting on the solid state reaction) promotes an increase of the rate of the movement. Times required to cross over a constant angle diminishe due to a faster increase in the concentration of the oxidation centers in the polymer (the other chemical constituent of the process).

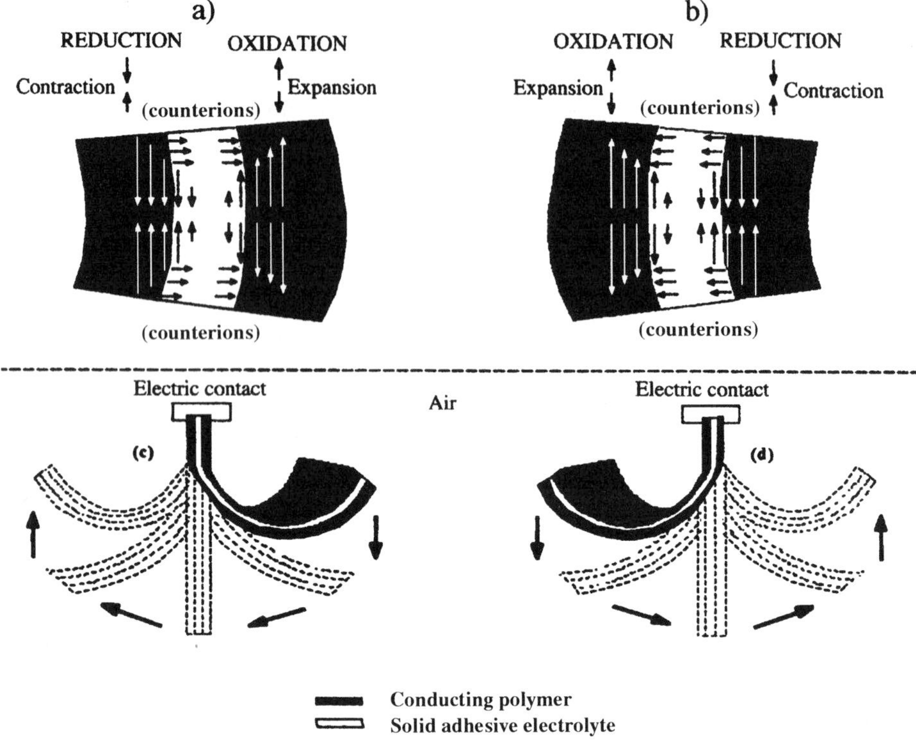

Fig. 7.9. A triple layer, polypyrrole/poly(epichloridrine-co-ethylene oxide)-$LiClO_4$/polypyrrole of counterions and local bending are represented at (a) and (b) under reverse senses of the current flow. The concomitant macroscopic movements are represented in (b) and (c).

On the other hand, movements related to anodic processes are always slower than these related to cathodic processes. This fact is related to the extra energy required to open the molecular entanglement and allow the penetration of counterions during oxidation. During reduction, on the contrary, counterions diffuse along the opened structure towards the solution without any resistance, giving a faster shrinking effect. In other words, conformational relaxation processes of the polymeric chains control oxidation, but not reduction.

The internal structure of the polymer plays an important role in determining the rate of movement: the appearance of stress gradients at the polymer-polymer interfaces requires an adequate crosslinking of the polymeric structure. This seems to be the main problem in developing artificial muscles from different conducting polymers. When the conditions of synthesis are restrictive, as in the case of the high anodic potential necessary to obtain polythiophene, dense crosslinking can occur. The resultant muscles have very slow movement, describing small angles around the vertical position.

All these effects indicate that a strong interrelation between electrochemistry and polymer science is required in order to explain redox processes in conducting polymers and related changes in properties (volume variations among them). In this way, a model for the opening and closing of the polymeric structure during redox switching controlled by conformational relaxation is giving good results in simulating electrochemical responses of polypyrrole-coated electrodes (Otero 1999). Models including mechanical components do not attain the same fit with experimental results.

7.3.11 Actuator and sensor

An artificial muscle works pushed by a constant current, keeping constant all the other electrochemical, chemical, and physical variables. If in successive experiments we hang increasing masses from the bottom of the muscle, increasing power is required to lift those masses. With a constant current density, the muscle responds with higher potentials and slower movements. So, a correlation exists between the lifted mass and the stationary potential of the working muscle: the muscle is at the same time an actuator and a sensor. In a similar way if a muscle moves under constant current in solutions containing decreasing concentrations of an electrolyte, increasing potentials are observed.

The oxidation depth controls the bending state of the device, so a bilayer can be used as a sensor in a gas or liquid phase able to detect the presence of any oxidising substance. If this is a reverse process, the sensor recovers the original position when the oxidant disappears from the ambient.

7.3.12 Life time and degradation processes

Artificial muscles degrade as they operate. In our laboratory, bilayers were checked over more than 150 cycles (a cycle is considered as a movement of the free end of the bilayer from -90 degrees, related to the vertical position, to +90 degrees and back). For a greater number of cycles (150-1000) the movement stops when a fissure appears close to the metallic clamp. The lifetime can be improved by modifying the synthesis and control conditions.

The key idea is that electropolymerization is a fast way through a complex mechanism to obtain mixed materials: linear and conducting chains, crosslinking points, chemically generated (and therefore non-conducting) polymer and partially degraded material. Through the conditions of synthesis we have a way to control the composition of the mixed conducting polymer and to obtain the best material for each application. Nevertheless, once made the polymer degrades in two main ways: Joule effect and overoxidation. As the neutral polymer is a semiconductor, there are difficulties in supporting high current densities when oxidation initiates. The flow of current through the high polymeric resistance produces heat (hot points can be observed in the film, mainly at the polymer/electrolyte interface), so fissures appear and the current flow stops. Overoxidation is related to chemical and physical variables. The flow of an anodic current requires an adequate concentration of counterions to allow the oxidation process to continue at low overpotential. Lower concentrations promote a thick diffusion layer and greater overpotentials: new reactions, as water discharge with formation of hydroxyl radicals, appear. These radicals give nucleophilic attacks on polarons with conjugation loss and slower movements (denser crosslinking).

Reverse oxidation and overoxidation (or degradation) processes can be followed as a function of the applied electric potential by voltammetry. A bilayer (3x1 cm), constructed with a 5 mg polypyrrole film is submitted to a potential sweep between -100 mV (vs. SCE) and 3000 mV in a 1 M $LiClO_4$ aqueous solution. In order to get an equilibrium state at every potential (the oxidation state of all the solid correlates with each potential), the sweep rate was slow: 3 mV s^{-1}.

The experimental voltammogram can be observed in Fig. 7.6. At -100 mV the polypyrrole film is reduced. Along the oxidation process until 700 mV a movement of 180° is observed. If the potential sweep is reversed from any potential previous to 700 mV the movement is reversed. At greater potentials than 700 mV an overoxidation-degradation process takes place and a slow reverse movement of the bilayer is observed, when the potential arrives to 2V. This fact points to a decrease in stress gradient at the polymer-polymer interface, probably due to an increase in crosslinking level. So all the electrochemical and mechanical processes become irreversible at high anodic potentials.

7.3.13 Mechanochemoelectrical devices

Most processes in nature can be reversed. Our electrochemomechanical devices are able to generate a mechanical energy by conformational movements stimulated by an electric current through an electrochemical reaction in an electrolytic medium. We can now imagine an oxidized polypirrole film in an electrolyte, which submitted to a mechanical deformation has to respond with a chemical reaction of reduction, decreasing volume with counterion expulsion, forcing the flow of an external current. A research team supervised by Kaneto (1995) designed and produced equipment able to measure the generated currents when different mechanical stresses were applied to the polymer.

7.3.14 Similarities with natural muscles

In a natural muscle an electric pulse arrives from the brain through the nervous system and triggers chemical reactions in the muscular cells, promoting conformational changes in myosin heads and concomitant mechanical forces. In artificial muscles constructed from conducting polymers, an electric pulse promotes electro-chemical reactions giving conformational changes of the polymer chains, which can be transformed into macroscopic movements. Moreover, natural muscles can be artificially activated through an electric pulse (remember Galvani's experiment).

Similarities between natural and artificial muscle based on conducting polymers can be summarized as follows. An electric pulse linked to a chemical reaction is involved. Conformational changes in polymeric chains are responsible for the mechanical work; all the processes occur in aqueous media. Flow of ions and water molecules through interfaces or membranes are required. A chemical reaction is present, being responsible for the generated mechanical energy. Strong chemical interactions between polymers and ions are formed and destroyed during muscle work. A change of volume is observed during work. Macroscopic mechanical movement is observed. Both natural and artificial systems work at constant temperature. A fraction of the involved energy is transformed into heat during work and this heat has to be eliminated. Both natural and artificial systems are three-dimensional molecular machines.

In spite of important improvements relative to previous molecular devices, some differences still persist between muscles and artificial muscles based on conducting polymers.

1. The driving power in muscles is the chemical energy produced by combustion, at constant temperature, of glucose. The nervous pulse acts as a trigger. The driving power in artificial muscles is the consumed electric charge. The polymer oxidation and reduction are mediators.

2. Muscles respond to ionic pulses. Artificial muscles respond to electronic pulses.

3. Muscles only work under contraction due to the irreversibility of the chemical reaction. The work of a second muscle is required in order to relax the first muscle to the original position. Artificial muscles constructed with conducting polymers are based on reversible electrochemical reactions. So they work under expansion as well as under contraction wen the direction of the current flow is changed.

7.4. ALL ORGANO-AQUEOUS BATTERY: ELECTRIC ORGANS

Oxidation or reduction of the neutral conducting polymer results in storage of positive or negative charges, respectively, along the polymers. So, polymeric electrodes for charge storage can be developed using a polymeric gel containing an electrolyte. An all organo-aqueous battery is obtained —a first approach to electric organs. The main technological advantage of such organic batteries, related to the inorganic ones is, as was remarked above, the use of three-dimensional electrodes where all the electroactive material is available simultaneously.

From an environmental point of view such ions as lithium, sodium, etc can be used as interchanging ions between anode and cathode, and polymeric materials which can be integrated in natural processes by biodegradation reactions, can be designed giving non-contaminating batteries. The final objective will be the use of proton interchanging biodegradable polymers as electroactive anode and cathode materials.

The availability of materials interchanging cations or anions during charge-discharge allows different designs for the positive and negative electrodes and for the electrolyte of the batteries (figure 7.10).

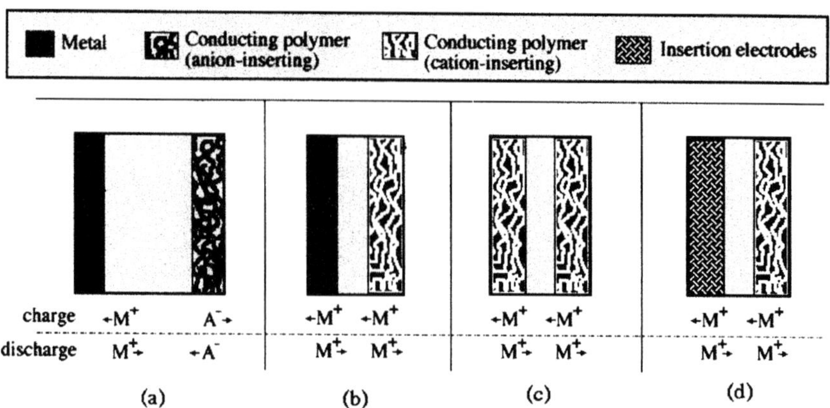

Fig. 7.10. Different electrode assemblies to make batteries using conducting polymers.

7.5. COLOR MIMICKING: SMART SKINS

If movements linked to electric currents are specific characteristics of living creatures, another important property of life is the ability to change color, or to develop filters of light under different conditions, like presence or absence of light. Nevertheless, the most attractive property related to color in nature is the ability to change color and thereby mimicking environmental conditions.

In order to be able to reproduce and control such ability, we need soft, wet and complex materials able to change color under control, similar to those employed by living creatures. Conducting polymers which fulfil these requirements are *electrochromic* materials. The color changes as the population of polarons and bipolarons rise. The intensity of the color is related to the oxidation depth i.e., with the population of polarons and bipolarons, and is controlled like the film volume by the potential or the charge, as can be observed on the "in situ" absorption-reflection UV-vis spectra from a polypyrrole film along a potential sweep (anodic). Any intermediate color and any intermediate adsorption can be attained. Applications to filters, smart mirrors and smart windows (figure 7.11) are already coming to the market.

7.6. TRANSDUCERS

During the electrochemical study of a conducting polymer the electric signal produced by the electrochemical equipment arrives at the polymer through a metal wire. The metal wire contacts the polymer and the polymer contacts the electrolyte. The system metal-conducting polymer-electrolyte forms a *transducer* from an electronic signal to an ionic (or chemical) signal. The direction of the concomitant movement through the two interfaces depends on the group of conducting polymers.

"SMART WINDOW"

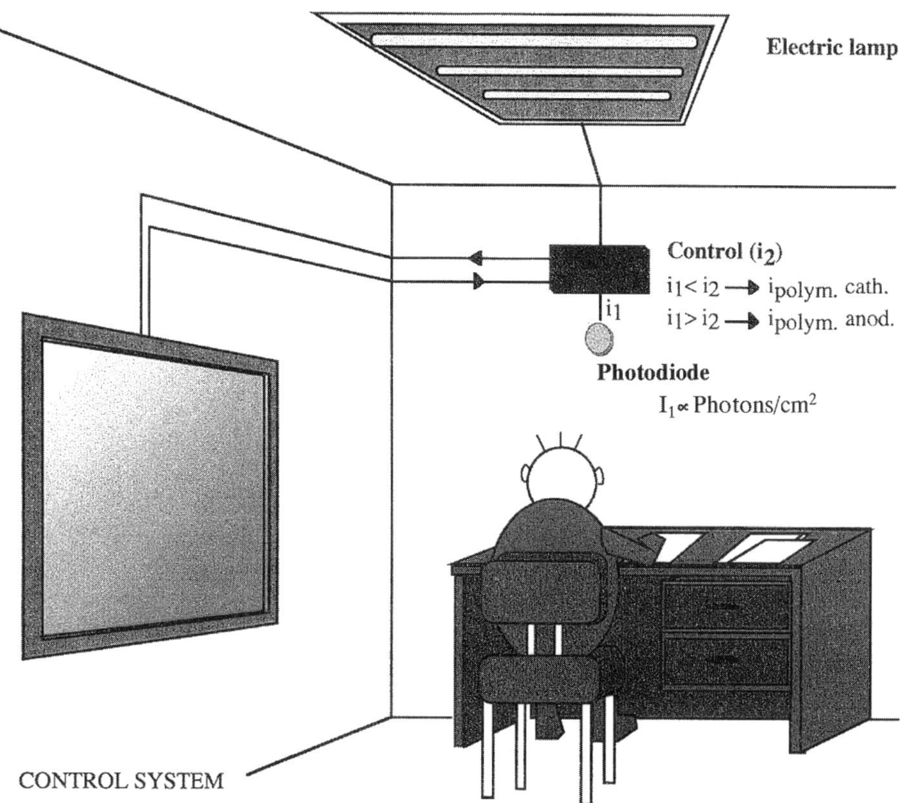

1. Reads the current i_1 produced by the photodiode
2. Compares i_1 with the desired level i_2
3. If $i_1 > i_2$ sends an anodic current through the polymer film which stops when $i_1 = i_2$
4. If $i_1 < i_2$ sends an cathodic current through the polymer film which stops when $i_1 = i_2$
5. If no responses to the cathodic current, then switch the electric lamp with adequate i_3 ($i_1 = i_2$)

Fig. 7.11. Automatic assembly to keep a constant luminosity

Basic conducting polymers, polyheterocycles and polymeric derivatives promote depletion-increase of the anion's concentration into the electrolyte side of the polymer/electrolyte interface during oxidation-reduction respectively. Self-doping polymers, composites and hybrid materials promote a rise/depletion of cations into the same interface during oxidation/reduction, respectively.

7.7. NERVOUS INTERFACES

Among the possible ionic-electronic transducers, *interfaces between nerves and electronic equipments* are the most specific. Electronic equipment mimicking eyes, ears, tongues, etc., are available in the market: video cameras, microphones and sensors. Most of such devices occupy less space and have greater sensitivity than the corresponding natural organs. But those devices give electronic signals, which cannot be understood by the nervous system. Nowadays, human technology is able to construct mechanical arms controlled electronically able to reproduce any of the movements of a natural arm. When implanted, these movements have to be harmonized and correlated with movements from all the other members of the body: it has to work under brain control. Brain orders arrive by ionic pulses, which must be separated, identified and converted to electronic signals. We need a biocompatible, organic base, soft, wet and complex transducer able to receive ionic signals and transduce then to electronic pulses.

Partial oxidized polyconjugated materials are membranes able to respond, at molecular level, to any ionic variation changing the membrane potential. So, they work as transducers from ionic to electronic signals. On the other hand, a partially oxidized conducting polymer responds to a cathodic current, or to a cathodic polarization, expelling a pulse of ions, acting now as transducers from electronic signals to ionic (and chemical) signals able to be understood by neurons through the dendrites.

A lot of work is being done in order to synthesize and characterize polyconjugated materials having specific ionic conductivities, being biocompatible and checking their abilities as nervous interfaces.

7.8. MEDICAL DOSAGE

Those states of the conducting polymers for which the material is full of the moving counterions (oxidized basic polymers, polymeric derivatives and polyheterocycles contain carrier anions, and reduced self-compensating polymers, polymeric composites and hybrid materials containing carrier cations) are chemical stores of those counterions. When the concomitant counterions are of pharmaceutical interest, they can be supplied to a patient under biological request. A system formed by a sensor indicates the drug level in the patient's body. When the level is below a set limit, an electric current is applied to the conducting polymer. The drug is released from the material, under control of the electric current, keeping the concentration in the body constant.

7.9. SMART MEMBRANES

From the point of view of the polymeric structure, the oxidation depth of a conducting polymer defines the degree of opening or compaction of this structure. Channel dimensions across the polymer film depend on this oxidation depth and the film can be used like a smart membrane. If we use an oxidized polymeric film, the presence of positive charges along the polymeric chains gives an anionic membrane, If the membrane is polarized at low potentials it attains a low oxidation depth and narrow channel allows the flux of small anions. A deeper oxidation enlarges the diameter of the channels and larger anions pass as well trough the membrane. The reversibility of the redox process allows a modulation of the dimensions of the anions able to cross the film.

A polymer like polythiophene can also be reduced at high cathodic potentials. So, using propylene carbonate as solvent we can reduce the polymer from the neutral state. Now negative charges are stored along the chains, giving a cationic membrane. Changing the potential we can move now from an anionic membrane to a cationic membrane and inside these regions we can modulate the dimensions of the channels.

7.10. THREE-DIMENSIONAL ELECTROCHEMICAL PROCESSES AND BIOLOGICAL MIMICKING

The approach performed in this chapter to electrochemomecanical devices based on conducting polymers uses a new concept: the electrochemically stimulated conformational relaxation processes of polymeric molecules. Related properties of the new three-dimensional electrodes, at molecular level, go beyond the limits of the chapter by mimicking biological processes, or being able to act as transducer between biological processes and electronic equipments.

Swelling and shrinking processes during reverse redox reactions occur in a three-dimensional electrode at molecular level where any segment of a polymeric chain reacts simultaneously (fig. 7.4). Molecular conformations change under influence of any of the variables acting on the electrochemical reaction, i.e., applied current, applied potential, electrolyte concentration, etc. Influences on the macroscopic movements of the electro-chemo-mechanical actuators experimentally proved this hypothesis. The swelling or shrinking processes, and the related movement occurs simultaneously at any point of the device.

We say that this is a new electrochemistry because all the electrochemical models developed until now are based on the existence of a two dimensional interface between a solution of a salt and a metal, or a semiconductor, or another solution. Even when the term "three-dimensional electrode" is usually found in the literature, it is related to fluidized baths, particles inside carbon paste, etc. That means that at microscopic level we have particles and on those particles a two-dimensional interface is present. When these particles are electroactive are consumed during electrochemical reactions, like in battery electrodes, atoms in the bulk are not available simultaneously to the atoms on the surface: a two-dimensional interface is formed between the electroactive material and the already consumed material, advancing inside the particle during work. Most of the technological advances in applied electrochemistry during the last century are based on treatments of the electroactive materials to get the maximum roughness. The limit of those advances arrives when every atom or every molecule of the electroactive material is available simultaneously and independently of their position at the surface or in the electrode bulk.

My point of view is that this is the main difference between traditional electrochemical systems and bioelectrochemical processes: they are a transition between two dimensional to three dimensional, at molecular level, processes. If we consider a potassium channel through a cell membrane there is interdependence between the electric field across the membrane, generated by the ionic concentration gradient, and the conformational structure of the macromolecules. Pores open, or close, in relation to a defined electric potential threshold through the membrane, promoting the concomitant conformational changes in the amorphous and electroactive biopolymers forming the pore. Electrochemical models, until now, do not include polymeric structures, surface structures of the electrodes or any other atomic or molecular structure of the electrode bulk.

This is the origin of difficulties in understanding ionic pulses, nervous transmission and, specially the generation of the nervous pulses inside neurons. Neurons act at the same time as impulse generators and ionic conductors; meanwhile in traditional electrochemistry batteries and fuel cells generate electronic currents, which are physically separated from external metal wires responsible for the electronic conduction. Generators are constituted by separated phases of electronic conductors and ionic conductors. Electronic conductors form the circuit. Using theoretical models based on these separate and well defined kind of systems, where the exploited result is the electronic power, scientists were trying to understand biological processes where generators and conductors coincide, resulting in independent, simultaneous and specifically modulated ionic and chemical fluxes.

In electric circuits we only have one kind of carrier (electrons) and any information produced or sent using this support has to be performed by modulation of this carrier. Intercellular and intracellular communications are based on ionic carriers. The number of organic and inorganic ions available in a biological medium is very high and probably unknown. Information can be sent using, simultaneously, different carriers each modulated in a different way. As a result of that, biological systems transfer information in both senses and the same charge flowing through a biological system contains several orders of magnitude more information than in electronic systems. Even higher orders of magnitude can be speculated about information storage. Those are the main differences between silicon-based computers and the nervous system, which could be the origin that the same amount of dry material performs either, many more, more complex and simultaneous operations, including emotions, in brain material than in silicon-based computers.

Coming back to the starting ideas of this section, bioelectrochemical systems are three-dimensional systems involving chemical and conformational changes in biopolymers, linked to ionic fluxes. The electrochemical behavior of conducting polymers is the origin of bilayer and multilayer arrangements related to artificial muscles.

7.11. THE FUTURE

Conducting polymers were envisaged here, under electrochemical interactions, like soft, wet complex and multifunctional materials. Large and reverse composition changes are bound to large and reverse changes on properties, which mimic most of the biological functions characteristic of the organs from mammals.

Advances related to developments on artificial muscles, all organo-aqueous batteries (mimicking electric organs) or electrochromic devices (mimicking smart skins) have been presented. Basic ideas and preliminary results related to nervous interfaces, smart membranes or medical dosage were stated. All these subjects constitute a new, emerging and fascinating field of biomimicking materials. Biomimetism is considered here as the study of materials and material properties able to reproduce biological functions in both dense and soft tissues and organs.

Fast muscular contractions, rapid color changes from electrochromic devices or high charge and discharge rates of the all organic batteries require a wet technology: water is a good plasticizer allowing fast conformational changes during electrochemical reactions. Inside other solvents having a lower polymer-solvent interaction the kinetics of the electrochemical processes occur under a slow conformational relaxation control giving low rates for the concomitant functions.

A rapid development of the new devices —nervous interfaces, specific sensors and transducers— requires a deep understanding and control of the organic stereosynthesis of the initial monomers. As increasing number of scientist come into those fields, surprising new developments and devices will appear during the next two decades based on the multifunctional properties from the different families and groups of conducting polymers, once synthetic tasks are undertaken.

From a practical point of view, the present state of the technology provides muscles for microrobotics, micromachinery or medical instrumentation. All organic batteries are coming to the market and smart mirrors, windows and filters are being tested for some specific applications.

ACKNOWLEDGMENTS

The Spanish Ministerio de Educación y Ciencia, the Basque Government and the Gipuzkoako Foru Aldundia have supported this work.

REFERENCES

Baugman, R.H. and Shaklette, L.W. (1990) *Science and Applications of Conducting Polymers*, eds. Salaneck, W.R., Clark, D.T. and Samuelsen, E.J.), Adam Hilger, New York.

Bourgmayer, P. and Murray, R.W. (1982) *J. Am. Chem. Soc.*, **104**, 6139.

Jeronimidis, G. and Atkins, A.G. (1995) *Proc. Instn. Mech. Engrs.* **209** p. 221.

Kaneto, K., Kaneko, M., Min, Y., and MacDiarmid, A.G. (1995) *Synth. Met.*, **71**, 2211.

Okabayashi, K., Goto, F., Abe, K. and Yoshida (1987) *Synth. Met.* **18**, 365.

Otero, T.F. (1997) in *Handbook of Organic Conductive Molecules and Polymers*, Vol 4. ed Hari Singh Nalwa. (John Wiley & Sons).

Otero, T.F. (1999) in *Modern Aspects of Electrochemistry*, Vol. 33, Eds. Conway, B.E., Bockris J.O'M and White, R. (Plenum Press).

Otero, T.F. (1999) in *Polymer Sensors and Actuators*. Eds. Rossi, D. de and Osada, Y. (Springer-Verlag) in press.

Otero, T.F. and Grande, H. (1997) in *Handbook of Conducting Polymers* eds. Stotheim, T., Elsenhaumer, R. and Reynolds, J. (Marcel Dekker).

Otero, T.F. and Rodríguez, J. (1993) *Intrinsically Conducting Polymers. An Emerging Technology*. (Kluwer Academic).

Slama, M. and Tanguy, J. (1989) *Synth. Met.* **28**, C171.

Tourillon, G. and Garnier, F. (1984) *J. Electroanal. Chem.*, **161**, 51.

Viney. C. (1993) *Mater. Sci. and Eng.* **10**, 187.

Chapter 8

Biological Fibrous Materials: Self-Assembled Structures and Optimised Properties

Chapter 8

Biological Fibrous Materials: Self-Assembled Structures and Optimised Properties

EMILY RENUART and CHRISTOPHER VINEY

8.1. INTRODUCTION

8.1.1. Background

A great variety of Nature's structural materials are deposited in fibrous form. Examples include: silk, keratin, collagen, viral spike proteins, tubulin and actin (all of which are proteins), cellulose and chitin (polysaccharides), and even mucin (a glycoprotein). All are characterised by *hierarchical molecular order*. As a result, the influence of individual molecules on bulk physical properties is exerted through the manner and patterns in which the molecules are able to *self-assemble* into larger structures. The *liquid crystalline state* (often supramolecular) plays a pivotal role in this self-assembly process (Neville 1993; Viney 1993; Viney 1997a; Goodby 1998). *Water* is also significant, not just in maintaining the structural and functional integrity of some fibres (e.g. in muscle or the cytoskeleton), but also in promoting liquid crystallinity and supramolecular self assembly (McGrath and Butler 1997).

Hierarchical molecular order enables fibres and other biological materials to exhibit several optimised properties simultaneously. Such a material is said to be *multifunctional*. The optimised properties need not all relate to mechanical behaviour; they include characteristics such as responsiveness to electrical stimuli (muscle fibres), to chemical information (insect antennae) or to ambient water (capture threads in spider webs). Multifunctionality is possible because different features, at different length scales, can be tailored to optimise the different properties.

The catalogue of fibre-forming biological polymers is extended if we include those that can be spun or drawn from solution artificially. Many derivatives and analogues of biological polymers are fibre-forming as well. Again, the liquid crystalline state and / or supramolecular assembly remain important to the process of fibre assembly, and so dictate final structures and properties. Included here are DNA (Strzelecka *et al.* 1988; Reich *et al.* 1994; Stryer 1995), filamentous phage and other viruses (Marvin 1966; Fraden 1995; Tang and Fraden 1995; Dogic and Fraden 1997), bacterial polyesters (Brandl *et al.* 1990; Kemmish 1993), synthetic polypeptides such as PBLG [poly(γ-benzyl-*L*-glutamate)] (Robinson 1966; Horio *et al.* 1985), cellulose derivatives (Atkins *et al.* 1980; Gray 1983; Gilbert 1985), and chimeric systems in which very small amounts of a rodlike species can be used to impose molecular order on adsorbed molecular coils (Huber and Viney 1998).

8.1.2. Technological interest

From the materials chemistry and materials engineering points of view, studies of natural fibres promise a number of potentially useful lessons. Nature's range of functional materials represents the success stories of four billion years of research and development. Nature has achieved programmed supramolecular self-assembly mechanisms, hierarchical microstructures, property combinations and durability that are beyond the current know-how of materials industries. Several examples will be discussed in detail later in this chapter. The ability to appreciate Nature's lessons on structural materials has advanced greatly as a result of parallel advances in materials characterisation and molecular biology. Because natural materials are evolved in a complex, interacting environment, it is often possible to appreciate Nature's solution to a materials problem while the problem itself remains difficult to identify (Bain 1994).

Nature's structural materials are often damage-tolerant; in some cases they are even self-repairing. Natural materials additionally offer the attractions of biosynthesis (they are produced from renewable resources), benign processing conditions (they are assembled and shaped in an aqueous environment and at mild temperatures) and biodegradability (they break down into harmless components when exposed to specific environments). In the particular case of proteins, each material has a rigorously defined, highly reproducible primary structure. The molecules are monodisperse and stereoregular. Such well-defined molecular characterisability contrasts with the statistical heterogeneity of the molecules in a conventional synthetic polymer.

For proteins as well as some polysaccharides, the techniques of molecular biology can be used to genetically engineer host cells or even multicellular organisms that are capable of producing economic quantities of the desired material (Steinbüchel 1991; Ferrari and Cappello 1997; Tirrell *et al.* 1997). Polymers that already exist in Nature, derivatised (chemically modified) natural molecules, and entirely new materials can be produced in this way. The last of these options – de novo polymer design and synthesis – is especially successful with proteins.

8.1.3. Proteins as versatile materials

The building blocks of proteins (Rawn 1989; Creighton 1993; Stryer 1995) are α-amino acids -(CO-CHR-NH)$_n$- . They are chiral (except in the case of glycine, when the side-group R is hydrogen), and have the stereochemical structure shown in Figure 8.1. Specifically, Figure 8.1 illustrates the *L*-configuration; its mirror image is known as the *R*-configuration. Since all natural proteins are constructed from glycine and *L*-amino acids, the explicit *L* designation is often dropped from the notation. All

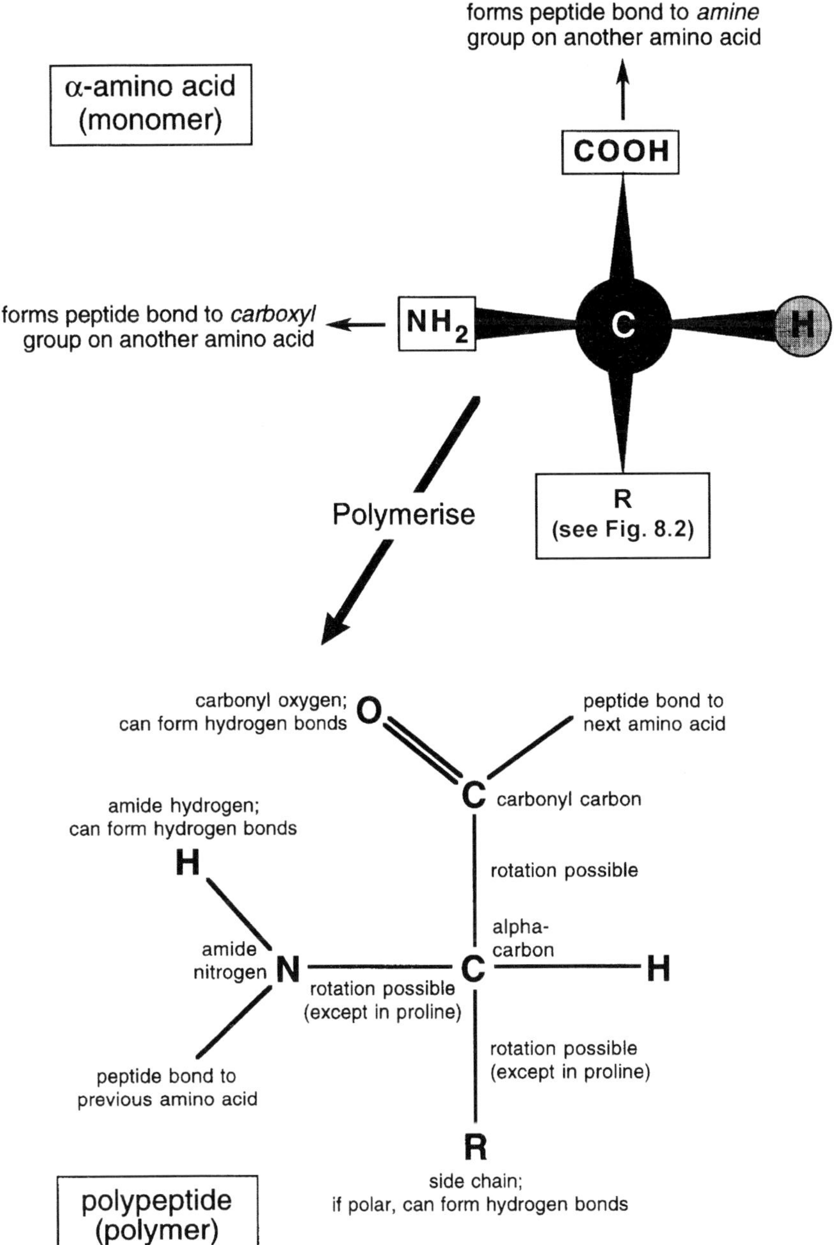

Fig. 8.1. Top: stereochemical configuration of a generic *L*-α-amino acid; examples of the side chain R are shown in Figure 8.2. Bottom: significant features of an amino acid residue in a polypeptide.

natural proteins are synthesized from only 21 types of amino acid, which are distinguished according to their R-group (Figure 8.2). Twenty of these amino acids are globally recognised in current textbooks; selenocysteine, the twenty-first, was identified relatively recently (F. Zinoni *et al.*, 1986; A. Bock *et al.*, 1991). In natural proteins, some of the amino acids undergo post-translational modification (i.e. chemical alteration subsequent to polymerisation), effectively increasing the number of different monomer types in the chain. Under contrived conditions, some bacteria can even be made to incorporate non-natural amino acids into protein chains, if these amino acids are closely related to naturally-occurring ones and are present in sufficient concentration in the culture medium. For example, the four non-natural amino acids shown in Figure 8.2 have been incorporated into proteins in this way; p-fluorophenylalanine can be substituted for phenylalanine, trifluoroleucine for leucine, norleucine for isoleucine, and selenomethionine for methionine (Dougherty *et al.* 1993; Yoshikawa *et al.* 1994).

Amino acids can be linked by peptide bonds, which join the amide nitrogen atom (Figure 8.1) of one residue to the carbonyl carbon atom (Figure 8.1) of another, accompanied by elimination of a molecule of water. The resulting polymers are called *peptides* if they are short chains of defined length and known amino acid sequence, *polypeptides* if they are longer chains with either the length or the sequence undefined, and *proteins* if they are long chains of specific length, sequence and three-dimensional folded conformation. Given (1) the large selection of available amino acids, (2) the fact that typical proteins contain around 500 amino acid residues (they can contain as many as 6000 in the case of some invertebrate collagens (Adams 1978)), it is clear that this family of molecules encompasses an extremely large number of possible primary structures. Included here are many biological fibrous materials, several types of non-fibrous connective tissue, enzymes, motor proteins, membrane proteins, proteins involved in the transport of metabolites, and all antibodies.

Why are these compounds so successful at providing the molecular basis of so many different functions?

Part of the answer lies in the intrinsic flexibility of the molecular backbones. While relative rotation of the molecular segments on either side of a peptide bond is inhibited by electron delocalization from the adjacent carbonyl group, rotation can in general occur about the other N-C bonds as well as the C-C bonds in a protein polymer backbone. (An exception occurs at proline residues, where the side-chain forms a ring structure with the amide nitrogen, leaving only the backbone C-C bond free to rotate.) The available rotational freedom imparts flexibility to the chain, so that proteins have the potential to fold into a large number of possible conformations. Main chain flexibility can be frustrated by steric interaction between (large) side groups, so the primary structure is a significant factor in determining the shapes which protein molecules can adopt.

Another source of the versatility of these molecules, and a principal factor determining the actual conformation of a given protein, is summarised in Figure 8.2. The behaviour of the R-groups in aqueous environments is extremely important. Non-polar side-groups will cause the chain to be locally hydrophobic, while polar side-groups will impart a hydrophilic character. Acidic side-groups will donate a proton to

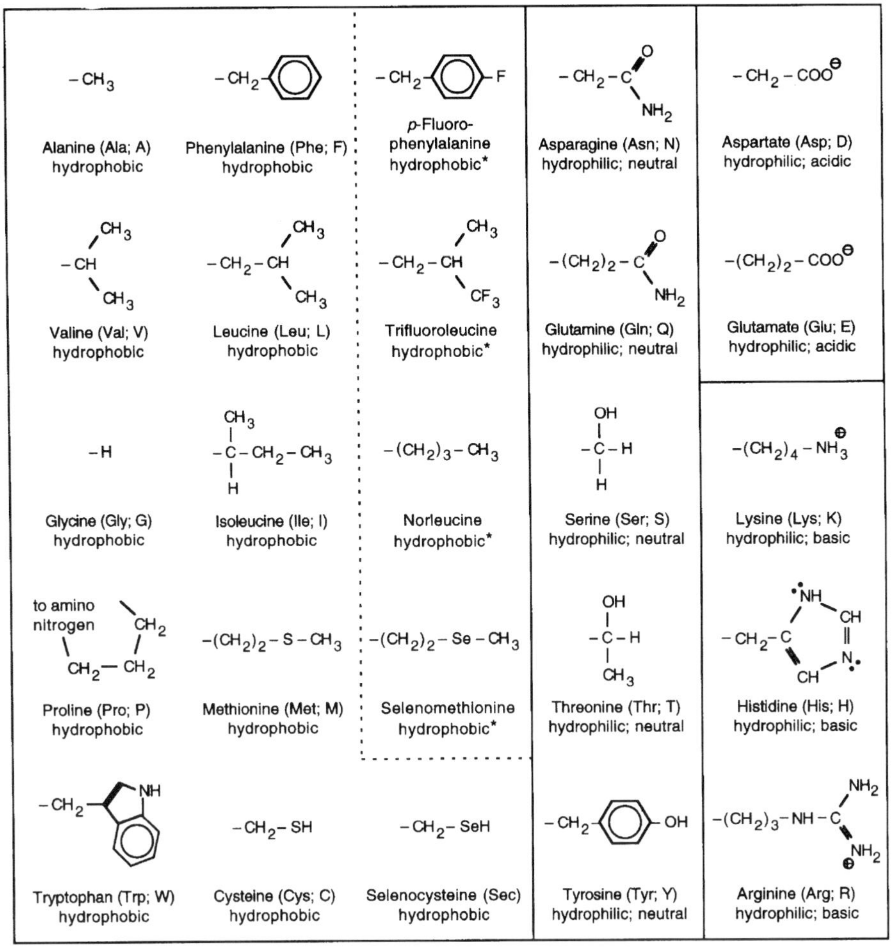

$-CH_3$ Alanine (Ala; A) hydrophobic	$-CH_2-$(ring) Phenylalanine (Phe; F) hydrophobic	$-CH_2-$(ring)$-F$ *p*-Fluoro-phenylalanine hydrophobic*	$-CH_2-C(=O)-NH_2$ Asparagine (Asn; N) hydrophilic; neutral	$-CH_2-COO^{\ominus}$ Aspartate (Asp; D) hydrophilic; acidic
$-CH(CH_3)(CH_3)$ Valine (Val; V) hydrophobic	$-CH_2-CH(CH_3)(CH_3)$ Leucine (Leu; L) hydrophobic	$-CH_2-CH(CH_3)(CF_3)$ Trifluoroleucine hydrophobic*	$-(CH_2)_2-C(=O)-NH_2$ Glutamine (Gln; Q) hydrophilic; neutral	$-(CH_2)_2-COO^{\ominus}$ Glutamate (Glu; E) hydrophilic; acidic
$-H$ Glycine (Gly; G) hydrophobic	$-C(CH_3)(H)-CH_2-CH_3$ Isoleucine (Ile; I) hydrophobic	$-(CH_2)_3-CH_3$ Norleucine hydrophobic*	$-C(OH)(H)-H$ Serine (Ser; S) hydrophilic; neutral	$-(CH_2)_4-NH_3^{\oplus}$ Lysine (Lys; K) hydrophilic; basic
to amino nitrogen $\backslash CH_2-CH_2-CH_2$ Proline (Pro; P) hydrophobic	$-(CH_2)_2-S-CH_3$ Methionine (Met; M) hydrophobic	$-(CH_2)_2-Se-CH_3$ Selenomethionine hydrophobic*	$-C(OH)(H)-CH_3$ Threonine (Thr; T) hydrophilic; neutral	$-CH_2-C$ (ring: NH, CH, N, CH) Histidine (His; H) hydrophilic; basic
$-CH_2-$(ring, NH) Tryptophan (Trp; W) hydrophobic	$-CH_2-SH$ Cysteine (Cys; C) hydrophobic	$-CH_2-SeH$ Selenocysteine (Sec) hydrophobic	$-CH_2-$(ring)$-OH$ Tyrosine (Tyr; Y) hydrophilic; neutral	$-(CH_2)_3-NH-C(NH_2)(NH_2^{\oplus})$ Arginine (Arg; R) hydrophilic; basic

Fig. 8.2. Structure of the R-groups (side chains) in each of the 21 L-α-amino acids from which the known natural proteins are synthesised. Four non-natural amino acids, marked with an asterisk, are included in the middle column; each is situated immediately to the right of the natural amino acid to which it corresponds most closely. The conventional three-letter and one-letter abbreviations for each natural amino acid are shown, as are the aqueous solution characteristics of the side chains.

an aqueous environment initially at pH 7, and basic side-groups will accept a proton from such an environment. The charge distribution along the molecules therefore will be sensitive to the presence of other charged species in their surroundings, and so will depend on pH and dissolved ions. The flexible protein chains will tend to fold in a way that allows hydrophobic segments to be screened from the water by the more hydrophilic segments; in turn this promotes the formation of noncovalent intramolecular and intermolecular bonds between positively charged and negatively charged sites.

So the three-dimensional structure of a protein depends on the nature and sequence of the amino acid side chains along the molecule, on the related backbone flexibility, on the characteristics of the aqueous environment, and on the proximity of neighbouring protein molecules.

8.1.4. Limitations of proteins in materials engineering

There are many factors that limit the viability of genetically altered organisms as a source of functional polymers: the stability of the altered gene (to mutation as well as to repair), toxic effects of the foreign protein on the host organism, intracellular degradation of the foreign protein by the host's enzymes, and the extent to which the desired protein can be recovered in useful amounts and in a processable form (Tirrell *et al.* 1991a; Tirrell *et al.* 1991b; Tirrell *et al.* 1994; Ferrari and Cappello 1997; Tirrell *et al.* 1997). The last factor often receives insufficient attention. If a natural protein contains sequences that constitute a significant microstructural feature in a biological material, the genetically engineered equivalent should not be based exclusively on multiple repeats of that sequence. More generally, it should not be assumed that final microstructure must directly reflect every detail of the primary structure. Some aspects of primary structure have evolved – and therefore must be considered when designing genetically engineered equivalents – to facilitate the protein's self-assembly into the desired material. Also, we have already noted that Nature does not achieve multifunctionality by relying on simple microstructures with significant features at just one length scale. In natural proteinaceous material, perfectly repeated structure can be assumed at the level of whole molecules (whose primary structure is controlled by DNA), but not at submolecular or supramolecular scales.

Enthusiasm for the positive attributes of biological materials must be tempered with realistic concessions to the limitations of Nature (Vogel 1992). Nature's technological success stories do not imply intrinsically superior design; rather, they simply represent the product of continuous evolution in response to changes in environmental conditions over very long periods of time. The necessary steps have been small and several. Nature has had more time than we do to solve materials problems, but other essential commodities (information storage capacity, energy supply rates, and diversity of available monomeric building blocks) are constrained in Nature. Many materials that engineers find invaluable have no counterpart in Nature, because natural selection exerted no pressure to evolve such materials. For example, modern technology needs fibres to reinforce composites that retain useful properties at high temperatures: consider the carbon-carbon composite in the brakes of a large aircraft, or ceramic-reinforced metal matrix composites proposed for use in jet engine turbine blades. Such materials have to survive for extended periods at 1000°C or more. No biological material with equivalent high temperature properties has been identified. However, bacteria have been found in the extreme environments that prevail near crustal cracks in the sea-floor (Barros and Deming 1983). Temperatures there can approach 350°C. Other bacteria thrive at high temperatures around sulphur vents on volcanoes, and in porous rocks thousands of meters below the earth's surface (Fredrickson and Onstott 1996). The resident bacteria must be able to synthesise and maintain thermally stable proteins, which suggests that genetically engineered proteins with similar (and perhaps greater?) stability should be attainable. The prospects of artificially evolving proteins for application in non-natural environments are encouraging (Arnold 1993).

Natural mechanisms of materials production are complex and/or slow in comparison to their *in vitro* counterparts and so appear economically unattractive. Spiders spin fibre at rates greater than any other organism, but even they can only manage semicontinuous production at 10 $cm.s^{-1}$, which is two to three orders of magnitude less than the rates which are typical of industrial dry solution spinning (Billmeyer 1984). One of the greatest challenges to implementing Nature's microstructural lessons in the context of artificial fibres relates to economical processing rates. It remains to be seen whether slow production is an inescapable price of Nature's advanced lessons for "green" materials processing and for achieving unrivalled combinations of optimised properties.

8.2. NATURE'S FIBROUS MATERIALS

8.2.1. ***Keratins*** (Rawn 1989)

8.2.1.1. Alpha-helices (Branden and Tooze 1991; Creighton 1993; Stryer 1995). The fundamental structural unit in keratin fibres is the α-helix. Individual, intrinsically flexible protein chains in keratin adopt a twisted conformation that exhibits the following characteristics:

a.- The twist is right-handed.

b.- Each turn of the helix requires 3.6 amino acids, i.e. 11 backbone atoms. The separation of adjacent amino acids, as measured in projection along the axis of the helix, is approximately 1.5 Å.

c.- The side chains extend outwards from the helix, and therefore interact with the environment.

d.- Stability is maintained by intramolecular hydrogen bonds; the carbonyl oxygen of residue i bonds to the amide hydrogen of residue $i+4$ (counting from the amino end towards the carboxyl end) along the length of the helix.

Throughout this chapter, a recurring theme is that hydrogen bonds provide necessary stability in many contexts of biological fibre self-assembly. While hydrogen bonds occur between partial charges, and so are individually weaker than covalent or ionic bonds, their effect becomes significant when it is possible for a large number of them to form.

The α-helix was first described by Pauling and Corey in 1951 (Pauling *et al.* 1951). It is one of the simplest regular conformations that a sequence of amino acids in a protein can adopt. It is also a common conformation, not limited to fibre-forming proteins, but equally not a prerequisite of fibre formation. When it does occur in fibre-forming proteins, it tends to account for all the secondary structure, i.e. the entire molecule is α-helical.

What factors stabilise α-helices? Attempts to state generalisations are made complicated by the delicate balance of intramolecular and intermolecular forces involved. Some trends include:

a.- Affinity between the solvent and the amino acid R-groups is required, otherwise the molecule will fold so as to protect these groups from the solvent. However, if the solvent is too polar, the helix will be denatured, because the intramolecular hydrogen bonds necessary for helix formation are replaced by polymer-solvent bonds.
b.- Proline is rarely found in α-helices, because its configuration generates a conformationally rigid kink in the molecule, that is incompatible with a smooth helical trajectory. Also, proline residues do not have an amide hydrogen, and so they cannot contribute fully to the hydrogen bonding pattern of an α-helix.
c.- Homopolypeptide sequences (e.g. consisting purely of alanine, leucine or phenylalanine) often form α-helices, unless the R-groups are highly charged (e.g. arginine or glutamate). This observation can be regarded as a corollary of the necessary solvent properties noted above. In the case of synthetic homopolypeptides, it is possible for *entire* molecules to adopt the α-helical conformation (Elliott and Ambrose 1950; Fasman 1991).
d.- If the protein contains both hydrophilic and hydrophobic residues, an α-helix on its own would not be stable in an aqueous environment. However, if the hydrophobic residues are concentrated on one side of the helix, then two or more helices can interact in a manner that places the hydrophobic surfaces in mutual contact. To test whether an amino acid sequence can form an α-helix with a hydrophobic stripe along one side, the sequence is plotted on a helical wheel (Branden and Tooze 1991; Creighton 1993) as shown in Figure 8.3. In non-aqueous environments, there are additional schemes for helix stabilisation and supramolecular ordering, especially if the environment is isotropic (Imanishi *et al.* 1996).

Alpha-helical structures have recently been identified in solutions of *polypeptoids* – polymers that are related to, but distinct from, polypeptides (Borman 1998). In polypeptoids, the side chains are attached to the amide nitrogens instead of the central (alpha) carbons. The lack of amide hydrogens precludes formation of the intramolecular hydrogen bonds that stabilise α-helices in proteins. Nevertheless, polypeptoids can adopt a right-handed α-helical conformation (Kirshenbaum *et al.* 1998). Polypeptoids are less susceptible to chemical degradation, and can be produced at one tenth of the cost, compared to polypeptides. They are of interest as novel polymeric materials with properties intermediate between those of proteins and engineering plastics.

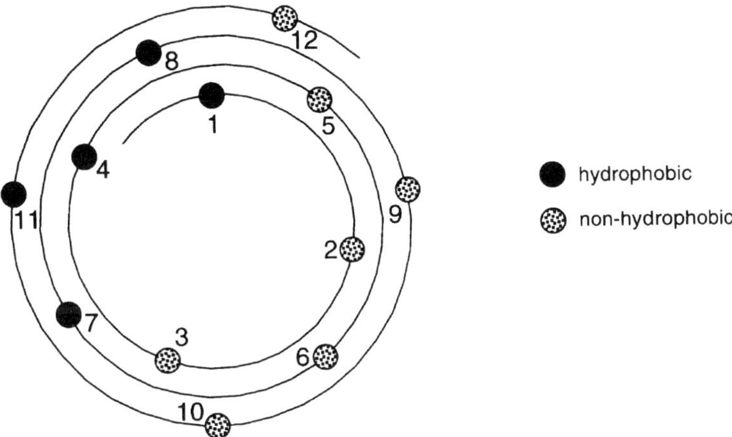

Fig. 8.3. Helical wheel (spiral) used to illustrate the distribution of side chain characteristics in polypeptide helices. The amino acids are plotted in sequence around the spiral, noting the polar or hydrophobic nature of each side chain. The angular separation of successive amino acids is preserved in the plot. In the specific example shown here, a hypothetical sequence of 12 amino acids in an α-helix is considered. Since an α-helix involves 3.6 amino acids per turn, the angular separation of successive amino acids is 100°. The α-helix is found to have a hydrophobic stripe along one side, and so would be a candidate for constructing a double helix or a supercoil stabilised by hydrophobic interactions.

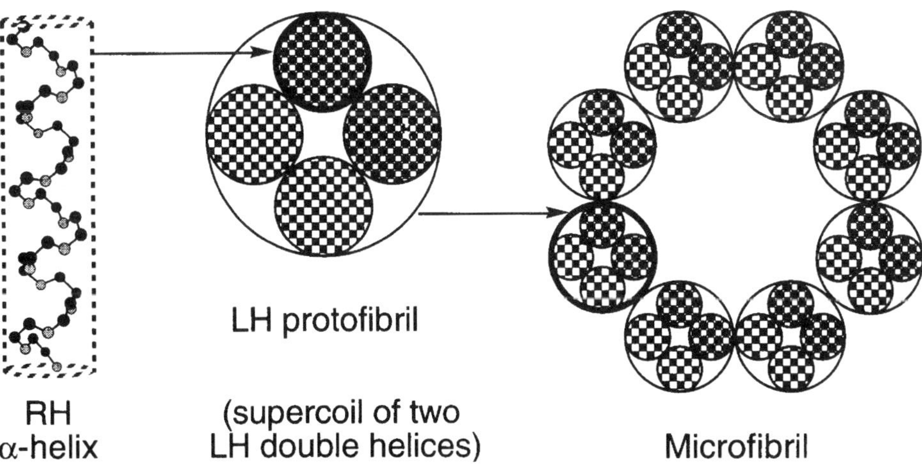

Fig. 8.4. Hierarchical structure of a keratin microfibril. The representation of a molecular α-helix shows only the $[\text{-N-C-C-}]_n$ backbone for clarity.

8.2.1.2. ***Supercoils*** (Branden and Tooze 1991; Stryer 1995). The next level of the hierarchical structure of keratin is formed by two right-handed α-helices winding into a left-handed double helix. Two of these double helices are combined in a left-handed supercoil, forming a keratin protofibril. Eight protofibrils are arranged into a microfibril (Figure 8.4). In some keratins, the microfibrils do not have a hollow core, but they still consist of eight protofibrils (Rawn 1989). The supercoils are stabilised by the juxtaposition of hydrophobic side chains over an extensive contact length. Intermolecular disulphide links, involving cysteine residues, confer additional stability.

8.2.1.3. ***Properties***. The bulk properties of keratin depend on the degree and nature of *cross-linking* within fibres, on the ambient *moisture* content, and on the relative amounts of *fibre and matrix*.

The molecular and supercoil twists in keratin occur in opposite directions. Attempts to unwind the left-handed twist will tighten the right-handed twist, and vice versa, so that fibres are stiff and resilient in tension. In this respect, the hierarchical microstructure of keratin is analogous to that found in a rope. At the same time, the hydrogen bonds and hydrophobic interactions that stabilise the supercoils permit intrinsic flexibility in bending, provided that there is little or no disulphide (covalent) cross-linking. The following list of materials, covering a very wide range of properties, is arranged according to increasing covalent cross-link density:

wool < hair < horn and tortoiseshell < beaks and claws

Hydrogen bonding makes keratin susceptible to moisture – hence the traditional use of hair in humidity-detecting "weather houses". The Young's modulus of hair can decrease by a factor of almost 3, and the shear modulus can decrease by a factor of 15, for a wet fibre in comparison to a dry one (Fraser *et al.* 1972). Indeed, all fibrous proteins have the potential to exhibit significant moisture sensitivity as a result of their hydrogen bonds; only extensive covalent cross-linking can reduce this sensitivity. Nevertheless, humidity often is not controlled or recorded at the time of mechanical testing, so the literature does not provide a consistent, reliable source of quantitative mechanical property data for fibrous proteins. (The comparison of published mechanical test data for biological materials in general can be haphazard. Not only moisture content, but also sample geometry, gauge length, strain rate, and temperature should at least be recorded, and if possible chosen relative to a known standard. Where standards do not exist, it would be valuable if agreed procedures were developed and adhered to.)

The keratin fibres are dispersed in a protein matrix. As is the case with artificial engineering composites, the mechanical properties depend on the volume fraction of the fibres, and on their orientation relative to the loading geometry. In fingernails, the fibres are deposited normal to the growth direction and parallel to the surface. In hair, the fibres are aligned parallel to the growth direction. Rhinoceros horn is reinforced by an interwoven network of fibres, to minimise the possibility of splitting (Fraser *et al.* 1972).

8.2.2. ***Collagens*** (Stryer 1988; Rawn 1989; Gorham 1991)

8.2.2.1 ***Collagen helices***. The individual linear unbranched polymer chains in collagen are called *procollagen*. Their general formula is (Gly-X-Y)$_n$, where many of the residues X and Y are proline.

The inflexibility of the backbone N-C bond within proline (Figure 8.2) promotes the formation of helical conformations that are more stretched out than the α-helix described above. Many of the prolines, and also some lysines undergo post-translational modification to 4-hydroxyproline (Hyp) and 5-hydroxylysine (Hyl) residues respectively (Figure 8.5).

The left-handed procollagen helices self-assemble into right-handed triple-helical supercoils. Assembly and stability are promoted by several factors:

a. The sequence of residues at the carboxyl end of procollagen contains cysteine, and therefore is capable of forming disulphide bonds with the corresponding sequence on an adjacent molecule. (The carboxy-terminal sequence is known as an *extension peptide*, because it is discarded at a later stage of collagen synthesis; its principal function appears to be the formation of disulphide bonds essential to triple-helix nucleation; the remainder of the procollagen sequence does not contain cysteine).

b. Intramolecular and intermolecular hydrogen bonding is extensive. Such interactions are promoted by the presence of the hydroxyl groups in hydroxyproline and hydroxylysine residues, which can hydrogen bond via bridging water molecules: -OH -- HOH -- HO-. Indeed, if procollagen is insufficiently hydroxylated, this seriously disrupts the ability of the protein to self-assemble into higher levels of structure. In humans, hydroxylation depends on the presence of ascorbic acid; deficiency leads to scurvy, which is characterised by fragile blood vessels, tendons and skin.

An alternative role for Hyp and Hyl in stabilising the collagen triple helix has been proposed (Holmgren *et al.* 1998; Roubi 1998). The immobilisation of bridging water to form hydrogen bonds – involving approximately 500 water molecules per collagen triple helix – represents a sizable entropy loss. Model triple helices made from (Gly-Flp-Pro)$_{10}$ strands (where Flp = fluoroproline; the 4-hydroxylation in Hyp has been replaced by 4-fluorination) are more stable than triple helices which consist of (Gly-Hyp-Pro)$_{10}$, even though the fluorine does not participate significantly in hydrogen bond formation. Both -OH and -F are electron-withdrawing groups, -F more so than -OH, and it is suggested that electron withdrawal from the backbone favours conformations which are characteristic of collagen triple helices.

c. The primary sequence and the conformation of procollagen together generate a hydrophobic stripe of glycine residues along one side of the helix. Glycine has a small side chain (hydrogen), so there is room to accommodate the glycine residues in the space between three close-packed helices (Figure 8.6).

Proline residue

4-Hydroxyproline residue

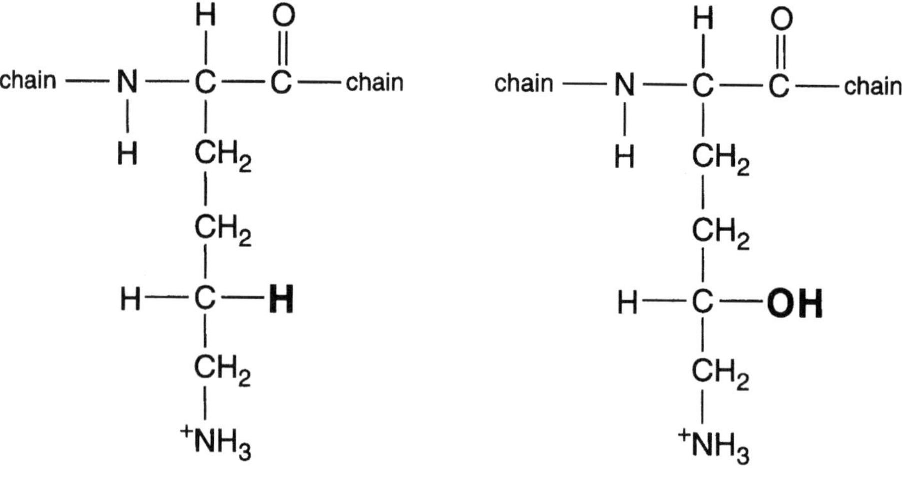

Lysine residue

5-Hydroxylysine residue

Fig. 8.5. Relationship of 4-hydroxyproline and 5-hydroxylysine to proline and lysine respectively. The numerical component of the full names identifies which carbon atom (counting sequentially from the carbonyl carbon in the main chain) has been hydroxylated.

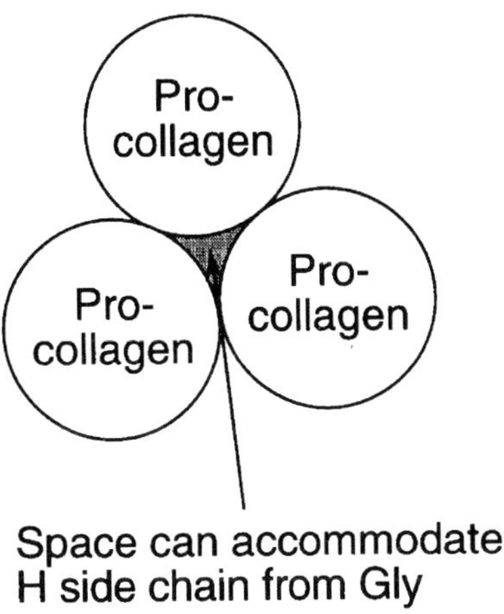

Fig. 8.6. Arbitrary transverse cross-section through a collagen triple helix, showing the local envelope occupied by each strand. Only glycine has a side chain (hydrogen) that is small enough to fit into the space between the individual strands.

We see that the interplay between bonding types and entropic effects, acting to stabilise fibrous structure in biological materials, is subtle and complex. Attempts to produce artificial analogues of such structure must recognise that there are several superimposed contributions to stability in the natural material.

8.2.2.2. Tropocollagen and collagen. Subsequent stages in the hierarchical assembly of collagen occur *outside* the cell. The extension peptides are cleaved off by enzymes, leaving *tropocollagen* triple helices. Tropocollagen then self-organises into a wide variety of structures, many of which exhibit features typical of liquid crystalline order: nematic (Gathercole *et al.* 1989), simple cholesteric (Bouligand and Giraud-Guille 1985; Giraud-Guille 1987), blue phase (Lepescheux 1988) and smectic (Hukins and Woodhead-Galloway 1977). The molecular order in these liquid crystalline phases is illustrated in Figure 8.7. Significantly for self-assembly at supramolecular length scales (Neville 1993), liquid crystalline order is also observed in solutions of collagen (Giraud-Guille 1989; Giraud-Guille 1992).

Several factors combine to stabilise collagen. Hydrophobic side chains are juxtaposed over an extensive contact length. Proline and its derivatives maintain the fundamental helix pitch. Two thirds of the amino acid residues are involved in hydrogen bonds (Stryer 1988). Covalent cross-linking occurs within and between tropocollagen triple helices: there are no disulphide bonds, due to the absence of cysteine, but lysine residues provide an alternative means of covalent bonding (Figure 8.8).

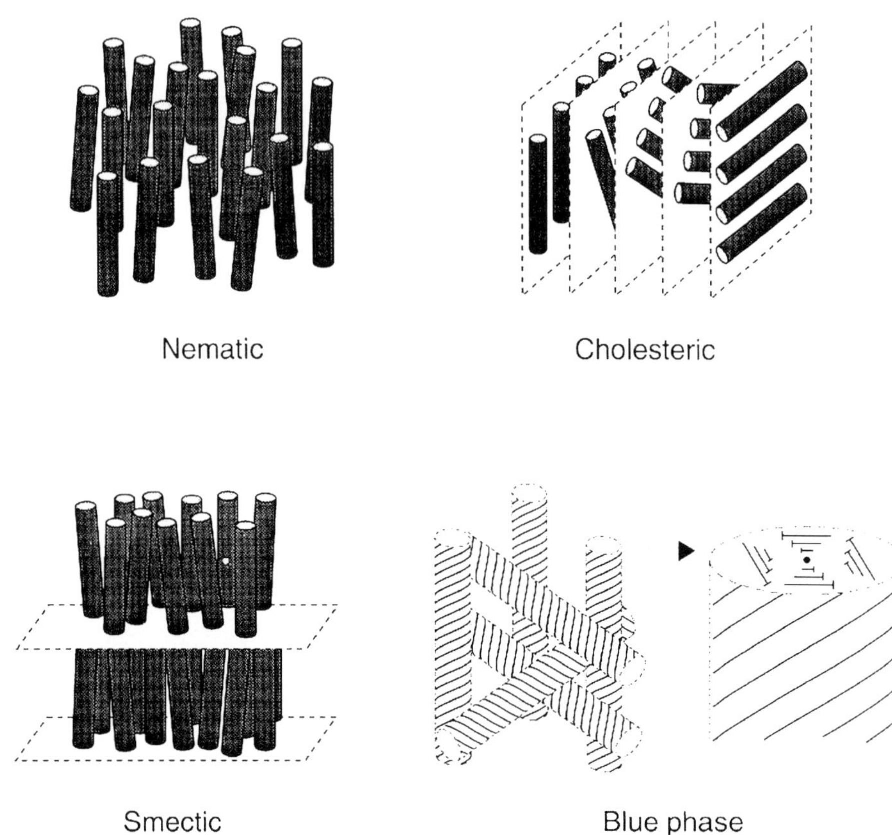

Fig. 8.7. Types of liquid crystalline order. In the illustrations of nematic, smectic and cholesteric order, local order of rod-like molecules is shown explicitly. For the blue phase, the solid lines and "nails" indicate the changing molecular orientation within more complex, cylindrical domains.

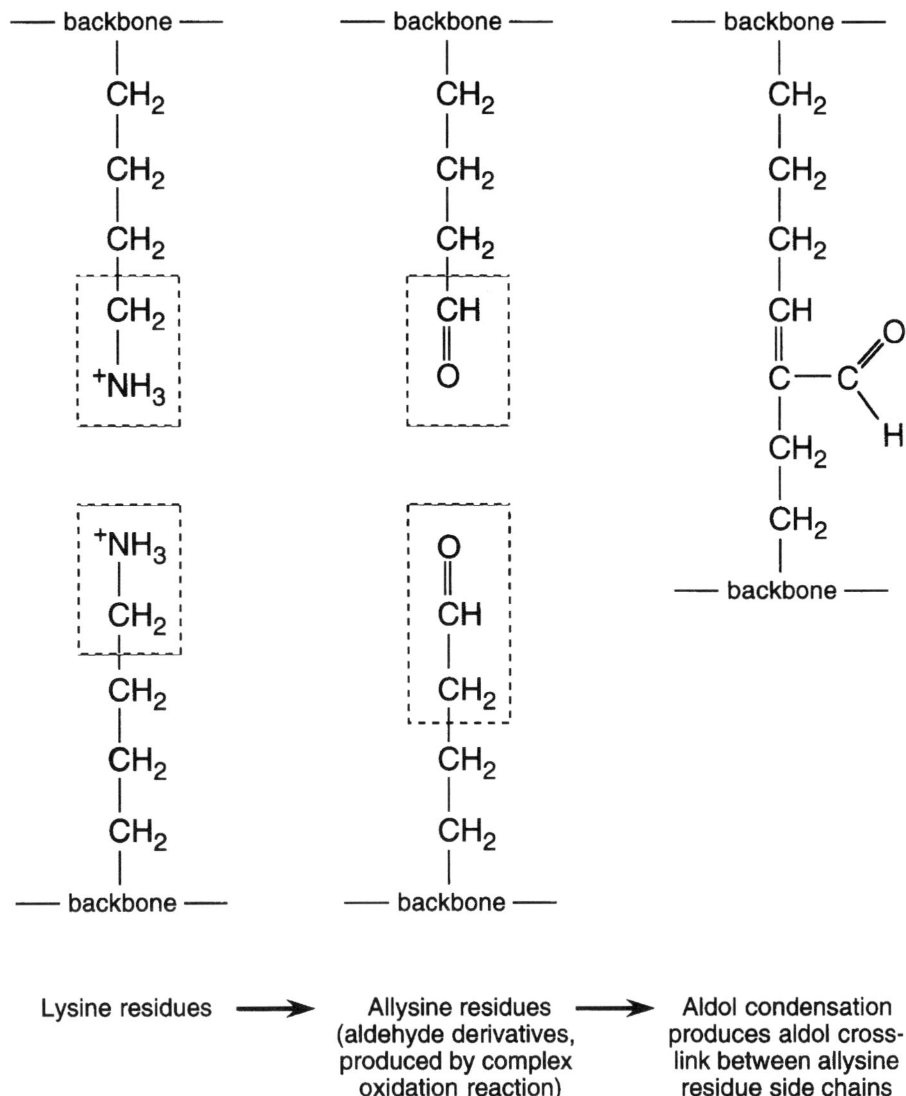

Fig. 8.8. An example of how lysine residues can react to form a covalent cross-link in collagen. Specifically, this diagram shows the formation of an *intra*molecular cross-link. More complex reactions, involving two hydroxylysines and one lysine, are involved in the formation of covalent *inter*molecular cross-links.

8.2.2.3. ***Properties.*** Collagens are the most abundant family of proteins in vertebrates. More than a quarter of the protein in mammals is collagen (Smith and Wood 1991). It is a versatile structural material, found in diverse contexts that encompass bone, teeth, cartilage, tendon, skin, and blood vessels. It is also the material from which the cornea of the eye is made; in this context its structure is optimised for optical as well as mechanical performance. The hierarchical microstructure of collagen confers outstanding damage tolerance and toughness.

The bulk properties of collagen depend on factors similar to those which affect keratin. The degree and nature of cross-linking within fibres (which increases with age), the ambient moisture content, and the relative amounts of fibre and matrix (in composite materials such as bones, teeth and cartilage) all have a significant effect. In addition, the mechanical properties of collagen depend on temperature.

Molecular and supercoil twists in tropocollagen occur in opposite directions. Tropocollagen therefore is stiff and strong in tension. At coarser length scales there can be additional levels of "rope-within-rope" structural hierarchy, as well as pleated structures (e.g. in tendon) that enhance extensibility without sacrificing ultimate tensile strength. The breaking strength of rat tail tendon is approximately 60 MPa, while the tensile modulus depends on the age of the rat (Woodhead-Galloway 1980). In the case of corneal tissue, the tropocollagen is arranged into 0°/90° "plywood" stacks, achieving high levels of crystallinity and optical transparency. Collagen is remarkably resilient: a human lifetime of 70 years and heart rate of 70 beats per minute equate to 2.6×10^9 heartbeats, each of which requires a reliable elastic response from the collagen-reinforced arterial walls.

The mechanical properties of collagen depend on the orientation of fibres relative to the loading geometry, and on the volume fraction and exact composition of any matrix phase. We have already noted the fibre orientation in tendons and corneas; in skin the collagen fibres are arranged in a pattern reminiscent of woven sheets. If the matrix can be made either stiff or fluid by tuning its ionic composition, highly aligned bundles of collagen fibres can either be locked in place or be allowed great freedom for relative displacement. This situation occurs in the "catch apparatus" – the ligament which stabilises the ball-and-socket joint between the shell and spine – of sea urchins (Trotter and Koob 1989). When the matrix is made fluid and the joint is unlocked, strains of over 200% are possible.

Non-covalent cross-linking is sensitive to temperature. Tropocollagen has a *melting temperature*, defined as the temperature above which more than half of the helical structure is destroyed (forming gelatin, which has a random coil conformation) (Stryer 1995). The melting temperature is an increasing function of the level of hydroxylation. Given the cost in material and energy, organisms will not perform more hydroxylations than necessary. Therefore hydroxylation levels are high in warm blooded animals, and low in arctic-dwelling cold blooded animals. Levels of covalent cross-linking are also lower in the collagen of cold blooded species, to retain flexibility.

8.2.3. Silks

Silks are described in detail elsewhere in this volume. However, for completeness in the context of fibre self-assembly, it is worth emphasising here that helices are not a fundamental structural requirement in fibre-forming systems.

8.2.3.1. ***Beta-strands, beta-sheets and beta-sheet crystals***. The ß-strand is another simple, regular conformation that can be adopted by a sequence of amino acids in a protein. Like the α-helix, it was first described by Pauling and Corey in 1951 (Pauling and Corey 1951). Individual, intrinsically flexible protein chains with this conformation exhibit the following characteristics:

a. The chains are almost fully extended. If there is a twist, it is right handed and gradual, ranging from an effectively infinite pitch in spider drag line silk (Thiel *et al.* 1997), to several hundred Ångstroms in many other protein crystals (Creighton 1993).
b. The separation of adjacent amino acids, as projected onto the axis of the strand, is approximately 3.5 Å.
c. Successive side chains extend in opposite directions, perpendicular to the strand (Figure 8.9), and therefore can interact with the environment.
d. Stability of the conformation is maintained by hydrogen bonds between the carbonyl oxygen and amide hydrogen on residues in different polypeptides (Figure 8.9). These polypeptides may belong to the same protein chain or to different chains, and they may run in the same (parallel) direction or in opposite (antiparallel) directions.

The preceding list is organised along similar lines to that in which the principal characteristics of α-helices were described.

Figure 8.9 shows that ß-strands follow a zig-zag trajectory. When hydrogen-bonded to neighbouring strands, they form pleated sheet-like structures, usually referred to as ß-sheets. The sheets can stack into three-dimensional ß-sheet crystals (Figure 8.9) in which the separation of the sheets is dictated by the size of the side groups that must be accommodated within that space.

8.2.3.2. ***Properties***. Silks exhibit a wide range of optimised tensile properties (Vollrath 1994): stiffness of the radial threads of spider webs, compliance of capture spiral of webs, and toughness of egg cocoons. Chapter 10 describes the relationship between primary structure, crystal architecture and properties of silks in detail, and provides representative values of silk tensile properties.

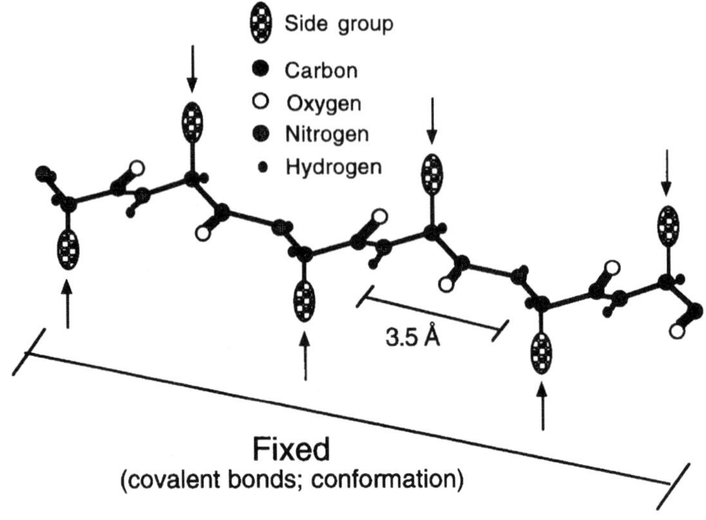

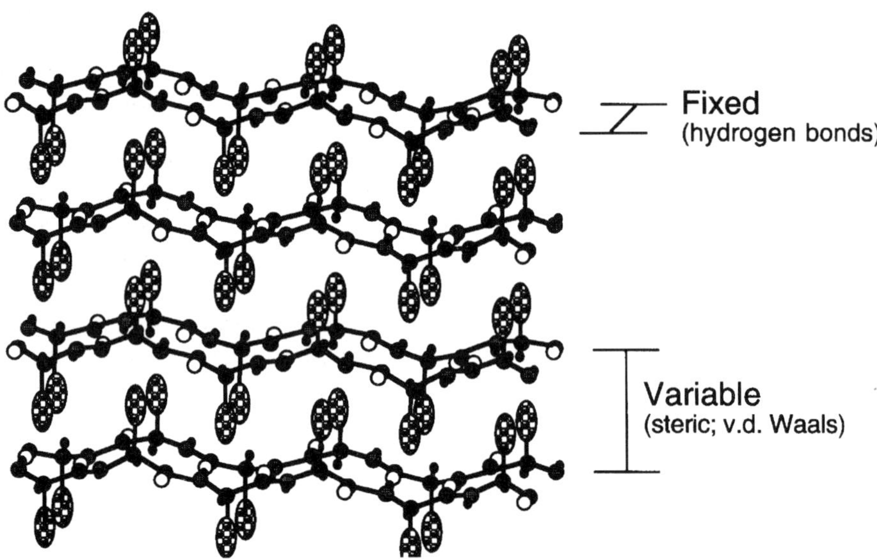

Fig. 8.9. Top: schematic representation of a generic ß-strand, viewed from a perspective that illustrates its zig-zag trajectory. Bottom: a ß-sheet crystal produced by stacking four ß-sheets. The factors that dictate the principal crystallographic separations within a ß-sheet crystal are identified.

Beta-sheet crystals reinforce silk fibres, conferring strength and stiffness due to the extended conformation of their constituent chains. Segments of the same polymer chains that build ß-sheet crystals also make up the amorphous phase, so that there is no discrete interface between these phases. As a result, the material can extend significantly once the yield strength imparted by the crystalline phase is exceeded. Silks therefore can exhibit high strains to failure. As is the case with all fibrous materials discussed in the present chapter, multifunctionality is achieved by microstructural complexity, which itself is the result of a complex primary structure (Thiel and Viney 1995b; Thiel and Viney 1995a; Thiel *et al.* 1997; Thiel and Viney 1997).

Hydrogen bonding and water are important to silk in several respects. The individual as-secreted protein molecules in silk have no regular elements of secondary structure and are folded into a globular tertiary structure; the conformation is stabilised by intramolecular hydrogen bonds which balance favourable interactions between water molecules and hydrophilic residues at the surface of the globular coils. At higher protein concentrations, the coils assemble into linear aggregates (Viney *et al.* 1994; Viney 1997b); the driving force for this process has not been quantified, but may be due to the greater entropy achieved when bound water is released from the surface of coils and replaced with coil-coil interactions. (Similar explanations for the aggregation of globular protein into linear supramolecular structures have been offered in the case of both actin and tubulin fibres, as will be discussed below.) The solution of linear aggregates forms a processable liquid crystalline phase (Kerkam *et al.* 1991), which spiders and silkworms use to produce water-insoluble fibre from water-soluble polymer. The intramolecular hydrogen bonding pattern is disrupted, chains are extended, and hydrophobic residues are exposed to water as the solution is spun; ß-sheet crystals develop from the more regular and hydrophobic amino acid sequences. Their hydrophobic side chain content, dense molecular packing, and extensive hydrogen bonding between backbones makes the crystals insoluble in water.

Water plays two important roles with respect to the macroscopic properties of silks. Spider drag line undergoes very large, non-volumetric dimensional changes that depend on moisture content, allowing spiders to achieve the correct tension in the web framework as it is spun (Work 1985). The energy dissipation mechanisms available to capture thread are partly the result of its microstructure (Gosline *et al.* 1995), and partly the result of a unique windlass mechanism, the latter depending on the presence of a water-based proteinaceous glue that coats the fibres (Vollrath 1994). The glue has a low surface energy with respect to the fibre, but a high surface energy with respect to air. Therefore, it favours maximum contact with the fibre and minimum contact with the air. A uniform thin coating of fluid glue on a straight fibre would be unstable (Stewart and Golubitsky 1992), so the glue exists as a series of discrete droplets. When the thread is extended by the impact of prey, the glue is spread out over its surface; subsequently the droplets re-form, slack thread is coiled into the droplets, and coalescence of droplets restores tension in the fibre.

8.2.4. Viral spike protein

The relatively small amount of genetic information stored in a virus means that simple and / or repeated motifs occur in the protein that makes up the surrounding capsid (coat). An analogy is provided by the "do loops" used in computer programming. The structural characteristics of virus coats are highly relevant to virus propagation, and therefore are the subject of intensive study – the coat must protect the nucleic acid (genetic) contents, be resilient against impact, be capable of broaching the outer wall of a target cell, and provide a secure pathway for conducting nucleic acid into the target. Hollow spikes on the capsid fulfil the latter two roles, from which it has been deduced that they must have unusually high strength and stiffness in axial compression (O'Brien 1993). Because compressive strength and stiffness have been a long-term elusive goal of polymer science (Santhosh *et al.* 1995; Sikkema 1998), the hierarchical structure of spike proteins deserves careful attention.

8.2.4.1. Cross-ß-sheets. Viral spike protein contains several repeats of relatively short ß-strand-forming amino acid sequences. The chain folds back and forth to assemble a ß-sheet, stabilised by intramolecular hydrogen bonds (Figure 8.10). Specifically, because the long axis of the sheet is transverse to the molecular backbone, this is known as a *cross-ß-sheet.*

8.2.4.2. Higher-order structure. Controversy still surrounds the detailed higher order structure of viral spikes, and there appears to be considerable diversity of structure between virus types (Green *et al.* 1983; DeGroot *et al.* 1987; Delmas and Laude 1990; Stouten *et al.* 1992; Mulvey and Brown 1996; Isa *et al.* 1997). It is not universally

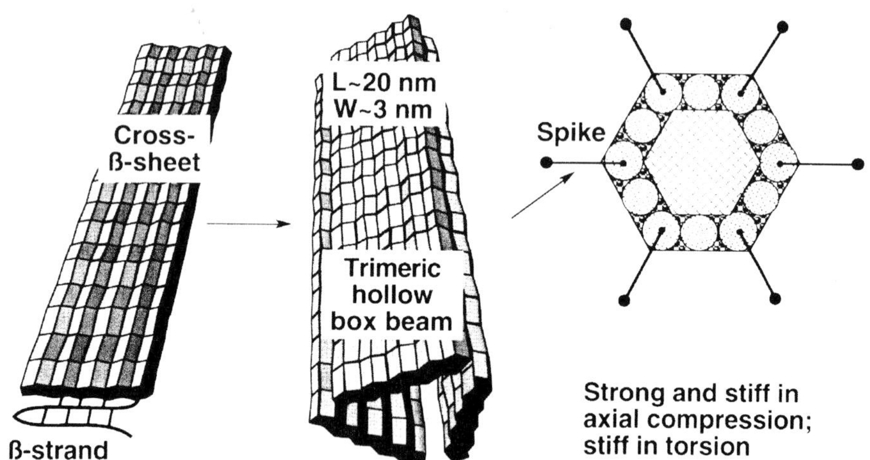

Fig. 8.10. Hierarchical structure of a viral spike.

accepted that the structure is based on cross-ß-sheets, although that model is well supported for both rotavirus (Isa *et al.* 1997) and human adenovirus (Chatellard and Chroboczek 1989; Hoess *et al.* 1992; O'Brien 1993; O'Brien *et al.* 1994; Hudson 1997). Three cross-ß-sheets are thought to interact to form a hollow trimeric box beam (Figure 8.10) that resists buckling in compression. Some researchers (DeGroot *et al.* 1987) describe the spike as having a triad of helices at its core – somewhat like the collagen triple helix, but with a continuous space enclosed between the three molecular helices. Compressive stiffness in this case is ascribed to opposite twists at the coil and supercoil levels.

Structural characterisation is hampered by the small size of individual spikes. Typically, dimensions do not exceed a length of 30 nm or a width of 5 nm. Attempts have been made to produce simple genetically engineered analogs, and to spin fibres for analysis by microscopy, diffraction or spectroscopy. However, these non-natural fibres are assembled under significantly off-equilibrium conditions, and so cannot be assumed to have the same internal structure as the native material. There may also be significant intrinsic differences between the architecture of spikes from different types of virus. Hydrophobic bonding is presumed to be important in stabilising their structure, since 70% of the amino acid residues are hydrophobic in representative cases (Estes and Cohen 1989).

Genetically engineered model polymers based on multiple consecutive copies of the principal repeated sequence in native adenovirus spike protein can self-assemble into fibrillar structures, which in turn can form a liquid crystalline phase in solution (O'Brien 1993). However, there is no evidence that fibres spun from this material contain trimeric box beams in their hierarchical microstructure (Gillespie *et al.* 1994).

8.2.4.3. Properties. The uniaxial mechanical properties of fibre spun from genetically engineered analog of spike protein have been disappointing. In tensile tests conducted on dry fibre, the breaking strength is ~0.3 GPa, the stiffness ~4 GPa, and the elongation to failure ~30 % (Hudson 1997). Realistically, this is not surprising. As already noted, the artificial microstructure is produced under significantly off-equilibrium conditions, compared to the near-equilibrium conditions that prevail during assembly of the native protein coat. One should not expect both processes to lead to identical microstructures and properties. The genetically engineered and artificially spun material contains only the repeated elements of the native sequence, and so is unlikely to be able to fold in the same way as the native protein. Hence our cautionary remarks in Section 8.1.4: some aspects of evolved primary structure facilitate the protein's self-assembly into the final material, and therefore must be considered when designing genetically engineered equivalents.

We also note the evidence that the native spikes rely on hydrophobic bonding to maintain their structure. Their mechanical properties, and the properties of properly assembled fibres based on analogous proteins, as measured in a hydrophobic environment are therefore likely to be inferior compared to results obtained in water. In other words, the natural material is designed to work in an aqueous medium, and attempts to mimic its properties must take this reality into account.

8.2.5. ***Actin*** (Kabsch and Vandekerckhove 1992; Furukawa and Fechheimer 1997; Steinmetz *et al.* 1997)

8.2.5.1. ***G-actin***. Actin is one of the principal constituents of muscle. Individual protein chains fold into a non-spherical globular conformation, that can fit into a space approximately 5.5 x 5.5 x 3.5 nm (Figure 8.11) (Kabsch and Vandekerckhove 1992). These globular molecules are conventionally referred to as *G-actin*. Two distinct domains can be identified in each; the gap between the domains is bridged twice by the protein backbone, forming a hinge that has important consequence for the mechanical properties of actin fibre. The inter-domain gap is also a binding site for ATP, which is significant to fibre formation (Lehninger 1975).

8.2.5.2. ***F-actin*** (Lodish *et al.* 1995). G-actin self-assembles into a right-handed, double-helical, elongated aggregate (Figure 8.11) that is referred to as *F-actin* in recognition of its fibrous structure. The rate at which F-actin forms is limited by nucleation: non-covalent association between just two G-actin molecules is much weaker than the interactions binding G-actin in a larger aggregate, because there are more nearest-neighbour interactions per G-actin molecule in the latter case. Self-assembly of F-actin is driven by several interlinked factors:

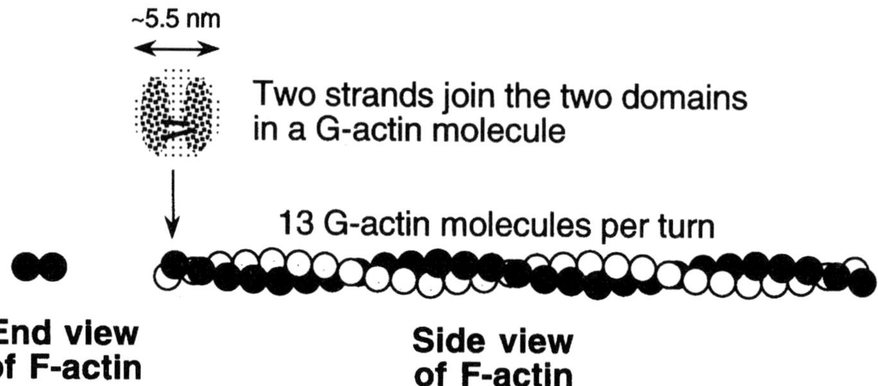

Fig. 8.11. Molecular and supramolecular features of F-actin.

a.- There are entropic considerations. G-actins that have become aggregated are able to bind significantly fewer water molecules compared to the same number of independent G-actins. Although G-actin aggregation is synonymous with an increase in G-actin order, the accompanying increase in the disorder of water is more than enough to compensate.

b.- The F-actin rods can become locally oriented, forming liquid crystalline domains. Within such domains, axial growth of the rods is favoured, and longer rods are in turn more successful at stabilising orientational order. Whether or not a fluid is able to exist in the liquid crystalline state is again an entropy-related issue, discussion of which will be reserved until later in this Chapter (Section 8.3.3.4). Also reviewed elsewhere is the evidence for liquid crystal formation by *actin* (Furukawa and Fechheimer 1997; Viney 1997a) and by *myosin* (Viney 1997a) (a protein that is closely associated with actin in muscle tissue).

Our focus at present is the synergism between liquid crystallinity and aggregate growth. Models of the liquid crystalline state (Chick and Viney 1993) predict a critical length-to-width ratio of the rods, below which liquid crystal formation is not possible. The simplest of these models (Onsager 1949) leads to the following requirement for liquid crystallinity:

$$c\,d\,L^2 \;>\; \text{constant} \qquad (8.1)$$

where c is concentration, d is the rod diameter, L is the rod length, and the value of the constant depends on the system of units. In practice, actin develops liquid crystalline order at concentrations significantly lower than implied by simple application of this formula (Furukawa and Fechheimer 1997). The model leading to Equation (8.1), along with other models that give analytical predictions of the relationship between rod dimensions and critical concentration, assumes that the rods are monodisperse. For polydisperse systems, such as solutions of F-actin, using the average rod length to substitute for L can be misleading. Because critical concentration is inversely proportional to the *square* of rod length, rods which are longer than the mean are more effective at lowering the critical concentration, compared with the ability of shorter rods to raise the critical concentration. In other words, a small number of longer rods can dramatically decrease the overall concentration needed for the phase transition to liquid crystalline order.

c.- Actin bundling proteins (ABPs) help to reduce the activity of G-actin in solution, allowing a greater concentration to accumulate in a particular location and thus enhancing the chances of contact and aggregation. By promoting aggregation, ABPs also enhance polydispersity, allowing liquid crystalline order to develop at lower F-actin concentrations.

d.- Aggregate formation is reversibly sensitive to the ionic strength of the surrounding medium. Aggregation as described in the following reaction (Lehninger 1975) is promoted by an increased concentration of cationic solutes:

$$\text{n(G-actin/ATP)} \rightarrow \underset{\textit{F-actin}}{\text{(G-actin/ADP)}_n} + \text{nP}$$

Cation-phosphate complexing will help to reduce the activity of phosphate in solution.

e.- The presence of globular proteins that are not attracted to actin can promote liquid crystalline phase separation, because mixing of rods and flexible coils is entropically unfavourable. This principle will be addressed in more detail below (Section 8.3.3.5.).

f.- F-actin growth can be enhanced by osmotically generated hydrostatic forces, which drive convective supply of G-actin to where it is needed. This factor is thought to be significant during the assembly of the acrosomal process (Oster *et al.* 1982). When sperm fertilises an egg, the sperm cell develops a protrusion (i.e. a process) which penetrates the egg cell and provides a conduit through which genetic material can be transferred into the egg. The process is constructed from actin, and, in the case of sea cucumber sperm, can grow by over 90 μm in less than 10 s – a rate that can be observed easily in real time in a light microscope (Tilney and Inoué 1982)! Diffusion-limited supply of G-actin to the process would be too slow to account for such a high growth rate.

8.2.5.3. Properties. Actin provides further examples of multifunctionality in a biological fibrous material. Its roles include muscle contraction, cell motility and barrier penetration (Lodish *et al.* 1995).

In many of these applications, it is necessary for actin to maintain rigidity under tension. If this were not the case, muscle and cytoskeletal actin fibres would simply stretch, rather than slide past neighbouring fibres as required. At the same time, actin fibres are flexible in torsion, allowing cells to change shape; this flexibility relies on the hinge between domains in the individual G-actin molecules.

The reality that cohesive, strong, durable, fibrous structures can assemble via non-covalent aggregation of globular chains has significant implications for the development of commercial polymers. The traditional view in polymer science and engineering has been that interpenetrating molecular coils (chain entanglements) are needed to maintain the cohesivity that allows processing of fluid polymer into useful fibres. Watching a weightlifter in action, one cannot dispute the cohesivity of fibres made from *non-covalently* associated, *non-interpenetrating* G-actin coils. What is less certain is whether it is possible to make analogous fibres that function in a dry environment.

8.2.6. Tubulin (Hyams and Lloyd 1994; Lodish *et al.* 1995)
Microtubules in flagella and actin filaments in muscle exhibit similar features of hierarchical structure. The most striking difference is that the tubulin-based structures are hollow.

8.2.6.1. Dimers, protofilaments and microtubules. Microtubules consist of two distinct types of globular protein, α-tubulin and β-tubulin (Figure 8.12). The first stage of microtubule assembly involves α-tubulin / β-tubulin dimerisation. A circular pattern of a third, related protein, γ-tubulin, occurs at the surface of microtubule organising centres (MTOCs), providing a template (Hyams and Lloyd 1994) to which the dimers are attracted and therefore on which the microtubules are nucleated. In animal cells, the MTOC is an organelle called the centrosome (Moritz *et al.* 1995; Zheng *et al.* 1995).

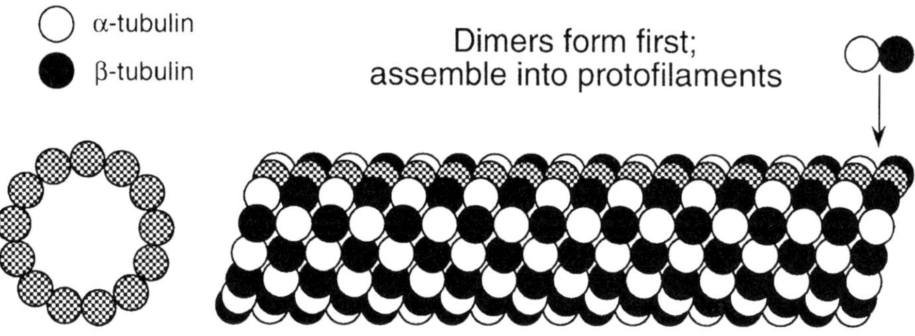

Fig. 8.12. Hierarchical structure of a microtubule. In the side view, the path of a representative protofilament is accented in grey.

A head-to-tail sequence of dimers forms a *protofilament*. The number of protofilaments in a microtubule can be as little as 7 or as many as 16, depending on the *in vivo* or *in vitro* environment in which the microtubule is formed. There are usually 13 protofilaments in natural microtubules. Longitudinal bonds between tubulin molecules are stronger than latitudinal ones (Hyams and Lloyd 1994), leading to the view that microtubules grow by the simultaneous, longitudinal growth of all the constituent protofilaments. Whether or not the protofilaments are parallel to the microtubule axis depends on how many protofilaments there are. Parallelism is obtained with 13 protofilaments (Wade and Chretien 1993); since this geometry should give the greatest axial strength, the natural preference for 13 protofilaments can be understood.

As was the case with actin, several factors combine to drive self-assembly:

a.- The number of protofilaments in the microtubule is dictated by the distribution of γ-tubulin in MTOCs.
b.- Each α/ß-tubulin dimer exhibits a charge dipole (Tuszynski *et al.* 1997), which helps it to assume the correct orientation to dock with a growing protofilament.
c.- The release of bound water from the aggregating tubulins can lead to a net increase of entropy in the solution (Tuszynski *et al.* 1997).
d.- Finally, liquid crystalline phase formation has been observed in vitro but not yet confirmed *in vivo*; evidence for liquid crystal formation by microtubules is reviewed elsewhere (Viney 1997a).

8.2.6.2. Properties. Like actin filaments, microtubules fulfil diverse roles. They are found in cytoskeletal fibres, flagella, cilia and mitotic spindles, and therefore are integral to maintaining cell structure, to cell motility, and to cell reproduction (Lodish *et al.* 1995). They also participate in material transport, signal transduction and (possibly) information storage (Tuszynski *et al.* 1997).

In all these applications, cohesive, strong, fibrous structures maintain rigidity under tension, again despite the fact that they consist of non-covalently aggregated globular chains. The non-covalent bonds are sufficiently numerous, and collectively strong enough, for the globular actin molecules to maintain their shape under load and to remain connected to their neighbours in the aggregates.

The tensile modulus of microtubules (Gittes *et al.* 1993) is approximately 1.2 GPa, similar to that of PMMA and other rigid plastics where significant molecular entanglements do occur (Billmeyer 1984). The flexural rigidity of microtubules is about 300 times greater than that of actin filaments. Microtubules therefore are rigid over cellular dimensions and can offer support to actin filaments in the cytoskeleton. Their rigidity is mainly due to their larger cross-section, achieved without unnecessary material expense by making the cross-section hollow. The principle of minimising deformation by placing as much of the structure as far away as possible from the neutral axis (Gordon 1978) was perfected by Nature long before it was established by engineers!

8.2.7. Cellulose

8.2.7.1. Hierarchical structure. Cellulose is one of the many possible polymers of glucose (Viney 1993), but the only one that forms structural fibres. The primary structure is shown in Figure 8.13. Each glucose residue contains three hydroxyl groups, providing extensive possibilities for intramolecular and intermolecular hydrogen bonds to form. Alternatively, these are all potential sites for chemical derivatisation.

A complex hierarchical microstructure exists in all natural cellulose materials, spanning over six orders of magnitude in scale (Krässig 1985). Each level of structure involves a well-defined pattern of hydrogen-bonded substructure. The assembly sequence is: molecules → elementary fibrils → microfibrils → fibrils → fibers → tissues. Some stages of this process may occur via a liquid crystalline phase. Evidence ranges from circumstantial (reviewed elsewhere (Neville 1993); some final structures, such as cell walls, have topological similarities with cholesteric liquid crystals), to direct observation of liquid crystalline order in cellulose-containing solutions in vitro (Gilbert 1985; Ritcey and Gray 1988) and *in vivo* (Willison and Abeysekera 1988).

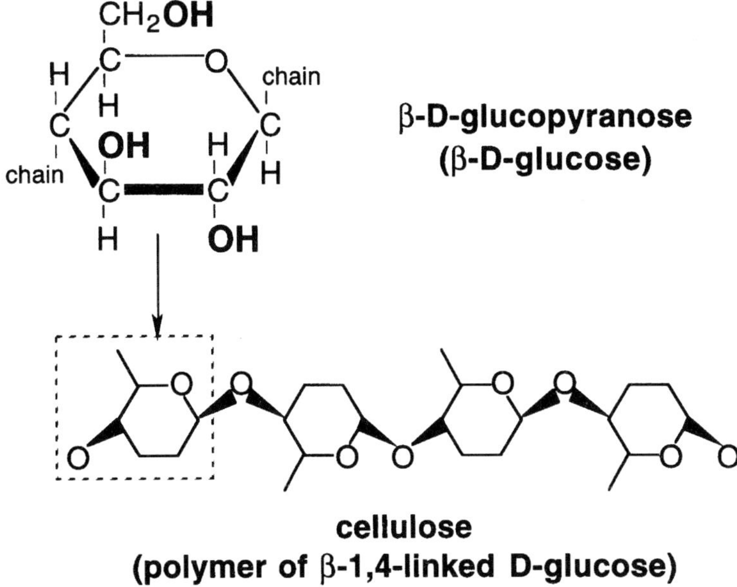

Fig. 8.13. The primary structure of a glucose residue, and its relationship to a cellulose molecule. Only carbon atoms and main chain oxygen atoms are shown in the framework representation of cellulose. Carbon atoms in each glucose residue are counted sequentially, starting with the carbon furthest from the $-CH_2OH$ side chain.

At the fibrillar scale of cellulose, the configuration of chains does not maximise hydrogen bonding or produce an energy-minimised microstructure. There are two useful reminders here:

The first is that Nature does not always aim for energy minimisation. In the case of cellulose-based structures, it is important for there to be flexibility as well as strength, so maximisation of hydrogen bonding is avoided. A corollary of this observation is that Nature has evolved pathways for building non-equilibrium microstructures *slowly*, without recourse to the rapid cooling or drying rates, or the mechanical deformation, that commercial processes use to achieve such microstructures.

The second reminder is that experimental data which relate to hierarchical structure should not be interpreted at inappropriate length scales. For the naturally occurring polymorph of cellulose, termed cellulose I, x-ray diffraction indicates that the chains in microfibrils are *parallel* (Gardner and Blackwell 1974). If cellulose is dissolved completely and then reconstituted from solution, the cellulose II polymorph is formed; it consists of *antiparallel* chains (Kolpak and Blackwell 1976). Cellulose II is also obtained if, instead of dissolving the native cellulose, one simply allows it to swell in dilute NaOH. Swelling affords the molecules little mobility, yet the polymorphic transition from cellulose I to cellulose II can be complete within a few minutes (Krässig 1985).

How is it that 50% of the chains in cellulose I are able to undergo an apparently head-over-heals inversion in so short a time under conditions of such limited mobility? The answer (Nishimura and Sarko 1987) becomes obvious if one recognises that "parallel" and "antiparallel" as deduced from x-ray diffraction are appropriate descriptions of the *local* orientation of chains only. The diffraction data should not be interpreted at too great a length scale. Within a given crystalline microfibril of cellulose I, all the chains can indeed be parallel. In another microfibril the chains can again be parallel to each other, while running antiparallel to those in the first. Swelling most readily occurs at the amorphous interface between microfibrils; small lateral displacement of chains can then effect intermixing of molecules from antiparallel *microfibrils*, producing a microstructure of antiparallel *chains* (Figure 8.14).

8.2.7.2 Properties. The combination of a hierarchical microstructure, structural anisotropy, and hydrogen bonding causes cellulose fibres to exhibit wide ranges of strength, stiffness and toughness in mechanical tests.

Humidity can affect the hydrogen bonding in accessible parts of the microstructure. Penetration by moisture occurs predominantly in amorphous regions, where chains have a relatively large specific volume and interchain hydrogen bonding is relatively weak. In crystalline regions, the packing is dense, and chains are closely and strongly hydrogen bonded to each other; water therefore has limited access, and polymer-solvent hydrogen bonds do not offer a significant lowering of energy compared to

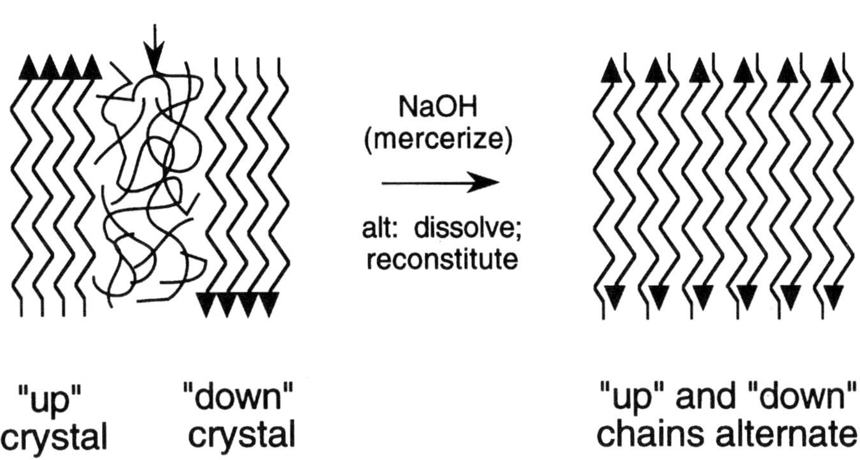

Fig. 8.14. Transformation of cellulose I (locally parallel chains) to cellulose II (antiparallel chains) can be achieved by lateral interdiffusion of chains from adjacent, oppositely oriented microfibrils. The necessary chain mobility can be provided by allowing the native cellulose to swell in warm dilute NaOH (a process referred to as mercerizing), or, alternatively, by dissolving and and then re-precipitating (reconstituting) the cellulose.

polymer-polymer hydrogen bonds. In addition, cellulose chains have only limited conformational flexibility, so the entropy difference between a chain in a crystal and the same chain in solution is small compared to the entropy that is sacrificed by water binding to the solvated chain. Cellulose therefore does not dissolve in water, instead requiring a solvent that is either more polar and/or more chaotropic.

The wet strength of cellulose is higher than the dry strength. When the amorphous regions are swelled by water, the local chain mobility increases. In turn, this enables tensile deformation to occur to larger strains, and therefore allows a greater degree of molecular order to develop in these regions, before the fibre can break (Hatakeyama 1989). In other words, greater chain mobility in wet amorphous material extends the range of the stress-strain curve in tensile tests.

8.2.8. Mucin

8.2.8.1. ***Structure.*** Mucin (Figure 8.15) is a glycoprotein which forms the macromolecular matrix of mucus, dominating its rheological properties. It consists of a protein backbone; segments that are heavily glycosylated (populated with polysaccharide side chains) alternate with naked segments (Bansil *et al.* 1995; Roberts *et al.* 1995). Individual mucin molecules are exported as compact packets (granules) by specialised secretory cells. The granules swell dramatically in appropriate extracellular environments: their volume can increase by a factor of 600 in 40 ms, implying that the initially condensed mucin must have been folded in an orderly way which enables unobstructed expansion (Verdugo *et al.* 1992). At concentrations above approximately 26 weight % in water and at physiological temperatures, pig stomach mucin forms a side-chain liquid crystalline phase (Davies and Viney 1998).

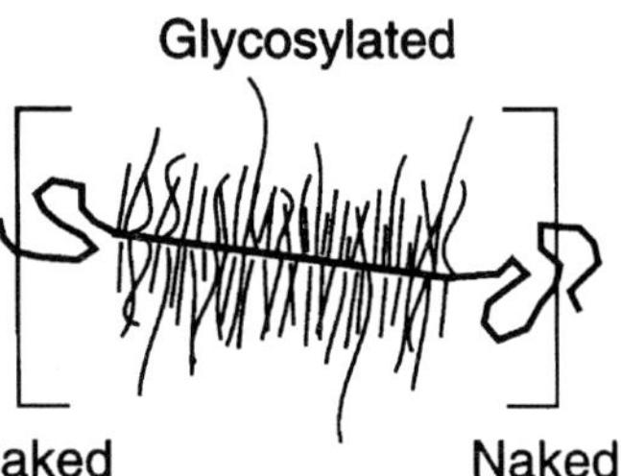

Fig. 8.15. Schematic illustration of mucin structure. Whole mucin can be regarded as a copolymer of relatively rigid (glycosylated) and relatively flexible (naked) moieties. Several molecules of whole mucin are exported in a single granule by mucin-secreting cells.

8.2.8.2. ***Properties.*** Mucus is used as an outstanding lubricant (giraffe tongues), a locomotion aid (slugs), a transport medium (mammalian lungs and female reproductive tract), and a selective barrier (stomach lining) – amongst a very large number of varied applications (Daniel 1981; Chantler and Ratcliffe 1989; Koch *et al.* 1991). It merits a mention in the present chapter because it can also be drawn into fibres; cohesivity in decondensed mucus is presumably maintained by main chain entanglements, as well as by the interdigitation of side chains in the liquid crystalline state. This property of mucus is exploited by some species of slugs when they mate: supported only by a strand of fibrous mucus, they descend by as much as 40 cm from a tree branch to avoid predators. Several species use mucus threads to descend from overhangs (South 1992). Fibrous strands are also found in the mucus under resting slugs (Denny and Gosline 1980). How this system of macromolecules, ions and water undergoes the change from a viscoelastic lubricant into a fibrous, load-supporting composite material is not yet understood.

8.2.9. ***Levan / DNA / water*** (Huber and Viney 1997; Huber and Viney 1998)

8.2.9.1. ***Structure***. Levan is a branched polymer of fructose (Han 1990; Simms *et al.* 1990). As with cellulose, there are several hydrogen bonding sites on each residue. Strong intramolecular hydrogen bonding causes each molecule to adopt a compact, spherically symmetrical globular conformation in aqueous solution (Stivala and Bahary 1978). The globular molecules do not interact with *each other* to form aggregates.

Dilute aqueous solutions of pure levan are isotropic, becoming gel-like as concentration approaches 10% w/w. Adding small amounts of DNA (of the order of 1 molecule of DNA per 180 molecules of levan) causes dilute solutions to become liquid crystalline; the exact levan:DNA ratio needed to stabilise liquid crystallinity depends on the average molecular weights of the levan and the DNA. The liquid crystalline solutions can be hand drawn into fibres. Several different experimental techniques point to the liquid crystal being formed by aggregates that consist of a dense layer of levan packed around a DNA core (Figure 8.16). No additional impurities are necessary to effect the binding between DNA and levan. The liquid crystalline phase in this system is novel in several respects:

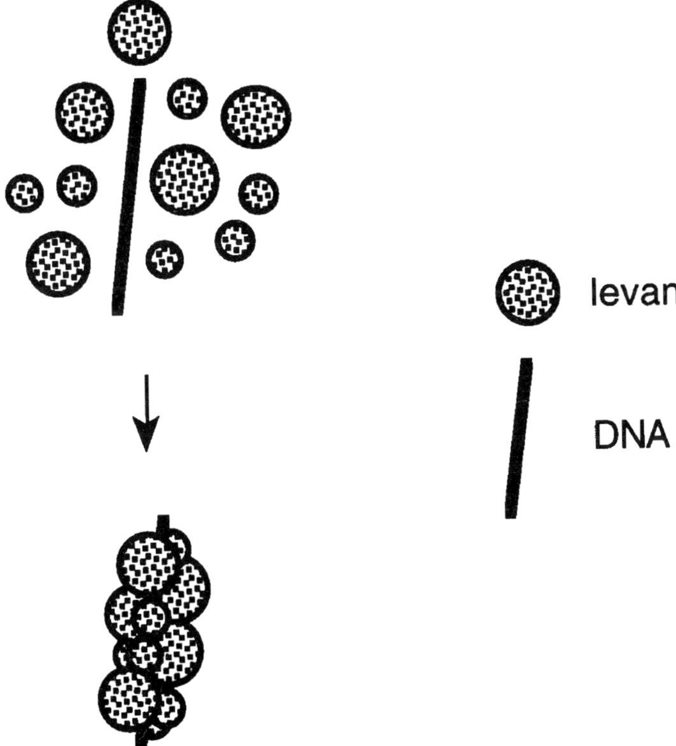

Fig. 8.16. Aggregation of globular (and polydisperse) levan molecules around a rod-like DNA core.

a.- The constituent supramolecular rods are constructed from two unrelated macromolecular species – hence the name "chimeric".

b.- Both types of macromolecule are needed to obtain the liquid crystalline phase. The globular levan does not associate to form rod-like structures in pure solutions. The DNA, though rod-like, is present in far too low a concentration to stabilise liquid crystalline order on its own. In the aggregates, DNA provides the necessary shape anisotropy, while levan raises the volume fraction of the rods to greater-than-critical levels.

c.- It is rare for rods and coils to coexist in the same phase, because rods can constrain the conformational freedom of coils (see Section 8.3.3.5, dealing with entropy). However, because this system is dilute, the levan coils need not be distorted significantly by packing constraints. Also, although the levan backbone is intrinsically flexible, the capacity for extensive intramolecular hydrogen bonding will preclude significant conformational freedom, so there is little conformational entropy to sacrifice when levan bonds to DNA. In other words, the levan behaves more like a rigid sphere than like a flexible coil. Binding of levan to DNA is strong as evidenced by the practical difficulty of ridding levan of DNA impurities. Enthalpic factors, dominated by the opportunity for non-covalent bonding, therefore override any entropy penalty associated with aggregation. Entropic factors then determine the concentration of *aggregates* needed to stabilise a liquid crystalline phase.

DNA has even been observed to induce complex levels of order in colloidal suspensions of synthetic polymer spheres, leading to the suggestion that such systems might be used to manufacture novel composite materials (Adams *et al.* 1998).

8.2.9.2. Properties. The levan/DNA/water system has been included here because it demonstrates again that a fibre-drawable liquid crystalline phase can be induced by appropriate supramolecular aggregation – even in systems that would not stereotypically be regarded as fibre-forming. What matters, is the pattern of non-covalent bonding that can develop within and between macromolecules in aqueous solution, and the magnitude of the entropy penalty for increased order.

Does the possible use of DNA as a processing aid to obtain fibres from non-traditional fibre sources bear consideration? Solution rheology may be a limiting factor. In conventional liquid crystals, alignment of "smooth" rods can be accompanied by a viscosity decrease of two decades or more (Prevorsek 1982). In the levan/DNA solutions studied thus far, viscosity *increases* monotonically as a function of aggregate concentration, and is also increased by shear. It remains to be seen whether these increases are due to the polydispersity of the levan (the aggregates are not molecularly smooth), or due to aggregates becoming rougher as they are partially dissociated by shear.

8.3. UNIFYING THEMES

We have now considered several examples of biological polymers that are able to form fibres by supramolecular self-assembly. The main practical consequences of self-assembly are a hierarchical microstructure and multifunctionality. Many of the physical principles of self-assembly are well-understood, even though it remains generally difficult to identify which element of detailed microstructure is associated with which optimised property.

In materials science, a correspondence between microstructure and properties is axiomatic: to mimic the properties of a natural material, it is necessary to emulate the natural microstructures – even if by a different processing route. Broad consideration of the preceding examples allows us to identify some common principles by which Nature achieves functional microstructures.

8.3.1. Types of bonding

Many properties of biological materials are affected directly by the type and distribution of bonds, both intramolecular and intermolecular. Compared to synthetic polymers, there is a greater reliance on non-covalent bonds and on interactions between the macromolecules and their environment. Table 8.1 summarises the bonding mechanisms that we have considered, and gives an example of each in the context of an optimised material property.

Table 8.1. Examples of structure-property relations

Bonding type	Material	Optimised property
Covalent (strongly directional)		
aligned chains	Silk	tensile stiffness (1-D)
extensive cross-linking	keratin (horn)	compressive stiffness (3-D)
Non-covalent (weakly directional)		
hydrogen bonds	cellulosics	wet strength
intermediate species (e.g. ABPs; ions)	actin	cohesivity under significant load
hydrophobic bonds	viral spikes	rigidity in aqueous environments

8.3.2. What drives fibre self-assembly?

Fibre self-assembly requires molecules that can serve as appropriate building blocks, a source of structural anisotropy, and an environment that promotes the self-assembly.

8.3.2.1. Sources of structural anisotropy. Most biological molecules are intrinsically flexible, but some can form anisotropic structures, such as helices or ß-sheet crystals, in water as a result of hydrogen bonding and/or hydrophobic interactions. Intrapolymer, interpolymer and polymer-water interactions can all contribute to stabilising structure at this level.

Globular molecules can form anisotropic structures by aggregation, either with other globular molecules or around existing rods. In the former case, anisotropic aggregation can be promoted by an asymmetric charge distribution (dipoles) on the interacting macromolecules, or by specificity of sites that take part in the intermolecular hydrogen bonds or hydrophobic bonds. Ions may also play a role in binding (Lehninger 1975; Thiel and Viney 1997).

Some globular molecules, in particular simple analogs of the fibrous protein elastin, can be made to adopt helical and therefore anisotropic conformations if the temperature is *raised* (Urry *et al.* 1997). This is a special case of the hydrophobic effect; the apparent decrease in entropy with increasing temperature is possible provided that other components in the system end up with increased entropy. We will consider these so-called *inverse temperature transitions* in Section 8.3.3.3.

Anisotropic structures can be promoted by templating, especially at the nucleation stage. The template may simply dictate the location and orientation of the anisotropic structure (for example, when cotton plants are genetically modified to precipitate polyester in the lumen of cellulose fibres (John and Keller 1996)), or it may impose stricter constraints on size and shape (as in the case of microtubule nucleation).

Liquid crystalline order can promote the aggregation of globular molecules into linear structures. In F-actin, in microtubules, and possibly in silk (before it is spun), synergism develops between alignment-enhanced assembly and shape-enhanced alignment. The assembling capacity of supramolecular liquid crystals transcends that of conventional molecular liquid crystals (Ciferri 1997; Huber and Viney 1998).

8.3.2.2. Self-assembly at greater length scales: Propagation of structural anisotropy. In an aqueous environment, helices can form superhelices as a result of hydrophobic bonding.

Superhelix (coiled coil) formation may alternatively be stabilised by electrostatic interactions (O'Shea *et al.* 1993).

We have noted the role of extension peptides in the assembly of collagen triple helices (Section 8.2.2): they interact to get the procollagen molecules started into a triple helical arrangement, and are subsequently discarded.

Liquid crystalline order can directly control the higher-level pattern into which rod-like structures become organised. There are many distinguishable schemes according to which rods can pack in a liquid crystalline fluid, and all the major cases have been detected in biological materials (Neville 1993; Viney 1993; Viney et al. 1993; Viney 1997a; Goodby 1998).

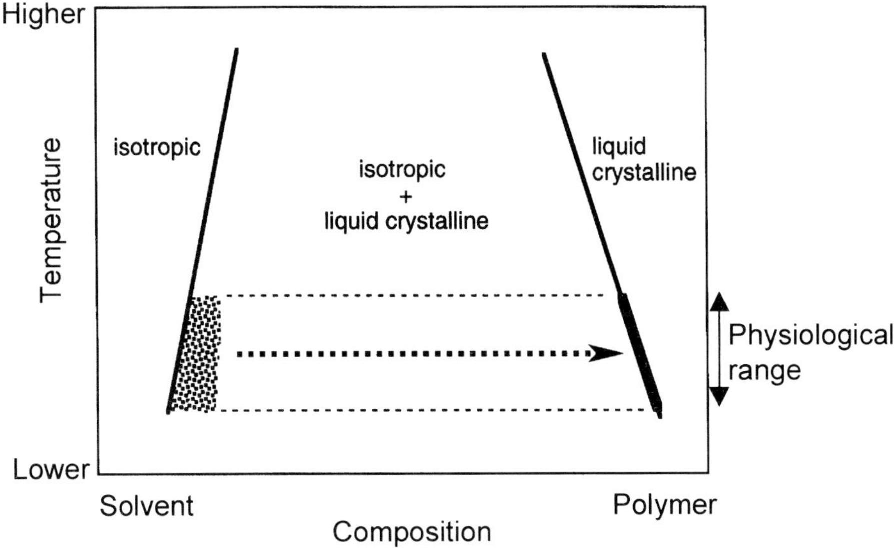

Fig. 8.17. A phase diagram with a wide biphasic (isotropic + liquid crystalline) regime. A dilute solution of rods (shaded region; restricted schematically to physiological temperatures) can exist in equilibrium with a concentrated liquid crystalline phase (thick segment of right-hand phase boundary).

Liquid crystalline phase separation can provide a pathway for achieving high *local* concentrations of the anisotropic fibre-forming species (Ciferri and Krigbaum 1981), even if (as is typical in living cells) these species are synthesised in dilute solution. Provided that the dilute solutions contain enough solute to enter the biphasic regime on the phase diagram, and provided that the biphasic regime is wide at the temperature of interest (Figure 8.17), a small amount of concentrated phase is produced. In a thermodynamically open system such as a living organism, newly synthesized polymer in dilute solution can be supplied at a rate that matches the removal of polymer into the liquid crystalline and then solid state.

Helical structures may favour particular patterns of dense packing (Rudall 1957; Bouligand and Giraud-Guille 1985; Neville 1993). Tightly packed helices in a plane (Figure 8.18) can generate a series of parallel, equidistant grooves that are oriented obliquely to the alignment direction of the helices. If the spacing of the grooves is similar to the lateral separation between helices, the grooves can serve as a template for a second layer of tightly packed helices. In this way, a supramolecular structure can self-assemble continuously in three dimensions. It is also possible for α-helices to pack in pairs such that the ridges formed by side chains on one helix fit into the ridges between side chains on the other, and vice versa (Branden and Tooze 1991).

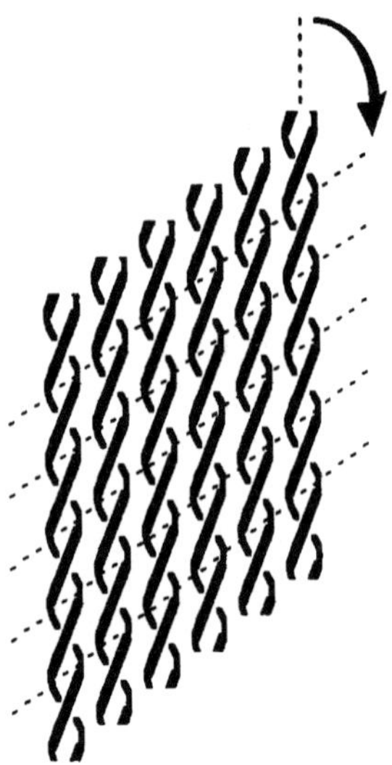

Fig. 8.18. Right-handed double helices packed in a plane. A series of grooves is created (oblique broken lines) which can accommodate another, similar layer of double helices. The second layer is related to the first by a left-handed twist (defined by looking from the first plane to the second, along their normal).

8.3.3. The role of entropy

Throughout this Chapter, we have encountered instances when entropy is the critical factor that decides whether or not a particular structure will form. Simplistic rules of preferred molecular association – such as "like prefers like" and "like avoids unlike" – are unreliable and are easily misapplied. In general, when macromolecular solutions behave in an apparently surprising way, it is because the role of entropy has been overlooked. We therefore provide here a concise treatment of entropy in the context of molecular self-assembly.

8.3.3.1. ***Types of entropy***. In simple theories of mixing, that describe (say) the interdiffusion of inert gases A and B, one is concerned only with the number of different ways in which the available atoms of A and B can be arranged in space. This gives a measure of *configurational* entropy, which can also be referred to as *translational* entropy or *positional* entropy.

If the system under consideration contains macromolecular species, it is additionally necessary to consider *conformational* entropy. A flexible backbone has the capacity to adopt a large number of different conformations; if it is constrained from doing so, there is an entropy penalty. The issue of constraint is important: just because a molecule adopts a conformation that resembles a random coil, it does not automatically follow that its conformational entropy is higher than that of a rigid or extended rod-like molecule. What matters is *whether the coil can readily undergo transitions to other conformations*, which may or may not themselves be random coils. If its conformation is stabilised by hydrogen bonds, it does not have high conformational entropy.

When macromolecules in suspension or solution have a rod-like conformation or some other anisotropic shape, a given positional distribution of rods can be associated with a variable level of *orientational* entropy, depending on how well aligned the rods are. Thus, in the most general case of macromolecular solutions, it is necessary to consider configurational, conformational and orientational contributions to entropy.

8.3.3.2. ***Decreasing solubility with increasing temperature***. Entropy is responsible for hydrophobic bonds (Stryer 1995). If a polymer contains both hydrophilic and hydrophobic segments, and if water is used as the solvent, a "cage" of water molecules is built around the hydrophobic segments. The water is locally structured to minimise unfavourable interactions between itself and the polymer. In other words, the local hydrogen bonding network of the water must become ordered to accommodate the hydrophobic sections of the polymer.

The entropy increase that accompanies mixing of polymer and solvent can be more than offset by the entropy decrease that accompanies this local ordering of the hydrogen bonds in water.* As temperature rises, the imposition of structure on water becomes increasingly unfavourable, and the solubility of the polymer decreases. The water molecule "cages" are collapsed at the higher temperatures.

8.3.3.3. ***Inverse temperature transitions*** (Urry *et al.* 1997). These transitions are a consequence of the hydrophobic effect in some polymer/water systems. It is not necessary for the polymer to be in solution; the inverse temperature transition can occur just as readily in a crosslinked polymer network in an aqueous environment (Urry 1988). The polymer must be slightly hydrophobic, must have a flexible backbone, and must be free to exploit this flexibility and undergo conformational changes.

Initially, the polymer is hydrated because, even though the polymer-water contacts are slightly unfavourable, the separated chains acquire greater free volume and conformational mobility. As temperature rises, polymer-polymer contacts become increasingly favourable compared to polymer-environment contacts, so the backbone conformation becomes more restricted. Some polymers can even undergo a disordered-to-helix conformational transition. Decreased entropy due to the higher degree of conformational order is compensated by the disordering of previously constrained solvent molecules, and by the increased freedom of ordered macromolecular segments to undergo small rotations and translations.

Cross-linked (Val-Pro-Gly-Val-Gly)$_n$ ($n \approx 100$) is a good example of a polymer network that exhibits an inverse temperature transition in an aqueous environment. The repeated sequence in this polymer is a common feature of elastin, a fibrous network protein that occurs in mammalian artery walls. The transition temperature can be raised or lowered by respectively decreasing or increasing the hydrophobicity of the polymer.

8.3.3.4. Formation of liquid crystalline phases. Entropy is significantly responsible for stabilising liquid crystalline phases. This fact can be appreciated by considering an increasing concentration of rod-like species in an initially dilute isotropic solution. A critical concentration is reached at which the addition of one more rod can only be accommodated if rods develop some degree of alignment. However, rather than all the rods sacrificing orientational entropy and developing a slight degree of partial alignment, it is entropically more favourable if a few rods become highly aligned, leaving the remainder of the system to be isotropic. The aligned fraction benefits from enhanced translational entropy, and the remaining fraction retains full orientational entropy. Further increases in rod concentration are accompanied by an increase in the amount of liquid crystalline material, until eventually a concentration is reached at which the entire solution is liquid crystalline.

Entropy considerations therefore explain how it is possible for small regions in even a dilute solution of rod-like species to spontaneously develop a high degree of molecular alignment. This is the physical principle that underlies Figure 8.17 and allows dense fibrous microstructures to evolve out of a dilute solution of rod-like moieties.

8.3.3.5. A final example. Although this example does not involve biological molecules, it illustrates many of the subtle relationships between primary structure, entropy considerations and molecular order. Also, this discussion will lead us to a simple liquid crystalline analog of muscle fibre contraction.

Decane is an oligomer of polyethylene, containing 10 carbon atoms in the backbone. Perfluorodecane is an oligomer of polytetrafluoroethylene (Teflon®), also containing 10 carbon atoms in the backbone. Both are fluids at room temperature. What happens if aliquots of both are poured into the same container? One might predict mixing on the basis of electronegativity differences: the net positive charges on the hydrogens in decane should attract the net negative charges on the fluorines in perfluorodecane. The observation that this enthalpic effect does *not* lead to miscibility implies that there must be one or more significant entropy-related effects driving phase separation. There would of course be an entropy penalty associated with aggregating oppositely charged molecules, there being no bound solvent to release in compensation. But if this were the whole story, one might expect mixing to occur at higher temperature. However, this is not observed either, because there are additional entropy effects to take into account:

Consider now a single molecule of decane, hypothetically surrounded by several perfluorodecane molecules. Decane is a flexible molecule, capable of adopting many different conformations. In contrast, perfluorodecane is conformationally rigid; the molecules are extended, linear and densely packed. The number of conformational states that could be occupied by the normally flexible decane would be constrained severely by any neighbouring, rigid, aligned perfluorodecane molecules. In other words, the perfluorodecane reduces the *conformational* entropy of the decane. At the same time, the flexible decane coil will tend to disrupt the alignment of the neighbouring perfluorodecane rods, which therefore lose some of their ability to undergo longitudinal translations. In other words, the decane reduces the *translational entropy* of the perfluorodecane.

Similarly, consider a single molecule of perfluorodecane, hypothetically surrounded by several decane molecules. Again, the presence of the rigid perfluorodecane rod would constrain the number of conformational states accessible to the normally flexible decane coils. Meanwhile, the decane coils would hinder translation of the perfluorodecane rod parallel to its axis.

So the decreases in conformational entropy and translational entropy on attempted mixing can be significant.

Decane and perfluorodecane moieties can however be forced to coexist in the liquid state if they are linked covalently to produce the semifluorinated alkane $F(CF_2)_{10}(CH_2)_{10}H$. This compound exhibits two smectic (layered) liquid crystalline phases (Viney *et al.* 1989a) (Figure 8.19) before melting to isotropic liquid. In both, the alkane segment is fully extended, i.e. it has the planar zig-zag conformation and is approximately as long as the fluorinated segment. In the higher-temperature liquid crystalline phase, alkane segments are juxtaposed with fluorinated segments. Even before interactions with neighbouring molecules are taken into account, the

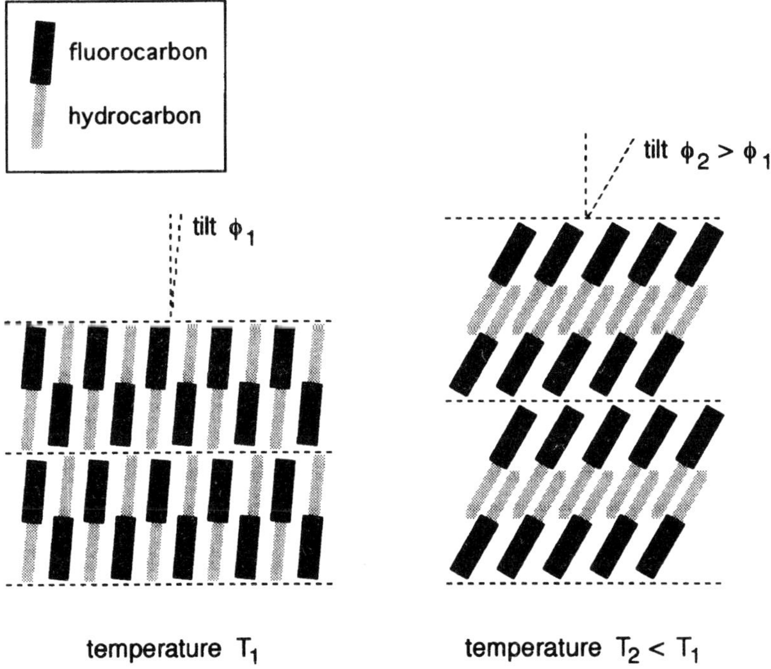

Fig. 8.19. Smectic liquid crystalline phases of $F(CF_2)_{10}(CH_2)_{10}H$ and its near homologues. Large changes in specific volume and molecular interdigitation occur at the transition temperature between the two phases.

conformational freedom of each alkane segment is curtailed by its attachment to a fluoroalkane segment which occupies space that might otherwise be accessible to the unattached end of the alkane. The further restriction imposed on the alkane by the fluorocarbon segments of neighbouring molecules does not represent a large additional entropy decrease, and the attraction between oppositely charged moieties is no longer offset by entropic factors.

In the lower-temperature liquid crystalline phase, the molecules apparently revert to a phase-separated arrangement – within the constraints allowed by the covalent pairing of alkane and fluoroalkane segments. At these temperatures, the molecules have lost freedom to undergo unrestricted rotation about their long axes. Because the alkane chains have an extended, planar zig-zag conformation, their cross-section is not circular, so loss of rotational freedom amounts to a decrease in orientational entropy. At the same time, the molecules are able to pack more efficiently in the new ordering scheme. A large specific volume difference between the two liquid crystalline phases is qualitatively evident (Viney *et al.* 1989b). The large change in the interdigitation of molecules at the transition temperature is analogous to the reversible, relative displacements that occur between actin and myosin filaments during the contraction / relaxation of muscle.

8.4. REPRISE AND OUTLOOK

Natural materials with optimised, reliable properties are produced by self-assembly in an aqueous environment, at or near room temperature. Self-assembly operates over an extensive range of structural length scales. It is achieved with complex molecules and subtle interactions. Interdisciplinary research strategies are required if one is to understand and then apply the technological lessons afforded by studying such materials.

This chapter has focussed on fibres and on fibrous materials. On Nature's scale of achievements, the object lessons chosen have been relatively simple. More challenging (and even more rewarding) systems await scrutiny by materials engineers. For example, insect antennae are self-assembled fibrous structures too, with the following additional attributes: they are small, they are mechanically robust, they are self-repairing, they can detect chemical and thermal information, they can convey this information for processing, and they can undergo controlled and rapid changes in shape and orientation.

Yet Nature's lessons do not stop even there. Self-organisation and self-assembly are used by Nature to produce *all* its structures and devices. The issue of shape and orientation control leads into the embryonic subject of Nature's nanomotors: how do they transduce energy (Urry 1993; Gruler 1998), and how are they linked to fibrous cilia, flagella and antennae (Howard 1997)? Single molecules rotating inside a supramolecular bearing have now been prepared artificially (Gimzewski *et al.* 1998). It is difficult to predict when a whole nanomachine will follow, but one can be confident that it will depend closely on self-assembly protocols learned from Nature.

REFERENCES

Adams, E. (1978) *Science* **202**, 591.

Adams, M., Dogic, Z., Keller, S.L. and Fraden, S. (1998) *Nature* **393**, 349.

Arnold, F.H. (1993) *FASEB Journal* **7**, 744.

Atkins, E.D.T., Fulton, W.S. and Miles, M.J. (1980). in *5th International Dissolving Pulps Conference*, TAPPI, Vienna, p. 208.

Bain, J. (1994) Personal Communication.

Bansil, R., Stanley, E. and LaMont, J.T. (1995) *Annual Reviews of Physiology* **57**, 635.

Barros, J.A. and Deming, J.W. (1983) *Nature* **303**, 423.

Billmeyer, F.W. (1984) *Textbook of Polymer Science*, John Wiley and Sons, New York.

Bock, A., Forchhammer, K., Heider, J., Leinfelder, W., Sawyers, G., Veprek, B. and Zinoni, F. (1991) *Molecular Microbiology* **5**, 515.

Borman, S. (1998) *Chemical and Engineering News* **76**(18), 56.

Bouligand, Y. and Giraud-Guille, M.-M. (1985) in *Biology of Invertebrate and Lower Vertebrate Collagens*, ed. Bairati, A. and Garrone, R. (Plenum, New York) p. 115.

Branden, C. and Tooze, J. (1991) *Introduction to Protein Structure*, Garland Publishing, Inc., New York, NY.

Brandl, H., Gross, R.A., Lenz, R.W. and Fuller, R.C. (1990) *Advances in Biochemical Engineering / Biotechnology* **41**, 77.

Chantler, E. and Ratcliffe, N.A., Eds. (1989) *Mucus and Related Topics*, Society for Experimental Biology, Cambridge, U.K.

Chatellard, C. and Chroboczek, J. (1989) *Gene* **81**, 267.

Chick, L.A. and Viney, C. (1993) *Molecular Crystals and Liquid Crystals* **226**, 25.

Ciferri, A. (1997) *Trends in Polymer Science* **5**(5), 142.

Ciferri, A. and Krigbaum, W.R. (1981) *Molecular Crystals and Liquid Crystals* **69**, 273.

Creighton, T.E. (1993) *Proteins*, W.H. Freeman and Company, New York.

Daniel, T.L. (1981) *Biological Bulletin* **160**, 376.

Davies, J.M. and Viney, C. (1998) *Thermochimica Acta* **315**, 39.

DeGroot, R.J., Luytjes, W., Horzinek, M.C., van der Zeijst, B.A.M., Spaan, W.J.M. and Lenstra, J.A. (1987) *Journal of Molecular Biology* **196**, 963.

Delmas, B. and Laude, H. (1990) *Journal of Virology* **64**, 5367.

Denny, M.W. and Gosline, J.M. (1980) *Journal of Experimental Biology* **88**, 375.

Dogic, Z. and Fraden, S. (1997) *Physical Review Letters* **78**, 2417.

Dougherty, M.J., Kothakota, S., Mason, T.L., Tirrell, D.A. and Fournier, M.J. (1993) *Macromolecules* **26**, 1779.

Elliott, A. and Ambrose, E.J. (1950) *Discussions of the Faraday Society* **9**, 246.

Estes, M.K. and Cohen, J. (1989) *Microbiological Reviews* **53**, 410.

Fasman, G.D. (1991) in *Materials Synthesis Based on Biological Processes,* ed. Alper, M., Calvert, P., Frankel, R., Rieke, P. and Tirrell, D. (Materials Research Society, Pittsburgh, PA) p. 49.

Ferrari, F.A. and Cappello, J. (1997) in *Protein-Based Materials,* ed. McGrath, K. and Kaplan, D. (Birkhäuser, Boston, MA) p. 37.

Fraden, S. (1995) in *Observation, Prediction and Simulation of Phase Transitions in Complex Fluids,* ed. Baus, M., Rull, L.F. and Ryckaert, J.P. (Kluwer Academic Publishers, Dordrecht) p 113.

Fraser, R.D.B., MacRae, T.P. and Rogers, G.E. (1972) *Keratins:Their Composition, Structure, and Biosynthesis*, Charles C. Thomas, Springfield, IL.

Fredrickson, J.K. and Onstott, T.C. (1996) *Scientific American* **275**(4), 42.

Furukawa, R. and Fechheimer, M. (1997) *International Review of Cytology - a Survey of Cell Biology* **175**, 29.
Gardner, K.H. and Blackwell, J. (1974) *Biopolymers* **13**, 1975.
Gathercole, L.J., Barnard, K. and Atkins, E.D.T. (1989) *International Journal of Biological Macromolecules* **11**, 335.
Gilbert, R.D. (1985) in *1985 Nonwovens Symposium*, TAPPI, p. 83.
Gillespie, D.B., Thiel, B.L., Trabbic, K.A., Viney, C. and Yager, P. (1994) *Macromolecules* **27**, 6177.
Gimzewski, J.K., Joachim, C., Schlittler, R.R., Langlais, V., Tang, H. and Johannsen, I. (1998) *Science* **281**, 531.
Giraud-Guille, M.-M. (1987) *Molecular Crystals and Liquid Crystals* **153**, 15.
Giraud-Guille, M.-M. (1989) *Biology of the Cell* **67**, 97.
Giraud-Guille, M.-M. (1992) *Journal of Molecular Biology* **224**, 861.
Gittes, F., Mickey, B., Nettleton, J. and Howard, J. (1993) *Journal of Cell Biology* **120**, 923.
Goodby, J.W. (1998) *Liquid Crystals* **24**, 25.
Gordon, J.E. (1978) *Structures (or Why Things Don't Fall Down)*, Penguin Books, Harmondsworth, UK.
Gorham, S.D. (1991) in *Biomaterials: Novel Materials from Biological Sources,* ed. Byrom, D. (Stockton Press, New York) p. 55.
Gosline, J., Nichols, C., Guerette, P., Cheng, A. and Katz, S. (1995) in *Biomimetics: Design and Processing of Materials,* ed. Sarikaya, M. and Aksay, I.A. (American Institute of Physics, Woodbury, NY) p. 237.
Gray, D.G. (1983) *Journal of Applied Polymer Science: Applied Polymer Symposia* **37**, 179.
Green, N.M., Wrigley, N.G., Russel, W.C., Martin, W.R. and McLachlan, A.D. (1983) *The EMBO Journal* **2**, 1357.
Gruler, H. (1998) *Liquid Crystals* **24**, 49.
Han, Y.W. (1990) in *Advances in Applied Microbiology,* ed. Neidleman, S.L. and Laskin, A.I., Vol. 35, (Academic Press, San Diego) p. 171.
Hatakeyama, T. (1989) in *Cellulose: Structural and Functional Aspects,* ed. Kennedy, J.F., Phillips, G.O. and Williams, P.A. (Ellis Horwood, Chichester, UK) p. 45.
Hoess, R.H., O'Brien, J.P. and Salemme, F.R. (1992) Structural Proteins from Artificial Genes. World Patent Application WO 92/09695.
Holmgren, S.K., Taylor, K.M., Bretscher, L.E. and Raines, R.T. (1998) *Nature* **392**, 666.
Horio, M., Ishikawa, S. and Oda, K. (1985) *Journal of Applied Polymer Science: Applied Polymer Symposia* **41**, 269.
Howard, J. (1997) *Nature* **389**, 561.
Huber, A.E. and Viney, C. (1997) *Macromolecules* **30**, 2662.
Huber, A.E. and Viney, C. (1998) *Physical Review Letters* **80**, 623.
Hudson, S.P. (1997) in *Protein-Based Materials,* ed. McGrath, K. and Kaplan, D. (Birkhäuser, Boston, MA) p. 313.
Hukins, D.W.L. and Woodhead-Galloway, J. (1977) *Molecular Crystals and Liquid Crystals* **41**, 33.
Hyams, J.S. and Lloyd, C.W., Eds. (1994) *Microtubules*, Wiley-Liss, New York, NY.
Imanishi, Y., Fujita, K., Miura, Y. and Kimura, S. (1996) *Supramolecular Science* **3**, 13.
Isa, P., Lopez, S., Segovia, L. and Arias, C.F. (1997) *Journal of Virology* **71**, 6749.
John, M.E. and Keller, G. (1996) *Proceedings of the National Academy of Sciences, USA* **93**, 12768.
Kabsch, W. and Vandekerckhove, J. (1992) *Annual Review of Biophysical and Biomolecular Structure* **21**, 49.

Kemmish, D. (1993) in *Biodegradable Polymers and Packaging,* ed. Ching, C., Kaplan, D.L. and Thomas, E.L. (Technomic, Lancaster, PA) p. 225.

Kerkam, K., Viney, C., Kaplan, D.L. and Lombardi, S.J. (1991) *Nature* **349**, 596.

Kirshenbaum, K., Barron, A.E., Goldsmith, R.A., Armand, P., Bradley, E.K., Truong, K.T.V., Dill, K.A., Cohen, F.E. and Zuckermann, R.N. (1998) *Proceedings of the National Academy of Sciences, USA* **95**, 4303.

Koch, E.A., Spitzer, R.H. and Pithawalla, R.B. (1991) *Journal of Structural Biology* **106**, 205.

Kolpak, F.J. and Blackwell, J. (1976) *Macromolecules* **9**, 273.

Krässig, H. (1985) in *Cellulose and its Derivatives,* ed. Kennedy, J.F., Phillips, G.O., Wedlock, D.J. and Williams, P.A. (Ellis Horwood, Chichester, UK) p. 3.

Lehninger, A.A. (1975) *Biochemistry*, Worth Publishers, Inc., New York, NY.

Lepescheux, L. (1988) *Biology of the Cell* **62**, 17.

Lodish, H., Baltimore, D., Berk, A., Zipursky, S.L., Matsudaira, P. and Darnell, J. (1995) *Molecular Cell Biology*, W.H. Freeman and Company, New York, NY.

Marvin, D.A. (1966) *Journal of Molecular Biology* **15**, 8.

McGrath, K.P. and Butler, M.M. (1997) in *Protein-Based Materials,* ed. McGrath, K. and Kaplan, D. (Birkhäuser, Boston, MA) p. 251.

Moritz, M., Braunfeld, M.B., Sedat, J.W., Alberts, B. and Agard, D.A. (1995) *Nature* **378**, 638.

Mulvey, M. and Brown, D.T. (1996) *Virology* **219**, 125.

Neville, A.C. (1993) *Biology of Fibrous Composites*, Cambridge University Press, Cambridge.

Nishimura, H. and Sarko, A. (1987) *Journal of Applied Polymer Science* **33**, 867.

O'Brien, J.P. (1993) *Trends in Polymer Science* **1**(8), 228.

O'Brien, J.P., Hoess, R.H., Gardner, K.H., Lock, R.L., Wasserman, Z.R., Weber, P.C. and Salemme, F.R. (1994) in *Silk Polymers - Materials Science and Biotechnology,* ed. Kaplan, D.L., Adams, W.W., Farmer, B.L. and Viney, C. (American Chemical Society, Washington, DC) p. 104.

O'Shea, E.K., Lumb, K.J. and Kim, P.S. (1993) *Current Biology* **3**, 658.

Onsager, L. (1949) *Annals of the New York Academy of Sciences* **51**, 627.

Oster, G., Perelson, A.S. and Tilney, L.G. (1982) *Journal of Mathematical Biology* **15**, 259.

Pauling, L. and Corey, R.B. (1951) *Proceedings of the National Academy of Sciences, USA* **37**, 729.

Pauling, L., Corey, R.B. and Branson, H.R. (1951) *Proceedings of the National Academy of Sciences, USA* **37**, 205.

Prevorsek, D.C. (1982) in *Polymer Liquid Crystals,* ed. Ciferri, A., Krigbaum, W.R. and Meyer, R.B. (Academic Press, New York, NY) p. 329.

Rawn, J.D. (1989) *Proteins, Energy, and Metabolism*, Neil Patterson Publishers, Burlington, NC.

Reich, Z., Wachtel, E.J. and Minsky, A. (1994) *Science* **264**, 1460.

Ritcey, A.M. and Gray, D.G. (1988) *Biopolymers* **27**, 1363.

Roberts, C.J., Shivji, A., Davies, M.C., Davis, S.S., Fiebrig, I., Harding, S.E., Tendler, S.J.B. and Williams, P.M. (1995) *Protein and Peptide Letters* **2**(3), 409.

Robinson, C. (1966) *Molecular Crystals* **1**, 467.

Roubi, M. (1998) *Chemical and Engineering News* **76**(18), 61.

Rudall, K.M. (1957) in *Lectures on the Scientific Basis of Medicine* Vol. V (Athlone Press, London) p. 217.

Santhosh, U., Newman, K.E. and Lee, C.Y.C. (1995) *Journal of Materials Science* **30**, 1894.

Sikkema, D.J. (1998) *Polymer* **39**, 5981.

Simms, P.J., Boyko, W.J. and Edwards, J.R. (1990) *Carbohydrate Research* **208**, 193.
Smith, C.A. and Wood, E.J. (1991) *Biological Molecules*, Chapman and Hall, London.
South, A. (1992) *Terrestrial Slugs*, Chapman and Hall, London.
Steinbüchel, A. (1991) in *Biomaterials: Novel Materials from Biological Sources,* ed. Byrom, D. (Stockton Press, New York) p. 123.
Steinmetz, M.O., Stoffler, D., Hoenger, A., Bremer, A. and Aebi, U. (1997) *Journal of Structural Biology* **119**, 295.
Stewart, I. and Golubitsky, M. (1992) *Fearful Symmetry*, Blackwell, Oxford, UK.
Stivala, S.S. and Bahary, W.S. (1978) *Carbohydrate Research* **67**, 17.
Stouten, P.F.W., Sander, C., Ruigrok, R.W.H. and Cusack, S. (1992) *Journal of Molecular Biology* **226**, 1073.
Stryer, L. (1988) *Biochemistry*, W.H. Freeman and Company, New York.
Stryer, L. (1995) *Biochemistry*, W.H. Freeman and Company, New York.
Strzelecka, T.E., Davidson, M.W. and Rill, R.L. (1988) *Nature* **331**, 457.
Tang, J. and Fraden, S. (1995) *Liquid Crystals* **19**, 459.
Thiel, B.L., Guess, K.B. and Viney, C. (1997) *Biopolymers* **41**, 703.
Thiel, B.L. and Viney, C. (1995a) in *Industrial Biotechnological Polymers,* ed. Gebelein, C.G. and Carraher, C.E. Jr. (Technomic, Lancaster, PA) p. 221.
Thiel, B.L. and Viney, C. (1995b) *MRS Bulletin* **20**(9), 52.
Thiel, B.L. and Viney, C. (1997) *Journal of Microscopy* **185**, 179.
Tilney, L.G. and Inoué, S. (1982) *Journal of Cell Biology* **93**, 820.
Tirrell, D.A., Fournier, M.J. and Mason, T.L. (1991a) *MRS Bulletin* **16**(7), 23.
Tirrell, D.A., Fournier, M.J. and Mason, T.L. (1991b) *Current Opinion in Structural Biology* **1**, 638.
Tirrell, J.G., Fournier, M.J., Mason, T.L. and Tirrell, D.A. (1994) *Chemical and Engineering News* **72**(51), 40.
Tirrell, J.G., Tirrell, D.A., Fournier, M.J. and Mason, T.L. (1997) in *Protein-Based Materials,* ed. McGrath, K. and Kaplan, D. (Birkhäuser, Boston, MA) p. 61.
Trotter, J.A. and Koob, T.J. (1989) *Cell and Tissue Research* **258**, 527.
Tuszynski, J.A., Trpisova, B., Sept, D. and Brown, J.A. (1997) *Journal of Structural Biology* **118**, 94.
Urry, D.W. (1988) *The Alabama Journal of Medical Sciences* **25**(4), 475.
Urry, D.W. (1993) *Angewandte Chemie International Edition in English* **32**, 819.
Urry, D.W., Luan, C.-H., Harris, C.M. and Parker, T.M. (1997) in *Protein-Based Materials,* ed. McGrath, K. and Kaplan, D. (Birkhäuser, Boston, MA) p. 133.
Verdugo, P., Deyrup-Olsen, I., Martin, A.W. and Luchtel, D.L. (1992) in *Swelling of Polymer Networks,* ed. Karalis, E. (Springer-Verlag, Heidelberg) p 671.
Viney, C. (1993) *Materials Science and Engineering R: Reports* **10**, 187.
Viney, C. (1997a) in *Protein-Based Materials,* ed. McGrath, K. and Kaplan, D. (Birkhäuser, Boston, MA) p. 281.
Viney, C. (1997b) *Supramolecular Science* **4**, 75.
Viney, C., Huber, A. and Verdugo, P. (1993) in *Biodegradable Polymers and Packaging,* ed. Ching, C., Kaplan, D.L. and Thomas, E.L. (Technomic, Lancaster, PA) p. 209.
Viney, C., Huber, A.E., Dunaway, D.L., Kerkam, K. and Case, S.T. (1994) in *Silk Polymers: Materials Science and Biotechnology,* ed. Kaplan, D.L., Adams, W.W., Farmer, B.L. and Viney, C. (American Chemical Society, Washington, DC) p. 120.
Viney, C., Russell, T.P., Depero, L.E. and Twieg, R.J. (1989a) *Molecular Crystals and Liquid Crystals* **168**, 63.
Viney, C., Twieg, R.J., Russell, T.P. and Depero, L.E. (1989b) *Liquid Crystals* **5**, 1783.

Vogel, S. (1992) *Biomimetics* **1**, 63.
Vollrath, F. (1994) in *Silk Polymers: Materials Science and Biotechnology,* ed. Kaplan, D.L., Adams, W.W., Farmer, B.L. and Viney, C. (American Chemical Society, Washington, DC) p. 17.
Wade, R.H. and Chretien, D. (1993) *Journal of Structural Biology* **110**, 1.
Willison, J.H.M. and Abeysekera, R.M. (1988) *Journal of Polymer Science Part C - Polymer Letters* **26**(2), 71.
Woodhead-Galloway, J. (1980) *Collagen : The Anatomy of a Protein*, Edward Arnold, London.
Work, R.W. (1985) *Journal of Experimental Biology* **118**, 379.
Yoshikawa, E., Fournier, M.J., Mason, T.L. and Tirrell, D.A. (1994) *Macromolecules* **27**, 5471.
Zheng, Y., Wong, M.L., Alberts, B. and Mitchison, T. (1995) *Nature* **378**, 578.
Zinoni, F., Birkmann, A., Stadtman, T.C. and Bock, A. (1986) *Proceedings of the National Academy of Sciences, USA* **83**, 4650.

Chapter 9

Computer Model for the Mechanical Properties of Synthetic and Biological Polymer Fibers

Chapter 9

Computer Model for the Mechanical Properties of Synthetic and Biological Polymer Fibers

YVES TERMONIA

9.1. INTRODUCTION

A general theoretical description of the mechanical properties of polymeric fibers is an extremely complex problem because of the need to consider a variety of parameters such as chain length and its distribution, inter- and intra-chain interactions, amorphous *vs.* crystalline content, etc. For that reason, analytical approaches are impossible and one needs to resort to computer simulation models. Most of the computer models introduced to date are essentially atomistic in nature in the sense that they focus on deformation of bonds and valence angles. These models are, in principle, exact if one knows the potential functions for inter- and intra-chain interactions. However, being on such a small scale, the largest system size and time that can be studied are extremely small. As a result, the atomistic models are often of little value for an understanding of macroscopic properties of experimental interest.

In view of these difficulties, we have introduced a series of molecular models which bypass details of the deformation on an atomistic scale and focus instead on a length scale of the order of the distance between entanglements, see Figure 9.1. This is of importance as entanglements constitute the actual load-bearing junctions in long chain systems which are characteristic of experimental situations. The objective of the present Chapter is to describe these models in some detail and to show their value in getting a better understanding of the factors controlling the mechanical properties of synthetic and biological fibers.

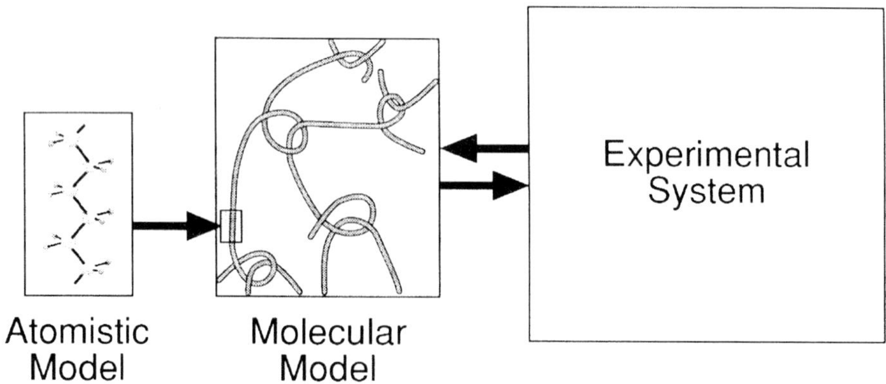

Fig. 9.1. Atomistic *vs.* molecular models.

Before introducing these models, it is important to briefly describe how fibers are being processed in industry and in most biological organisms such as the abdominal glands in the spider.

Immediately after polymerization, polymer chains are in a random coil configuration and they can be compared to an agglomerate of "cooked spaghetti", see Fig. 9.2a. The mechanical properties of these systems are extremely poor as any applied load is carried essentially by the weak attractive bonds between chains with little contribution from the strong chain backbone.

For that reason, these agglomerates are further processed by drawing into a fiber form wherein the polymer chains are now perfectly ordered and extended along the fiber axis (Fig. 9.2b). In such a configuration, the strong covalent backbone chains play a crucial role and tensile mechanical properties are optimized. Experiments clearly indicate that the higher the draw applied to the macromolecular chains of Fig. 9.2a, the better their orientation in Fig. 9.2b and the higher the fiber tensile strength.

9.2. MOLECULAR MODEL

Our molecular model for a dense network of polymer chains prior to drawing is depicted in Fig. 9.3. In our representation, the entanglements (symbol ●) are initially placed at the sites of a regular 2-dimensional diamond lattice. Thus, the unit lattice length is set by the chain length between entanglements, M_e. The entanglement points are connected by chains, which are, prior to deformation, in a random coil configuration. Chain ends account for the finite molecular weight of the sample. In addition to being entangled, chains also interact via weak attractive forces which are also taken into account, see Fig. 9.3.

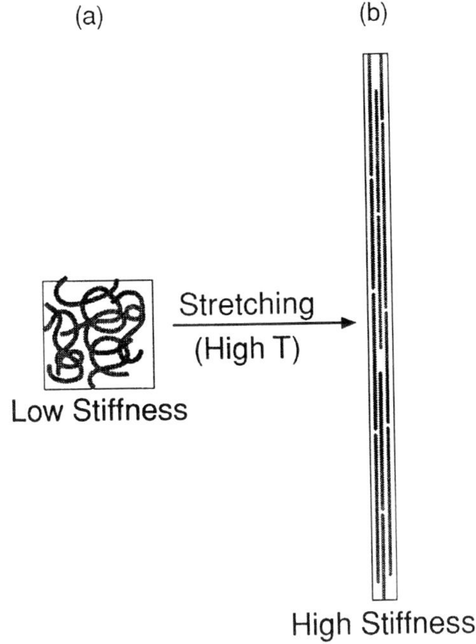

Fig. 9.2. (a) Network of polymer chains after polymerization. (b) Same network after drawing during spinning.

In the following paragraph, we describe in some detail our procedure for building the dense network of chains in Fig. 9.3.

We start with an empty 2-dimensional diamond lattice, the sites of which are occupied by "future" entanglement points. We pick a length M for the first chain to be build, according to the desired molecular weight distribution. That chain is then constructed through a random walk of m $(=M/M_e)$ steps, as follows:An unoccupied bond is first selected at random and partially filled-in with a chain end of molecular weight $M_e/2$. From that end, we then build a random walk of m steps, the last one of which representing the other end of the chain. Multiple occupancy of a lattice bond by more than one chain strand is forbidden. Hence, in order to facilitate our construction procedure, the direction for each step is chosen from a set of probabilities obtained from a "looking forward" procedure which calculates the number of chains of $b < m$ steps that can be constructed along a given direction without overlapping previously generated chains.An example of our procedure is illustrated in Figure 9.4 for the construction of a chain (labeled d) having $m = 5$ steps. Clearly, the larger the number b of "looking forward" steps, the closer the actual molecular weight distribution to its prescribed value.

Upon connecting all entanglement points with polymer chains, we superimpose on the network of chains a second lattice of "overall" attractive bonds further connecting each entanglement to its nearest neighbors, see Fig.9.3b.

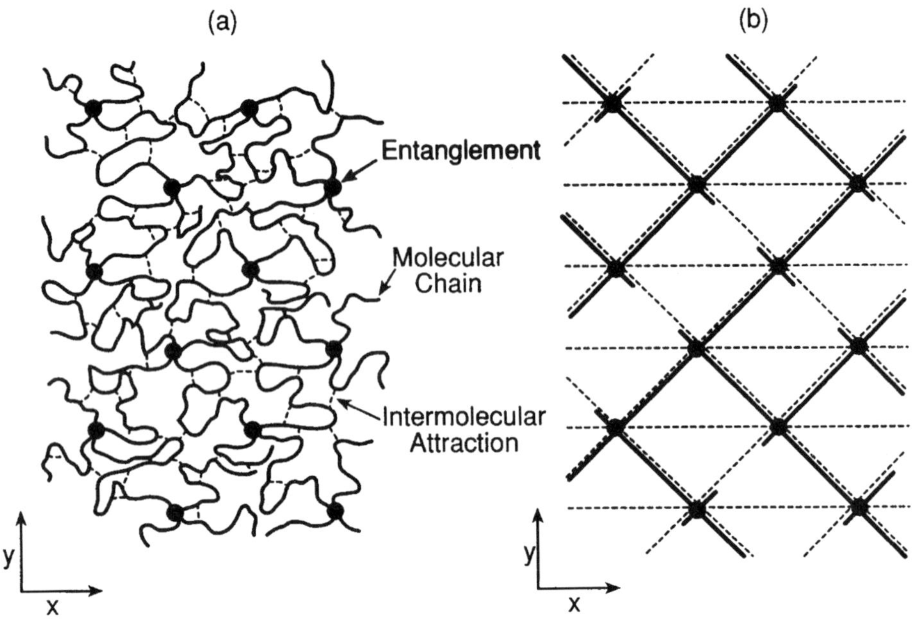

Fig. 9.3. Molecular model for an aggregate of polymer chains. (a) Dense system of chains prior to drawing. The heavy black circles represent entanglement loci and the dotted lines denote the attractive bonds between and within chains. (b) More schematic representation of the network. The heavy solid lines indicate chain vectors between entanglements; chain ends are represented by shorter solid lines. Individual attractive bonds have been replaced by "overall" bonds (dotted lines) joining each entanglement to its nearest neighbors.

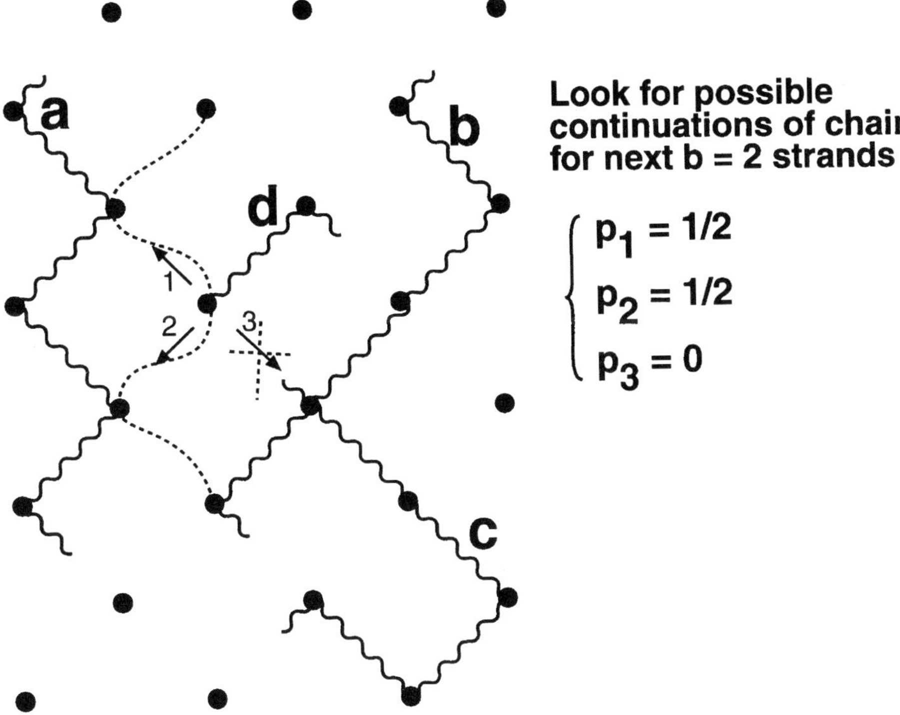

Fig. 9.4. Illustration of our technique for constructing a chain d having m = 5 steps. The figure is for a "looking forward" procedure which counts the number of future chains of b = 2 steps. There are 3 possible directions for the third step of chain d. One chain of b = 2 steps can be generated starting along direction 1; another along direction 2. Clearly, any chain continuing along direction 3 would overlap previously constructed chains b and c. Hence, $p_3=0$ whereas $p_1=p_2=1/2$.

After completion of the network construction, the regular lattice of Fig.9.3b is deformed at a constant temperature and rate of strain. That deformation is performed in a succession of very small length increments δL, determined by the strain rate $\varepsilon/\delta t$, in which $\varepsilon = \delta L/L_o$ and L_o is the initial length. In that process, we start by moving the upper row of entanglement points a distance δL along the positive y-axis, while the bottom row is held fixed. The positions of the entanglements in between these two rows are then readjusted by an iterative relaxation procedure which minimizes the net residual force acting on each lattice site (for details, see process (*iv*) below). After each strain increment and upon complete relaxation of all lattice sites, individual bonds and entanglement points are visited at random by a Monte-Carlo lottery and four processes are allowed to occur:

(i) Breaking of the attractive bonds between chains.
We assume that the process is thermally activated and its rate ν can be described using the relation (Kausch 1978).

$$\nu_i = \tau \exp[-(U - \beta \sigma_i)/kT] \tag{9.1}$$

In Eq. (9.1), the index i refers to the particular bond being considered, τ is the thermal vibration frequency, U and β are, respectively, the activation energy and volume whereas

$$\sigma_i = K \varepsilon_i \tag{9.2}$$

is the local stress acting on bond i. Here, ε_i is the local strain and K is the elastic constant. Use of Eqs. 9.1-9.2 within the framework of a Monte-Carlo lottery is performed as follows. The probability p_i for breaking bond i is first calculated from (Termonia and Smith 1987, 1988).

$$p_i = \nu_i / \nu_{max} \tag{9.3}$$

in which ν_{max} is the rate of breakage of the most strained bond in the array. We then generate a random number normalized between 0 and 1. If the number happens to fall below p_i, we break the bond. If not, the bond stays intact. After each visit of a bond, the "time" t of our simulations is augmented by $1/[\nu_{max} \cdot n(t)]$ where $n(t)$ is the total number of intact bonds at time t. The process is stopped once the simulation time t is increased by the preset δt interval (see above). Note that the bond breakages lead to a release of the underlying chain strands, which are now to support the external load. Once-broken, attractive bonds are assumed not to reform.

(ii) Slippage of chains through entanglements
As the stress on the "freed" chain strands increases, slippage through entanglements is assumed to set in at a rate that has the same functional form as that for the attractive bond breakings (Eq. 9.1), but with different values for the activation energy U and volume β. Also, σ_i now denotes the difference in stress in two consecutive chain strands that are separated by entanglement i. This stress difference is calculated using the classical treatment of rubber elasticity. According to this theory, the stress on a stretched chain strand having a vector length r is given by (Treloar 1985).

$$\sigma = \alpha k T \mathcal{L}^{-1}(r / n\ell) \tag{9.4}$$

Here, n is the number of statistical chains segments of length ℓ in a strand, $\mathcal{L}^{-1}$ is the inverse Langevin function and α is a proportionality constant which depends on the number N of chain strands per unit volume. The latter is obtained from

$$\alpha = \left(N/3\right)\ n^{1/2} \tag{9.5}$$

The chain slippage process described by Eqs.(9.1) and (9.4-9.5) is executed by a Monte-Carlo technique similar to that used for process (*i*). Here, however, ν_{max} (see Eq.9.3) denotes the highest rate of slippage and $n(t)$ is the total number of entanglements at time t. In accordance with reported experimental data for viscous flow of paraffins, we assume that the unit length for chain slippage is of the order of a statistical segment.

(iii) Chain breakage

The slippage process described above leads to a change in the number of statistical chain units between entanglements, and occasionally, to chain disentanglement. If the rate of chain slippage is too low, maximum elongation of the chain strands between entanglements can be reached and chain fracture is allowed to occur at a local draw ratio $\lambda = \sqrt{n}$. Alternatively, one could also assume that the process is thermally activated and occurs at a rate similar to that of Eqs.9.1-9.2 using different values for the activation energy and volume; for more details see (Termonia, Allen and Smith 1985).

(iv) Network relaxation

The three processes described above -again- perturb the mechanical equilibrium existing among the various entanglement points. That equilibrium is then restored by minimizing the residual force acting on each entanglement. That minimization is executed using a series of fast computer algorithms, described in (Termonia and Smith 1987, 1988) and (Termonia, Meakin and Smith 1985), which steadily reduce the net residual force acting on each entanglement point. This leads to displacements of the entanglement loci along the x- and y- axis. In order to save computer time, only displacements along the y-axis of draw are explicitly calculated. Distances in the transverse x-direction are assumed to be contracted homogeneously by a factor $\lambda^{-1/2}$, where $\lambda = 1 + \varepsilon$ is the overall draw ratio along the y-axis. After these relaxation steps, which constitute the most computer-time consuming processes in the simulation, the axial nominal stress at one end of the network is calculated.

After the network of entanglements has been fully relaxed towards mechanical equilibrium, an additional elongation increment δL is applied to the network and the four processes described above are restarted for another time interval δt. And so on and so forth, until the network fails. A brief flow chart of the network construction and of its subsequent deformation process is given in Table 9.1.

Table 9.1. Flow chart of our algorithm for network construction and its subsequent deformation

---

NETWORK CONSTRUCTION

- Generate 2-dimensional diamond lattice of entanglement points
- Connect entanglements with chains according to prescribed molecular weight distribution
- Superimpose a second lattice of "overall" attractive bonds

NETWORK DEFORMATION

(0) set value for strain rate $\varepsilon/\delta t$ in which $\varepsilon = \delta L/L_0$ and set overall time $t = 0$

(1) elongate network by increment δL
- move top row of entanglements by δL along y-axis
- relax remaining entanglements towards mechanical equilibrium (bottom row fixed)

(2) break attractive bonds for time interval δt
- select bond i at random
- calculate $p_i = v_i/v_{max}$ using Eqs. 9.1-9.3
- generate random number and check for breaking
- increase process time by $1/[v_{max} \cdot n(t)]$

(3) slip chains for time interval δt
- select entanglement i at random
- calculate $p_i = v_i/v_{max}$ using Eqs. 9.1 and 9.3-9.5
- generate random number and check for slippage
- increase process time by $1/[v_{max} \cdot n(t)]$

(4) break chain strands
- select chain strand i at random
- break strand if local draw ratio $\lambda_i > n_i^{1/2}$

(5) relax entanglements towards mechanical equilibrium

(6) set overall time $t = t + \delta t$

(7) return to (1) and repeat the sequence until overall network breaks

---

9.3. APPLICATION

We now turn to application of our model to a detailed study of the factors controlling the drawability of polyethylene (PE).

PE is a semi-crystalline polymer in which the crystallites are held together by attractive bonds of the van der Waals (vdW) type. These bonds are rather weak and they easily break at the high temperatures (100-120°C) used in drawing. For that reason, we may neglect in the present section the effects of initial crystallinity and crystallite size present in the polymer prior to deformation. (In our approach, crystallinity is, in fact, smeared homogeneously over the whole lattice.) Details of the values of the model parameters can be found in (Termonia and Smith 1987, 1988).

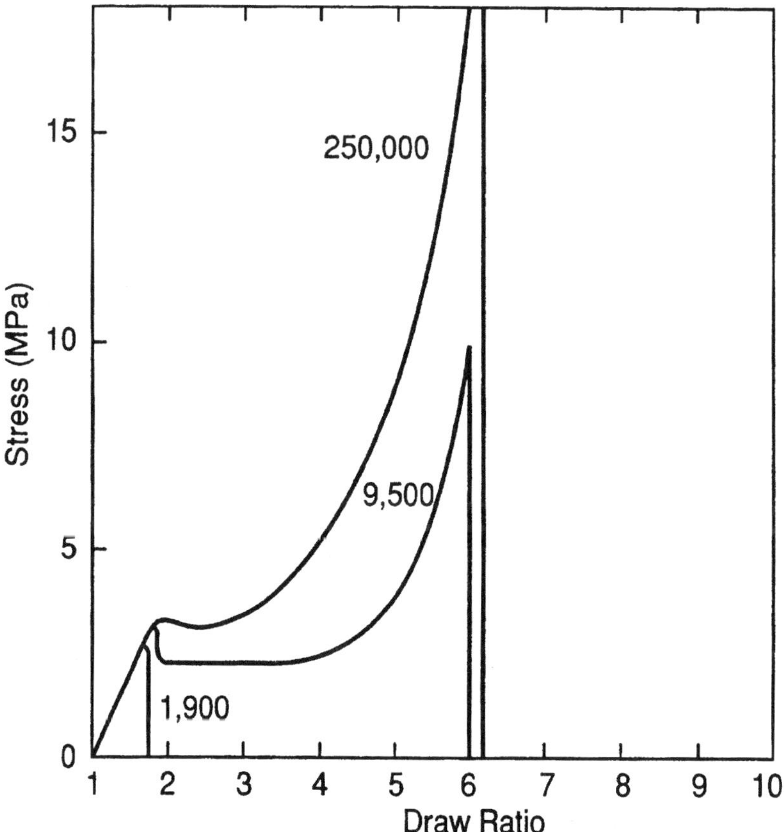

Fig. 9.5. Effect of molecular weight, M, on nominal stress-draw ratio curves for PE. The deformation temperature was 75°C and the rate of strain was 500%/min.

9.3.1 Effect of molecular weight

Figure 9.5 shows a series of stress-draw ratio curves calculated with our model for molecular weights M = 1900, 9500 and 250000.

To recall, the draw ratio is defined as $\lambda = 1 + \delta L / L_o$ in which δL is the elongation and L_o is the initial length of the sample. Note that the molecular weight between entanglements in the melt for PE has value M_e^{melt} = 1900. For simplicity, we have assumed no entanglement slippage. All three curves show an initial linear regime, which extends to draw ratios $\lambda = 1.7$, and is characterized by straining of the network of vdW bonds. At $\lambda = 1.7$, these bonds start to break and the stress-strain curves become strongly dependent on molecular weight.

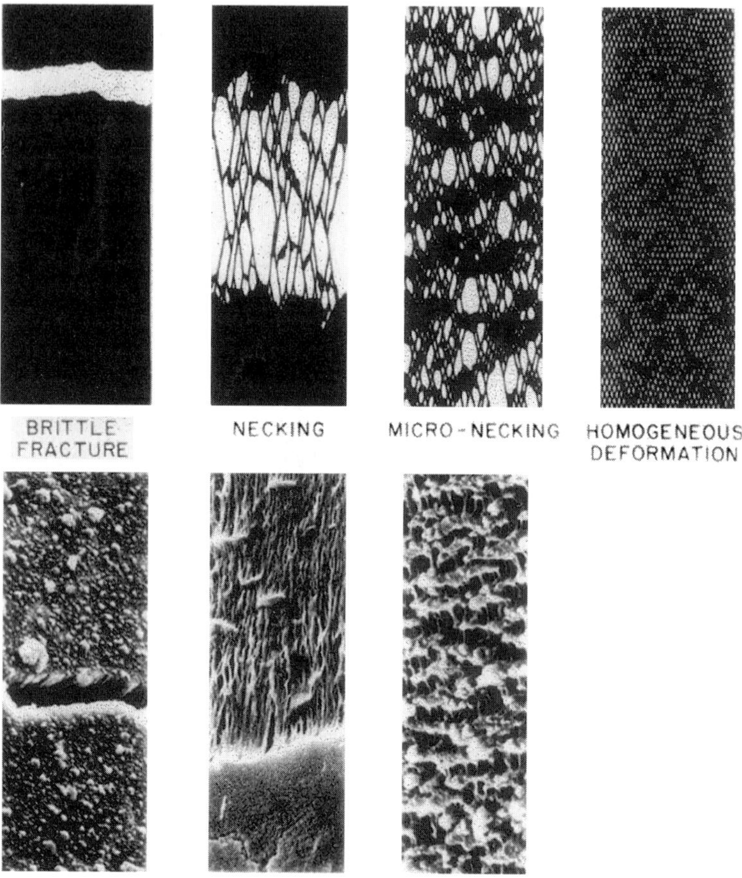

Fig. 9.6. Top: Typical morphologies obtained with the model for polyethylenes having molecular weights (left to right): M=1,900, M=9,500, M=20,000 and M=250,000. Bottom: Experimentally observed morphologies obtained at similar molecular weights.

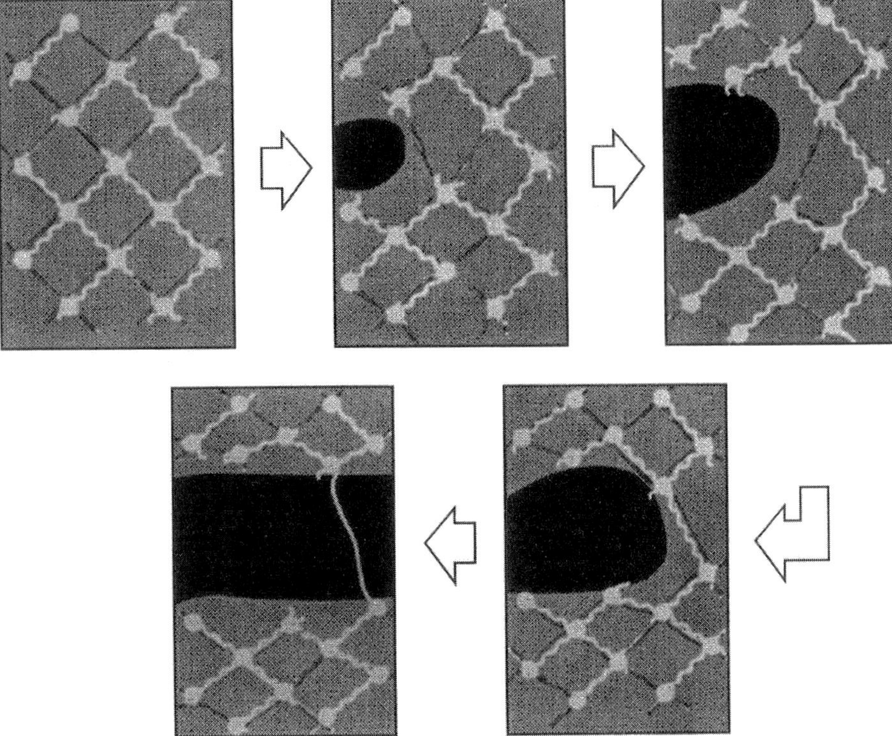

Fig. 9.7.a Schematic model representation of the deformation behavior of small molecular weight polyethylenes. Neck formation.

Figure 9.6 (top) displays a schematic illustration of the morphologies obtained with the model for the various molecular weight values studied in Fig. 9.5. At M = 1,900, brittle fracture is observed; at M = 9,500 a well-defined single neck appears which then propagates along the sample; at M = 20,000 several micro-necks are formed; and at M = 250,000 the deformation appears to be homogeneous.

The bottom of Fig. 9.6 shows some typical experimental morphologies obtained at comparable molecular weight values. An excellent agreement with the model predictions is found.

A careful analysis of our model results gives the following insight into the strong dependence of morphology of deformation on molecular weight. We start by studying the case of low M < 10,000. For those systems, the concentration of chain ends is high. As a result, the early breaking of vdW bonds leads to the formation of a microcrack which quickly propagates transversally, meeting occasionally a few load bearing chain

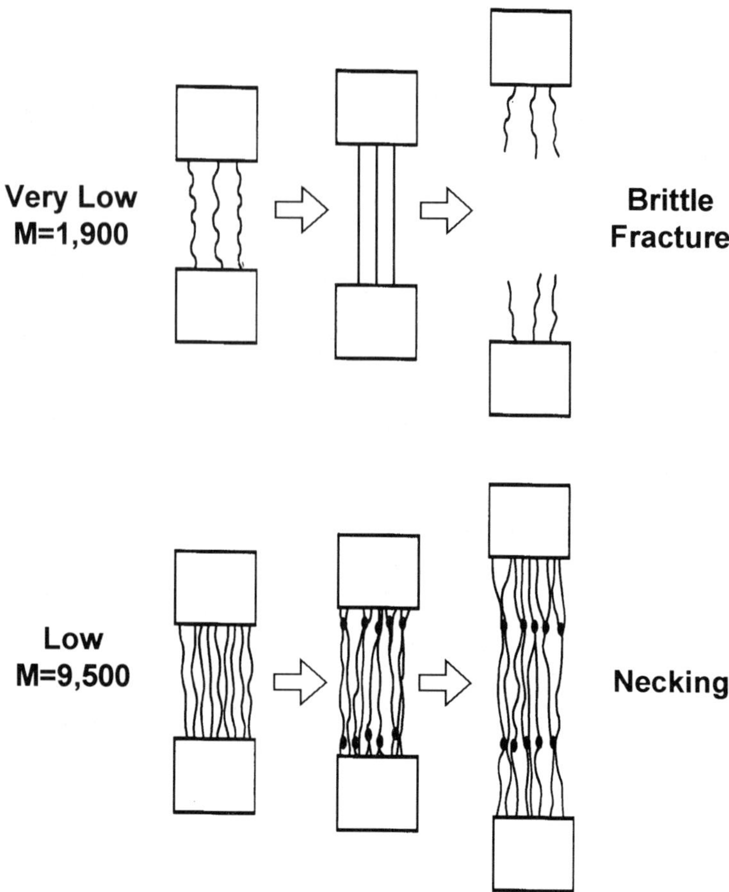

Fig. 9.7.b Schematic model representation of the deformation behavior of small molecular weight polyethylenes. Neck propagation.

strands (see Fig. 9.7a). At this stage of the deformation, two possibilities arise, see Fig. 9.7b.

At very low $M = 1900$, there are not enough chain strands bridging the initial crack. These chain quickly stretch to maximum extension and break, leading to brittle fracture.

At higher $M = 9{,}500$, the number of chain strands extending across the crack is high enough to overcome the yield stress at the interface with the undeformed material. As a result, more chains are pulled into the deformed region and a "neck" easily propagates along the sample.

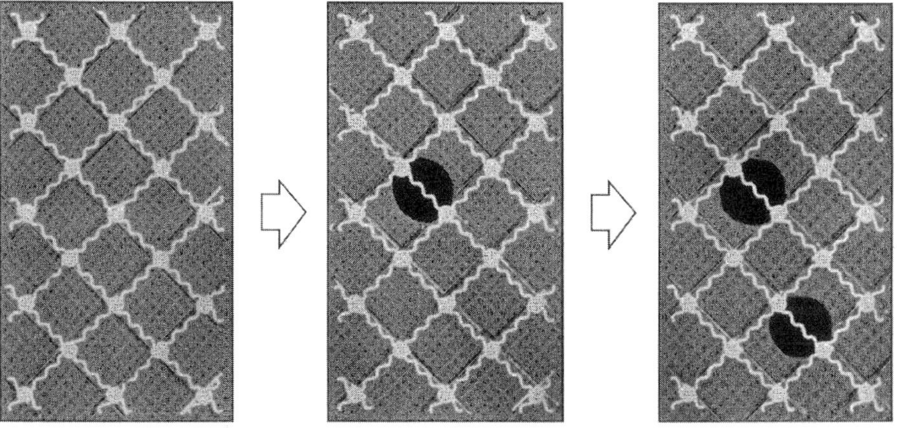

Fig. 9.8. Schematic model representation of the deformation behavior of very high molecular weight polyethylenes

We now turn to high molecular weight samples, see Fig. 9.8. In these systems, the load carried by broken vdW bonds is easily transferred to an underlying chain strand and no local stress concentration is generated. As a result, vdW bonds break at random throughout the sample and the deformation remains homogeneous at all times.

9.3.2 Effect of entanglement spacing

In order to vary the entanglement spacing, we introduce the factor ϕ defined as

$$\phi = (M_e/M_e^{melt})^{-1} \tag{9.6}$$

The selection of the spacing factor ϕ is, of course, not coincidental. It is well known that entanglements can be spaced apart experimentally through dilution of the polymer. The molecular weight between entanglements in solution is approximately given by the relation (Graessley 1974).

$$(M_e)^{soln} \sim (M_e)^{melt} / \phi \tag{9.7}$$

where ϕ is the volume fraction of the polymer.

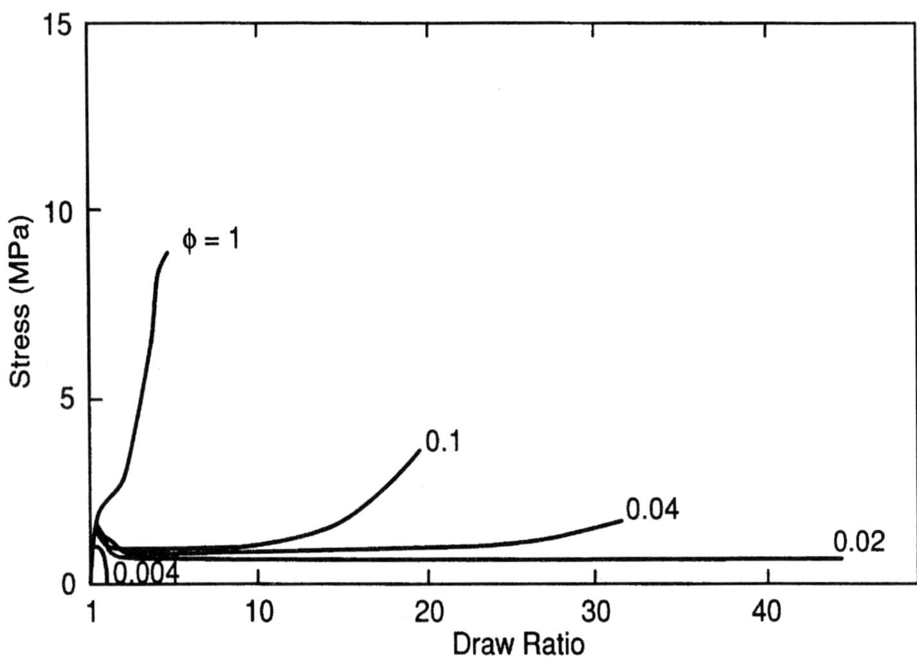

Fig. 9.9. Calculated stress-draw ratio curves for PE at different values of ϕ (Eq.9.6). The figure is for a molecular weight M=475000. The deformation temperature was $109^{o}C$ and the rate of strain was 500%/min.

Figure 9.9 shows a series of stress/draw ratio curves calculated for monodisperse polyethylene of M = 475,000 at 5 different values of the entanglement spacing factor ϕ(1, 0.1, 0.04, 0.02 and 0.004). The deformation temperature was taken to be 109°C. This figure reveals the dramatic effect of the entanglement spacing on the deformation characteristics, notably on the post-yield strain hardening and on the strain at break. At decreasing values of ϕ, the rate of strain hardening, i.e. the post-yield modulus, rapidly dropped to reach a negative value at ϕ= 0.004.The strain at break, on the other hand, drastically increased from 4.5 to 45 when ϕ decreased from 1 to 0.02. At much lower values of ϕ, e.g. 0.004, the plastic deformation leading to high values of the strain at break no longer occurred as a result of continued strain softening and ductile failure was observed. The latter result is, of course, due to the fact that, at ϕ= 0.004, the molecular weight between entanglements is 1,900/0.004 = 475,000, which equals the molecular weight of the polyethylene in the simulation. Accordingly, transfer of applied load, in this special case, occurs only from one chain to its nearest neighbors through weak vdW bonds and stress concentrations arising from vdW-bond breaks are not distributed uniformly throughout the entanglement network. As a result, very little

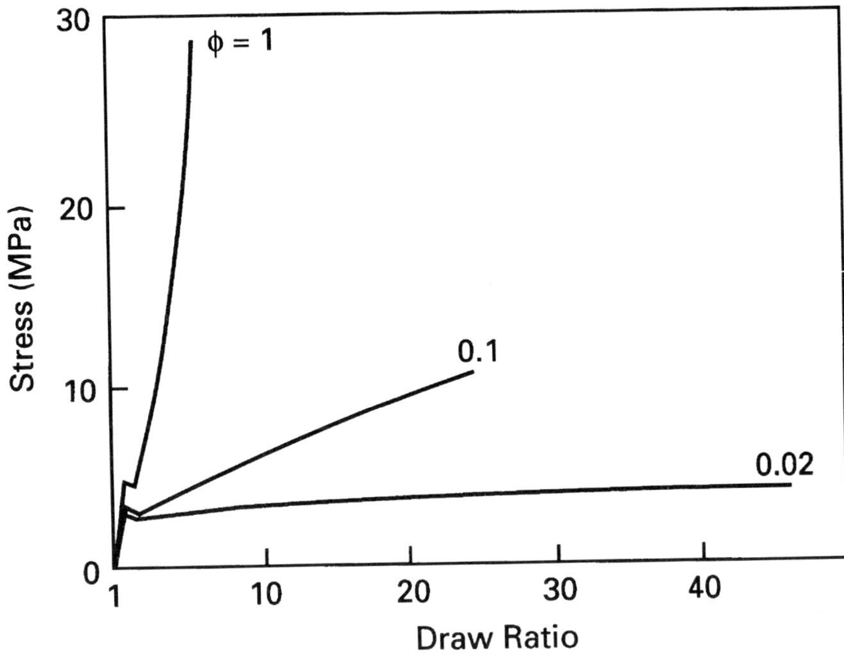

Fig. 9.10. Experimental stress-draw ratio curves for PE at different values of the dilution factor ϕ. The figure is for M_W=1.5x10^6. The data are taken from (Smith, Lemstra and Booij 1981).

deformation occurred and failure was highly localized. The situation is very similar to that described previously in a melt with M = 1900 (see Fig. 9.5).

Figure 9.10 shows a series of experimental stress-draw ratio curves taken from (Smith, Lemstra and Booij 1981). The curves are for a polydisperse system with M_w = 1.5 x 10^6. The experimental data compare very well with our calculated predictions of Fig. 9.9, which leads to confidence in the validity of our model. Note also the good quantitative agreement between calculated and observed values for the dependence of the maximum draw ratio on ϕ.

Figure 9.11 compares calculated (right) and experimental (left) morphologies obtained for a high molecular weight polyethylene at various ϕ values. Agreement is -again- judged to be excellent. Note also that the sequence of morphologies obtained at decreasing ϕ is very similar to that observed when lowering the molecular weight in the solvent-free polymer (see Fig. 9.6). This is understandable because both a decrease in ϕ and in molecular weight lead to a reduction in the number of entanglements which, as was stressed in the Introduction, fully control the deformation behavior.

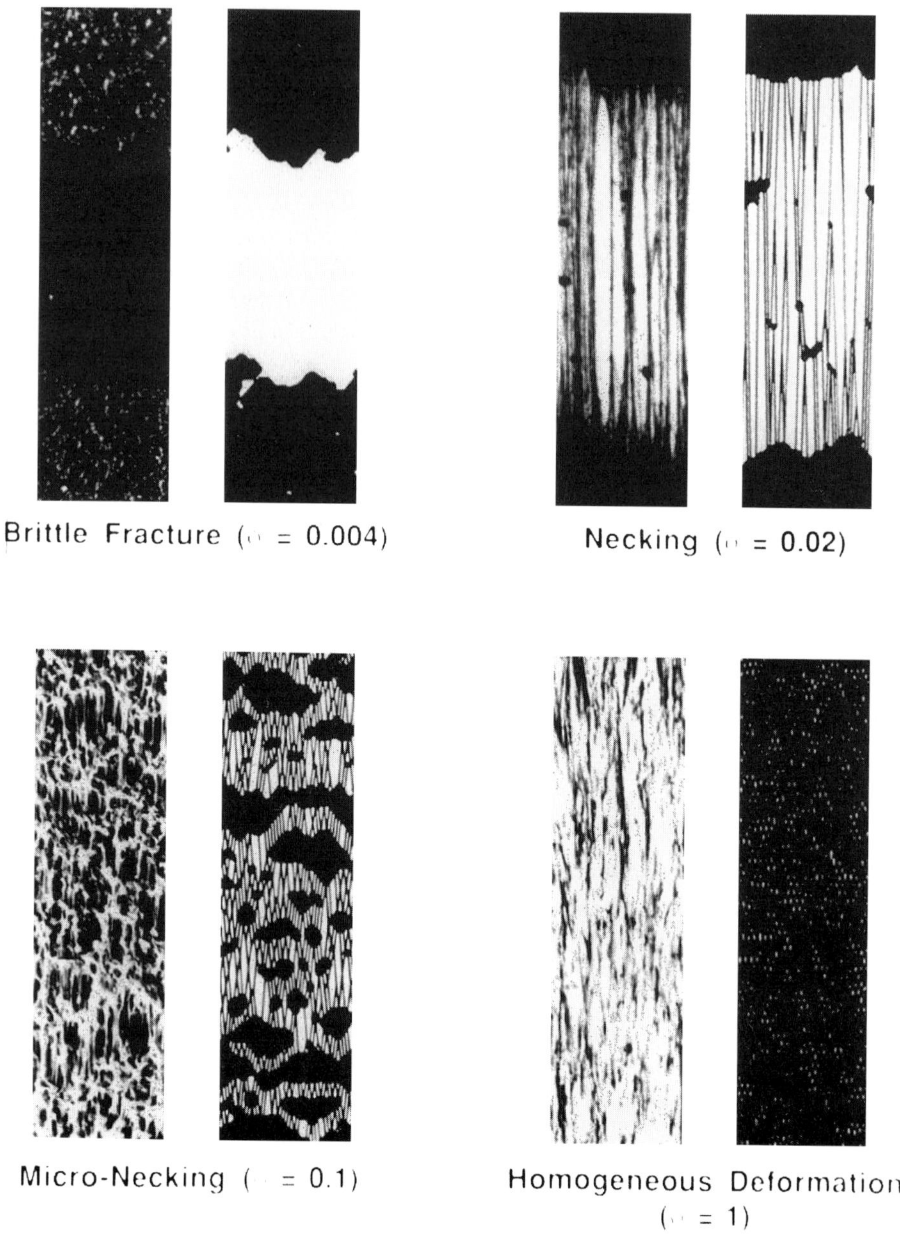

Fig. 9.11. Calculated (right) and experimental (left) morphologies obtained for high molecular weight polyethylene at various values of ϕ. For more details, see (Termonia and Smith 1988).

9.3.3 Effect of drawing conditions

Figure 9.12 shows a series of stress-draw ratio curves for monodisperse polyethylene (M = 143,000) calculated at different temperatures of deformation (Termonia, Allen and Smith 1988; Termonia and Smith 1992). The strain rate was kept constant at 625%/min.

At low temperatures (T<100°C), the computer results show an important strain-hardening effect immediately after the yield point. This effect is due to a straining of the molecular chain strands between entanglements, which break, at their maximum draw ratio. When the temperature is increased (T=120°C-130°C), a smoothening of the strain-hardening effect is observed. Inspection of the computer results shows that this smoothening is a result of slippage of chains through entanglement points: a process that is exacerbated at elevated temperatures. Chain slippage leads to an effective increase in the number n of statistical segments between entanglements and, therefore to an increase in the draw ratio at break. Simulations carried out at temperatures exceeding 130°C show that chain slippage becomes substantially faster than the strain rate. This causes a continuous decrease of the stress past the yield point and to a lowering in the largest attainable draw ratio. The results described above point to the existence of an optimum temperature for the achievement of maximum draw. For monodisperse polyethylene of M = 143,000 elongated at a rate of 625% min^{-1}, this temperature is predicted to be around T = 130°C.

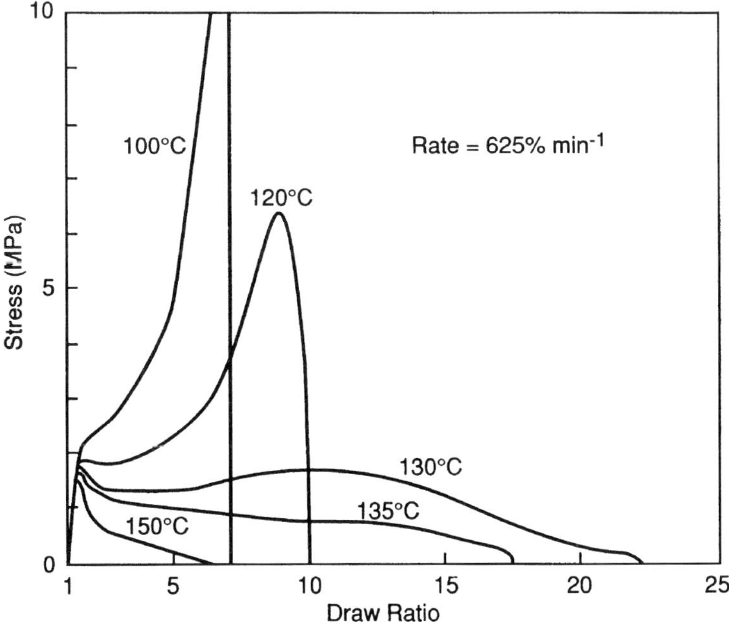

Fig. 9.12. Effect of temperature of deformation on nominal stress-draw ratio curves for PE. The figure is for a molecular weight M=143000.

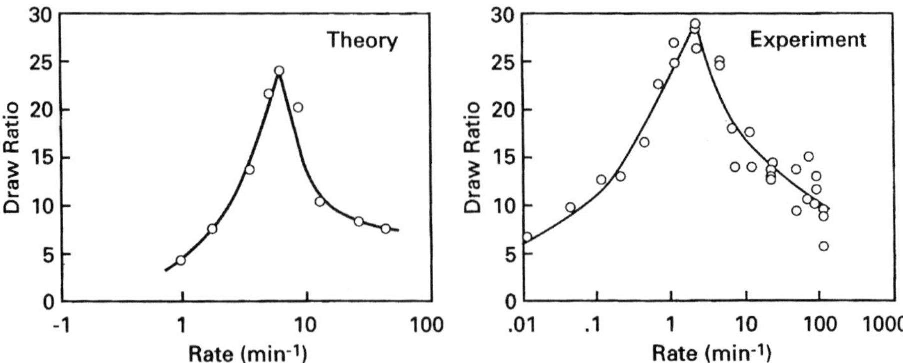

Fig. 9.13. Calculated and experimental dependence of the maximum draw ratio on rate of deformation for polyethylene. For more details, see (Termonia, Allen and Smith 1988).

Note that, since our approach is based on a thermally activated rate theory, results similar to those of Fig. 9.12 can be obtained by varying the rate of deformation, keeping the temperature constant. This is clearly demonstrated in Fig. 9.13 which gives our model predictions for the dependence of maximum draw ratio on deformation rate at M = 143,000. As in Fig. 9.12, we observe the presence of a well-defined rate window within which drawability reaches a maximum. Also represented in the figure (rhs) are actual experimental data for NBS SRM 1484 which has a close-to monodisperse molecular weight distribution with M_n = 111,000 and M_w = 125,000. Agreement between theory and experiment is judged to be excellent. Note that a better fit between theoretical and experimental optimum rate windows could have been obtained by adjusting our values for the activation energy for chain slippage, which was not attempted in the present calculations.

A further experimental confirmation of our prediction of an optimum rate (or temperature) window for drawing can be found in Fig. 9.14. The figure shows actual NBS SRM 1484 samples drawn to break at different temperatures. Optimum drawing around T=75°C is clearly observed.

The results presented above conclusively indicate that the optimum window for drawing is controlled by the rate of slippage of chains through entanglements. Since the latter is controlled by chain length, we also expect that window to be strongly dependent on molecular weight (see Figure 9.7, Chapter 11). Thus, every molecular weight value has its own optimum rate or temperature for drawing and, as a result, the narrow windows observed in Figs. 9.13-9.14 are expected to be more diffuse in polydisperse samples. This is more clearly exemplified in Fig. 9.15 which shows the effect of the polydispersity index M_z/M_w on the dependence of maximum draw on testing conditions, see also (Termonia and Smith 1992). Both theory and experiment confirm the progressive disappearance of an optimum drawing rate, which is also associated with a lower drawability of the sample.

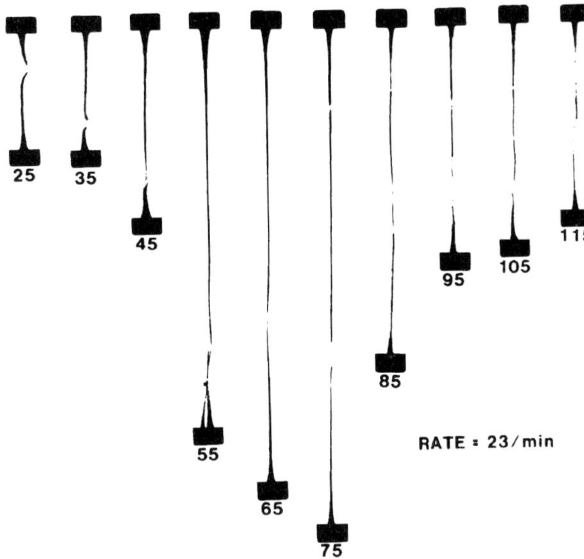

Fig. 9.14. Actual polyethylene samples drawn to break at different temperatures. The strain rate was 23/min.

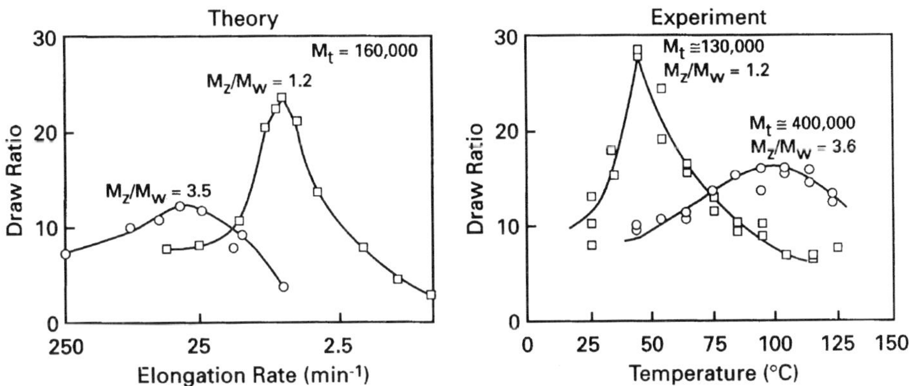

Fig. 9.15. Effect of polydispersity on the dependence of draw ratio on testing conditions.

9.3.4 Ultimate tensile strength

In this section, we assume that the PE fiber has been successfully drawn to very high draw ratios so that the macromolecules are perfectly oriented and extended along the fiber axis, as in Fig. 9.2b. In order to study the so-called ultimate strength of these fibers, we use a model similar to that described above, in which vdW bonds and covalent backbone bonds are broken using a thermally activated process. For details on the activation energies and volumes for these processes, the reader is referred to (Termonia, Meakin and Smith 1985). For simplicity, we assume that the fiber is free of entanglements.

Figure 9.16 show a series of stress-strain curves for various molecular weights ranging from $M = 1.4 \times 10^3$ to 3×10^5. The strain is defined as $\varepsilon = \delta L/L_o$. At low molecular weights ($M < 8 \times 10^4$), our results indicate a substantial amount of breaking of vdW bonds with little or no rupture of covalent backbone bonds. Under such circumstances, plastic deformation is observed and the curves are bell-shaped with a very slow decrease in the stress towards the breaking point. At higher molecular weights, we observe rupture of both vdW and covalent backbone bonds and, as a result, the fracture of the sample seems more of a brittle nature. Inspection of the figure reveals

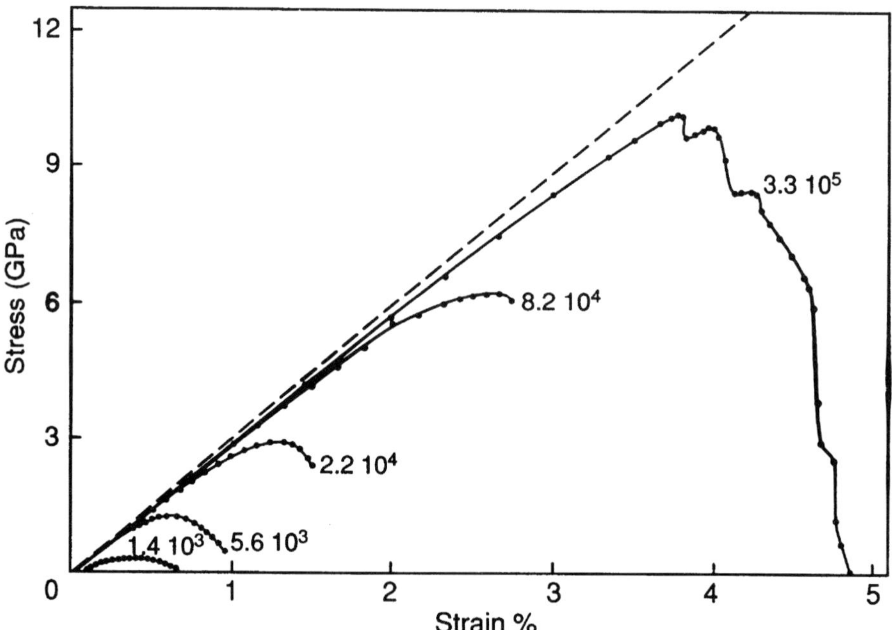

Fig. 9.16. Ultimate stress-strain curves for perfectly ordered and oriented PE fibers. The curves are for different molecular weights. The figure is for room temperature and a rate of strain 100%/min.

a rather weak dependence of the initial modulus on molecular weight. The tensile strength (maximum of the curves), on the other hand, is seen to increase with molecular weight. Results (not reproduced) indicate that, in the range $2 \times 10^4 < M < 10^6$, the ultimate tensile strength increases as $M^{0.4}$.

9.4. CONCLUSIONS

In summary, we have presented a Monte-Carlo model for the study of the mechanical properties of synthetic and biological polymer fibers. Our description is in terms of molecular parameters such as molecular weight, density of entanglements, crystalline fraction, etc. which can be easily determined from experimental data. As a first step towards a basic understanding of the factors controlling the mechanical properties of fibers, our model has been applied to polyethylene (PE) which represents the simplest and most extensively studied synthetic polymer. PE is a semi-crystalline material in which the flexible chains interact through weak van der Waals (vdW) bonds. As a result, the initial crystallinity is of minor importance in studies of drawability, which allows to better isolate the effects of molecular weight, molecular weight distribution and density of entanglements.

REFERENCES

Graessley W.W. (1974), *Adv. Polym. Sci.* **16**, 3.
Kausch H.H. (1978) Polymer *Fracture,* Springer-Verlag. Berlin.
Smith P., Lemstra P.J. and Booij H.C. (1981), *J. Polym. Sci.: Polym.Phys.Ed.* **19**, 877.
Termonia Y., Meakin P. and Smith P. (1985), *Macromolecules*, **18**, 2246.
Termonia Y. and Smith P. (1987) *Macromolecules*, **20**, 835.
Termonia Y. and Smith P. (1988) *Macromolecules*, **21**, 2184.
Termonia Y., Allen S.R. and Smith P. (1988) *Macromolecules*, **21**, 3485.
Termonia Y. and Smith P. (1992) *Coll.Polym.Sci.* , **270**, 1085.
Treloar L.R.G. (1985) *The Physics of Rubber Elasticity,* 2nd ed. (Clarendon. Oxford).

Chapter 10

Silk Fibres: Origins, Nature and Consequences of Structure

Chapter 10

Silk Fibres: Origins, Nature and Consequences of Structure

CHRISTOPHER VINEY

10.1. BACKGROUND

10.1.1 Introduction

Natural silks have evolved towards the simultaneous optimisation of several significant properties. These include (i) unrivalled *combinations* of high strength, stiffness and toughness, in both tension and compression (Zemlin 1968; Kaplan *et al.* 1991; Kaplan *et al.* 1994; Kaplan *et al.* 1997), (ii) *smart processability* (Thiel and Viney 1997; Viney 1997) from aqueous solution at ambient temperature, and (iii) *reliability* (the silk performs regardless of the temperature and humidity that prevailed during spinning). Features of the complex molecular and microstructural architectures, which underlie these properties, will be discussed below. Exploitation of silks in textiles has developed over several millennia (Hyde 1984), and interest has expanded recently to include load-bearing or impact-resistant engineering materials. From an engineering perspective, silks are additionally attractive because they are processed from renewable resources, and, though durable in many environments, they are biodegradable: spiders are highly effective recyclers of their web and dragline fibre (Foelix 1982).

Engineering applications of natural silks are limited by a poor tolerance of high temperatures, and by their large spread in mechanical property values (silkworm silk has Weibull characteristics close to those of glass (Pérez-Rigueiro *et al.* 1998)). The latter problem is in part a consequence of poorly reproducible cross-sectional geometry. Developments in biotechnology offer the tools for synthesising large quantities of polymer with a complex primary structure identical or related to that of silk. However, the success of such ventures will depend on whether the microstructures and multifunctional properties of silk can be replicated in fibre that is spun at economic rates.

10.1.2 Diversity of silk-producing organisms and their silks

All spider species (of which there are more than 30,000 (Foelix 1982)) and a very large number of insect and myriapod species (Lucas and Rudall 1968; Case *et al.* 1994; Craig 1997) are able to produce silk. Insect silk is well known for its use in making cocoons in which pupae or eggs are protected against predators and the elements. The fibre harvested from the cocoons of silkworms, especially *Bombyx mori*, has been indispensable to textile manufacture for over 4000 years. Some insects use silk to build or reinforce their habitat, typified by the underwater dwelling tubes constructed by caddis fly larvae. Water-dwelling insect larvae may additionally rely on silk to produce filters that can trap food.

Spiders put silks to even more diverse uses (Foelix 1982; Hillyard 1994). At least three silks are involved in the construction of orb webs alone: the supporting radii (frame silk; equivalent to dragline), the core fibre of the capture thread, and the attachment pads at the outer ends of the radii. Each is secreted by uniquely specialised glands. It is thought probable that the "cement" at junctions between radial thread and capture thread is made from the same secretion as the attachment pads (Tillinghast and Townley 1987; Tillinghast and Townley 1994). Yet another proteinaceous secretion – in this case a low molecular weight silk – is an essential ingredient of the sticky fluid with which the capture thread is coated. Once a spider has snared prey, the victim may be further immobilised in swathing silk: the struggling prey becomes enmeshed in this material, and the spider is able to restrain catches which might otherwise pose a danger or break free of the web. Some spiders which do not spin orb webs produce instead a cobweb, consisting simply of a tangled mass of threads. More unusual snares produced from silk include the bolas of *Mastophora* spiders; this is a sticky ball of ancestral capture thread, swung at the end of a single fibre (Vollrath 1994).

Not all spider silks are dedicated to prey capture. Spiders use silk to produce cocoons around clusters of eggs; typically the cocoon comprises distinct inner and outer layers spun from different kinds of silk. Toughness and resistance to photochemical degradation are necessary properties in this application. Silk is also used as a locomotion aid, for making controlled descents as well as for ballooning; the latter term describes the process whereby spiders ride air currents on a "parachute" of silk (Hillyard 1994).

Spiders therefore display a high level of specialisation in the utilisation of silk. Each application appears to be associated with a specific type of silk, produced in a unique set of glands. There is, however, an exception to this one-to-one correspondence. The same material (principally Major Ampullate Silk, MAS) which constitutes the radial fibres of orb webs is also used by the spider to achieve vertical descents when escaping predators. In its "abseiling" application, MAS is spun at approximately ten times the rate as in web building. The mechanical properties required in the two applications are different, but in either case the properties must be reliable (Gosline *et al.* 1996). In the web, the dragline fibres function rather like the guy ropes holding up a TV mast; they provide support for the capture thread and they carry the static weight of the spider. In addition, they transmit vibrations signalling to the spider that prey has been caught (Foelix 1982). A high modulus is useful for these purposes, as is high strength. The kinetic energy of trapped prey is dissipated in the threads of the capture spiral. In contrast, when a spider uses its dragline to arrest a fall (which may sometimes be preceded by a running jump), it relies on the dragline alone to limit and dissipate kinetic energy. In such circumstances, a more compliant fibre is needed. From measurements of thermal expansion coefficient (Guess and Viney 1998), it has been shown indirectly but unambiguously that MAS spun at "abseiling" rates (approx. 10 $cm.s^{-1}$) is less stiff than silk spun at web-building rates (approx. 1 $cm.s^{-1}$ (Foelix 1982)). Depending on the speed at which it is spun, and on the probably synergistic control of other processing variables such as spinneret geometry (Wilson 1962a; Wilson 1962b) and the ionic composition of the silk secretion (Thiel and Viney 1997), MAS caters to divergent design criteria. At their present stage of evolution, therefore, it is efficient for spiders to optimise silk properties by differentiated *synthesis* in most cases, though they rely on tailored *processing* to enable the dual functions of MAS. This observation both develops and restricts the principle of "design is cheaper than material" (Vincent 1993), applied by Nature in products as different as nutshells and hedgehog spines. The processes underlying the evolution of the spider silk gene family remain poorly understood at present (Hayashi and Lewis 1998).

10.1.3 Scope and limitations of this chapter

This chapter will highlight specific characteristics of silks that provide insight into how the synthesis, processing, hierarchical microstructure and mechanical property control of industrial fibres might be advanced or refined. Throughout, the specific ideas stimulated by studies of MAS from *Nephila clavipes* (golden orb weaver) spiders will be regarded as generalisable in the context of lyotropic polymer fibre production. However, there is no guarantee that similarly detailed consideration of the MAS from a different type of spider (there are more than 2500 orb-weaving species worldwide) would lead to exactly the same lessons being learned. Also, while partial information is known about the tensile properties of many different silks, very few of these materials have been characterised thoroughly in consistent, well-documented detail. It is still too early to say confidently whether, for example, the draglines from a representative sampling of spider species have comparable compositions, protein primary structures, molecular order, and tensile properties.

Textile silks have enjoyed a long history of mechanical property evaluation. They were also one of the first materials to be subjected to structural analysis by x-ray methods (referenced in (Becker *et al.* 1994)). Yet, subsequent to the seminal x-ray work of Pauling and co-workers in the 1950s (Marsh *et al.* 1955a; Marsh *et al.* 1955b), the microstructure and nanostructure of larval silks have received relatively little attention. Most notably, the techniques of analytical electron microscopy that might provide unambiguous information about the spatial distribution, size, shape, orientation and internal order of individual crystallites have not been applied to silkworm or related silks. The structure of silkworm silk as determined by x-ray diffraction (XRD) is relatively simple, and has, unfortunately, tended to colour the interpretation of spider silk microstructures – even though the protein sequences are markedly different.

Spider MAS, which exhibits tensile properties that surpass those of textile silk, began to occupy the interest of polymer scientists much more recently, coinciding with widespread availability of powerful, complementary microanalytical techniques. Several investigators have attempted to characterise the hierarchical molecular order in this material (Nguyen *et al.* 1994; Thiel *et al.* 1994; Simmons *et al.* 1996; Vollrath *et al.* 1996; Bram *et al.* 1997; Grubb and Jelinski 1997; Parkhe *et al.* 1997; Thiel *et al.* 1997; Thiel and Viney 1997) and to relate molecular order to mechanical properties (Cunniff *et al.* 1994; Gosline *et al.* 1995). A particular focus of these studies, and therefore of the present chapter, is the MAS from *N. clavipes* spiders.

Some interpretations of experimental data pertaining to MAS structure remain controversial. Disagreements arise when interpretation is not matched to the length scales (or time scales) over which an experimental technique samples a microstructure. It can be misleading to rely on any one analysis technique while attempting to construct a microstructural model for materials in which there is a hierarchical arrangement of supramolecular components. When dealing with such complex microstructures, it is especially important to keep in mind the fundamental tenets that different characterisation techniques may (i) depend on physically different types of specimen / probe interactions, (ii) alter specimen microstructures in different ways, and (iii) be strictly valid only for materials similar to those used in calibration data sets. The last point is exemplified by molecular modelling, or by a chemometric technique such as Raman scattering (Gillespie *et al.* 1994), when used to determine the distribution of secondary structures in a protein. If a purported secondary structure is under-represented in the basis set, an erroneous picture of molecular order in the sample may be obtained: a fibrous protein such as silk is not well represented by calibrations derived from globular proteins. A final structural caveat is that there is no justification for seeking to associate microstructural features with *every* detail of primary structure. Some aspects of primary structure may be there simply to help the microstructure to develop. In other words, their main function is that of internal *processing* aid rather than *building* block.

10.2. MECHANICAL PROPERTIES OF SPIDER SILKS

10.2.1 Characterising the uniaxial tensile behaviour of silk fibres

10.2.1.1 The absence of standardised test procedures. Many native silks are available in short lengths only. Although silkworm cocoons are constructed from continuous filament, they have to be de-gummed before the filament can be reeled. De-gumming typically involves exposure to 100°C temperatures and alkaline environments, which must change the microstructure and properties. If the cocoon is not de-gummed, the practical length of fibre that can be teased from the surface is limited to a few centimetres. MAS can be reeled mechanically from restrained spiders, but there is evidence that the tensile properties of such material are inferior and more variable compared to results obtained from radial threads in webs built by the same spiders (Work 1976; Vollrath 1994). Other spider silks, for example capture thread, do not lend themselves to reeling directly from the animal; the spider is able to shut off the flow of silk through the spinnerets. If silks are recovered from webs, the unencumbered length for testing is restricted to the length of thread between junction points.

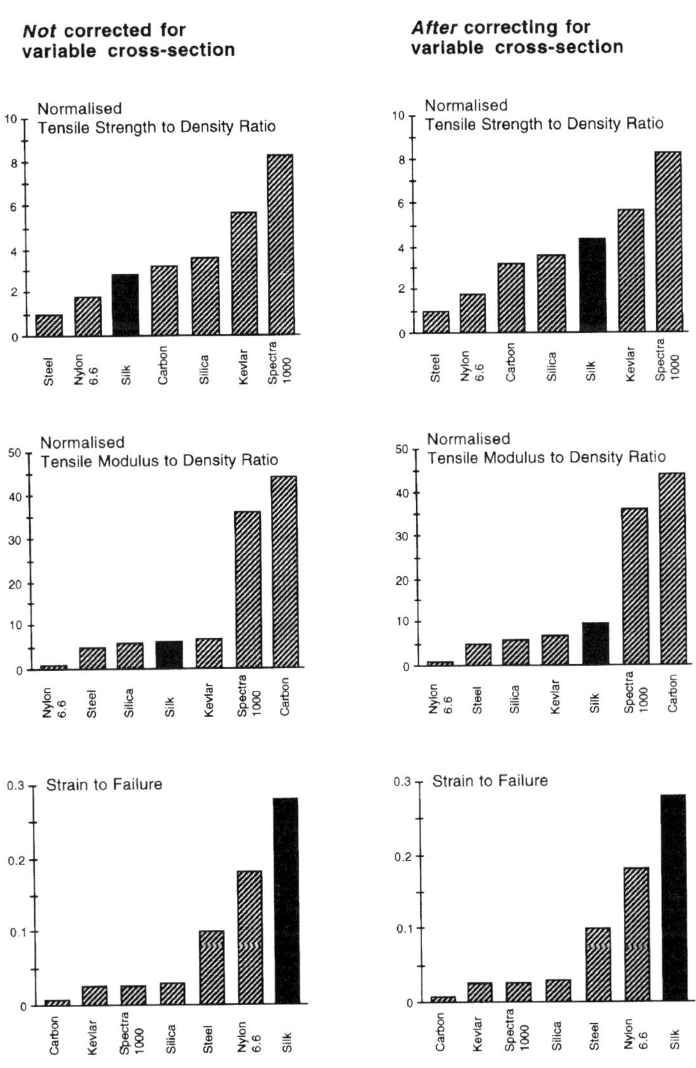

Fig. 10.1. Comparison of MAS and other high-tensile materials. Data for the different materials were compiled from several sources (Zemlin 1968; Gosline *et al.* 1986; ACerS 1990; Prevorsek 1995), and pertain to comparable (but not identical) test conditions. The charts for strength and modulus are normalised relative to steel piano wire and high-modulus nylon 6.6 fibre respectively; in each case these materials were assigned a property-to-density ratio of 1. MAS differs from the other materials in that its cross-sectional geometry is highly non-uniform along the length of the fibre. Charts on the left of the Figure show data as assembled from the literature, while charts on the right of the Figure give a more accurate picture of MAS behaviour by recognising that MAS deformation will be dominated by regions of small cross-section.

The small diameter of spider silks, a few micrometers at most, necessitates testing at low loads. This has led individual research groups to develop in-house testing hardware, which, together with the restrictions on available specimen length, has resulted in a proliferation of protocols. Differences in specimen gauge length, strain rate, test temperature and ambient humidity make it difficult to achieve meaningful cross-laboratory comparison of results. For example, studies of spider silk tensile properties have included tests performed on gauge lengths of 5 mm (Vollrath and Edmonds 1989), 12.5 mm (Dunaway *et al.* 1995b), or 25 mm and 40 mm (Stauffer *et al.* 1994).

10.2.1.2 Fibre cross-section. In order to quantify the stress in a fibre, and hence to determine parameters such as yield strength, breaking strength and Young's modulus, it is necessary to divide measurements of force by a measurement of cross-sectional area. Accurate characterisation of cross-sectional area is difficult in the case of silks. Single fibres are not adequately represented by a long thin cylinder; the apparent diameter of *N. clavipes* MAS can vary by as much as 20% relative to the mean within a mere 0.6 mm length of fibre, and the cross-section is approximately oval (Dunaway *et al.* 1995a). The cross-sectional geometry of silkworm silk is even less regular (Fouda and El-Tonsy 1990; Dunaway *et al.* 1995b).

An average diameter of the MAS reeled from mature specimens of intrinsically large spiders such as *Nephila* can be determined at the resolutions afforded by light microscopy. Even so, the average cross-sectional area calculated from such a measurement is not a reliable indicator of the initial area at the point of failure, as failure is likely to occur where stress is concentrated due to the initial area being *smaller* than average. On this basis, the tensile strength and stiffness of silk in most studies will be seriously underestimated ($1 / 0.8^2 \approx 1.56$). In Figure 10.1, which provides a comparison of some high-tensile materials, the data for silk have been corrected accordingly.

Other methods for characterising the cross-sectional geometry of silk include:

a.- The mass of a known length is measured accurately with a balance, and a gradient column is used to measure density (Stauffer *et al.* 1994). These data are used to calculate an average cross-sectional area that is not sensitive to the actual shape of the cross-section. It is assumed that the samples do not imbibe any of the fluid in the density gradient column.

b.- The profile of the fibre is projected optically onto a digital measuring pad (Stauffer *et al.* 1994).

c.- A laser beam, incident normal to the length of the fibre, is used to obtain optical diffraction patterns, and the separation of maxima in these patterns is measured (Dunaway *et al.* 1995a; Dunaway *et al.* 1995b). The fibre is mounted to enable rotation about its long axis, so that several readings of diameter can be taken at a given position along the fibre.

d.- The diameter can be measured by scanning electron microscopy (Dunaway *et al.* 1995a; Dunaway *et al.* 1995b) (spider silk), (Pérez-Rigueiro *et al.* 1998) (silkworm silk).

10.2.1.3 Reproducibility of results. Stress-strain curves obtained from MAS samples reeled at a fixed rate (e.g. 6.1 $cm.s^{-1}$ (Cunniff *et al.* 1994) or 10.3 $cm.s^{-1}$ (Dunaway *et al.* 1995b)) exhibit significant variability. If curves for MAS spun at one fixed rate (e.g. 1.5 $cm.s^{-1}$) are averaged, and compared to the averaged tensile test data for MAS spun at another fixed rate (e.g. 12.2 $cm.s^{-1}$), the difference is not significant on the scale of the variability within either data set (Cunniff *et al.* 1994). The aforementioned uncertainties in characterising the cross-sectional area of MAS are a significant source of the noise in all such comparisons.

Some reduction of variability in the tensile modulus obtained from MAS (Work 1976; Work 1977; Dunaway *et al.* 1995b) and *B. mori* cocoon silk (Pérez-Rigueiro *et al.* 1998) can be achieved by using a series of *adjacent* samples cut from the original fibre. Further decreases in the spread of modulus data can be realised by characterising the cross-sectional area of each individual sample, instead of using a more global average. The scatter in tensile fracture strength of MAS and *B. mori* silk is even more pronounced than the variability in elastic modulus (Dunaway *et al.* 1995b): it is sensitive not only to cross-sectional area but also to the distribution of microstructural flaws (Pérez-Rigueiro *et al.* 1998). The Weibull modulus of *B. mori* silk is found to be similar to that of glass! In other words, despite its attractive combination of strength, stiffness and toughness, the failure predictability of silkworm silk is similar to that of a brittle material. Fortunately, silk synthesised by genetically modified bacteria and spun under controlled conditions through an artificial spinneret should have a more uniform cross-sectional area, more reproducible molecular alignment, and fewer microstructural flaws compared to the native material.

10.2.1.4 The usefulness of thermal expansion data. It is clear that standard tensile tests do not provide an unambiguous, ready means of finding correlations between spinning rate and mechanical properties. Reeling silk at web-building rates and "abseiling" rates yields material with distinguishable microstructures (Thiel and Viney 1997), so one should expect these materials to exhibit distinguishable mechanical properties in tensile tests. However, any trend is masked by the difficulties of characterising cross-sectional geometry. What is needed, is a method of characterising stiffness which is insensitive to sample cross-section.

One solution is provided by measuring thermal expansion coefficient (Guess and Viney 1998), which can be accomplished with a dynamic mechanical analyser (DMA). Thermal expansion data obtained with the DMA are highly reproducible below the glass transition of MAS (approximately 160 °C) and they show a marked dependence on the rate at which the silk was reeled. Results are not sensitive to residual moisture. It is possible to use specimens that consist of a bundle of fibres as the specimen, without having to worry about energy loss due to friction within the bundle. The data confirm that the highest intrinsic stiffness of MAS is realised at spinning rates used in web construction, and that the spider spins MAS that is more compliant when it must elude a predator.

10.2.1.5 Handling silk specimens. In tensile tests performed on *B. mori* cocoon silk at 0.00017 s^{-1} and interrupted by unload / reload steps, the tensile modulus on reloading is insensitive to the cumulative deformation experienced by the specimen (Pérez-Rigueiro *et al.* 1998). The stress-strain relationship is also found to be insensitive to strain rate. Measurements of tensile modulus should therefore not be influenced by accidental stretching introduced while the specimen is being handled.

10.2.2 Major Ampullate Silk (MAS) from spiders

10.2.2.1 Properties of dry silk. All studies of tensile behaviour have revealed at least two regimes in load-extension or stress-strain curves (Figure 10.2a and Table 10.1). Initially the material is stiff; yield occurs at a few per cent strain. The plots then exhibit a more gradual slope, which remains approximately constant until the fibres break. In some cases, continued drawing causes the fibres to work harden (presumably due to chain alignment), and there may then be a second yield point (Dunaway *et al.* 1995b) (Figure 10.2b). The breaking strength of single fibres from both species addressed in Table 10.1 is statistically identical, but the *Nephila* MAS is significantly more ductile than the *Araneus* MAS. Inter-species differences in the mechanical properties, exhibited by the (nominally) same functional silk, make it difficult to deduce generalised structure-property correlations from studying only a few examples.

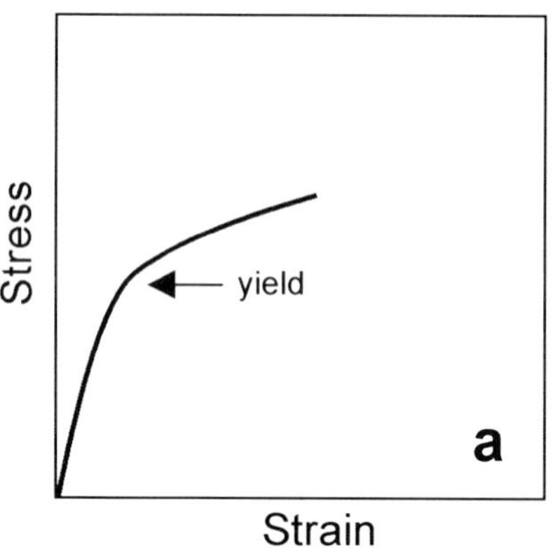

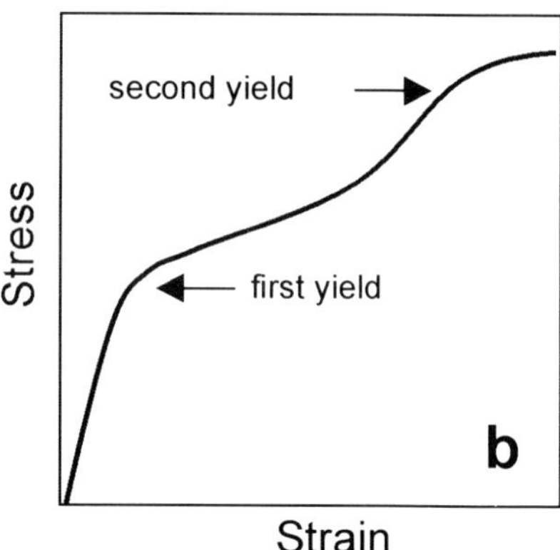

Fig. 10.2. Schematic stress-strain curves for dry MAS.
Either single yield (a) or double yield (b) behaviour is observed.

Table 10.1. Tensile properties of two types of silk, in each case from two different species of spider.

Spider	*Silk*	*Yield strain*	*Breaking strength**	*Breaking strain*
Nephila clavipes	major ampullate	0.04 – 0.05	4.6 ± 0.2	0.23 ± 0.05
	cocoon	0.04 – 0.05	1.3 ± 0.2	0.24 ± 0.02
Araneus gemmoides	major ampullate	0.04 – 0.05	4.7 ± 0.5	0.15 ± 0.02
	cocoon	0.04 – 0.05	2.3 ±0.2	0.19 ± 0.02

Single-fibre data, collated from ref. (Stauffer et al. 1994). Average values and standard deviations in the last two columns are calculated from 10 readings. * Breaking strength in GPa.

The existence of a second yield point (Figure 10.2b) has not been observed in all studies. One possible explanation is that this is an artifact of test specimen gauge length: a longer sample has a greater probability of containing two regions that can form necks; the weakest one deforms first and then work hardens, until deformation of the second weak region can be triggered. There are, however, several observations, which countermand this interpretation:

a.- Sample diameters in tensile tests decrease uniformly along the length of the fibre; i.e. deformation is not restricted to well-defined necks (Carmichael and Viney 1997).

b.- The second yield is sometimes exhibited by samples that consist of a *bundle* of fibres (Stauffer *et al.* 1994). With as many as 100 fibres in a sample, it should not be possible to reproduce two distinct yields if they depend on statistical weak links.

c.- The second yield has been observed in samples of widely differing gauge lengths, i.e. 40 mm (Stauffer *et al.* 1994) and 12.5 mm (Work 1976; Dunaway *et al.* 1995b).

d.- There are either one or two yields, but never more.

e.- The number of yields observed is consistent among different pieces of silk collected in one reeling from a given spider. However, the number can be different for silk reeled from a different spider, or for silk reeled from the original spider on a different occasion (Dunaway 1994).

f.- Each yield is associated with a distinct range of strains (Dunaway *et al.* 1995b), suggesting that it may be a critical level of molecular *orientation* that is required to trigger each process.

A microstructural basis for the double-yield behaviour is implicated; this point will be addressed again later in the Chapter. Whether or not the second yield is accessible depends on the sample not breaking first, which in turn may be affected by the distribution of flaws (Pérez-Rigueiro *et al.* 1998).

The shape of the single-yield stress-strain relationship for MAS can be predicted closely by a computer model (Termonia 1996 and Chapters 9 and 11) which places small deformation-resistant crystals in a rubbery matrix and invokes a thin, stiff interphase region at the boundaries between crystals and the matrix. This simple representation does not take account of the hierarchical nature of the microstructure, nor the existence of more than one type of crystalline reinforcement (section 10.3). It therefore does not predict the second yield point or the dual functionality of MAS.

10.2.2.2. Supercontraction. Dragline silks undergo contraction when immersed in water (Work 1981; Work and Morosoff 1982; Fornes *et al.* 1983; Gosline *et al.* 1984; Work 1985; Gosline *et al.* 1995) or salt solutions (Vollrath *et al.* 1996). The effect is so dramatic – an axial shrinkage by up to 40% of the original length, and radial swelling to as much as twice the original thickness – that it is referred to as *supercontraction.* The hydrated, contracted silk can be regarded as a composite in which a cross-linked network of elastomeric random coils is filled with reinforcing particles. XRD indicates that the crystalline components of dry fibre remain intact (though they may have rotated) after hydration, so it is the amorphous regions which swell to form the elastomer. This picture is consistent with the model (Thiel and Viney 1995a; Viney 1997) of MAS microstructural evolution where crystallisation from silk secretion is driven by hydrophobic interactions between shear-straightened chains. One possible use of supercontraction to the spider (Work 1977; Work 1981; Tillinghast and Townley 1987) is that it helps the web to support the added weight of rain or dew. The same retractive forces which produce supercontraction would also oppose the extensional forces due to the weight of water. The water in turn fulfils useful functions as detailed in the section on capture thread below.

10.2.3. Spider cocoon silk

Some tensile data for cocoon silk are included in Table 10.1. For both species of spider considered, the breaking strength of cocoon fibre is substantially lower than that of MAS. Qualitatively, it is apparent from comparing stress-strain curves (Stauffer *et al.* 1994) that cocoon silk has a lower tensile modulus than MAS. The same authors also report that the cocoon fibre exhibits "brittle" behaviour when attempts are made to tease fibre from cocoons. This comment would appear to conflict with the 20% extension to failure recorded in tensile tests, but may simply reflect weakness in deformation that involves significant torsion and / or bending. In any case, it is clear that cocoon silk is less effective than MAS at resisting deformation and fracture, which leads to the question of whether MAS might not in fact do a better job of protecting spider eggs. Given the way in which cobwebs work (Section 10.2.5) it may be that a mass of broken cocoon fibres is an effective deterrent to a predator, which might risk entanglement if it persists in attempting to break through the wall of a cocoon.

10.2.4. Capture thread (viscid silk)

The energy dissipation mechanisms available to capture thread are partly the result of its elastomeric, non-crystalline microstructure (Gosline *et al.* 1995), and partly the result of a unique "windlass" mechanism, the latter depending on the presence of a water-based proteinaceous glue that coats the fibres as they are spun (Vollrath and Edmonds 1989; Vollrath 1994).

When dry, *Araneus* capture thread has an initial modulus of 1 GPa (versus 10 GPa for MAS) and a failure strain of approximately 200% (versus 20% for MAS) (Gosline *et al.* 1995). Both silks have similar amino acid composition and *potential* for crystallisation, yet one is clearly more rubber-like in its mechanical behaviour. Viscid silk contains a non-volatile, water-soluble component that inhibits crystallisation during fibre formation (Gosline *et al.* 1995). Further study of this component may lead to a processing aid for use when protein solutions are spun into fibre artificially.

The water-based proteinaceous glue performs several functions:

a.- It is hygroscopic (Edmonds and Vollrath 1992); i.e. it can attract water from the atmosphere, and therefore can maintain its properties over several hours.

b.- The glue plasticises the capture silk, allowing reversible extensions of up to 500% that exhibit hysteresis and therefore enable energy dissipation. In contrast, uncoated capture thread (Vollrath and Edmonds 1989) extends to less than 200% in reaching its maximum load bearing capacity. Nuclear magnetic resonance (NMR) spectroscopy shows that the water confers mobility at the level of individual protein molecules in the fibre, specifically in the non-crystalline regions (Bonthrone *et al.* 1992). A corollary of this NMR study is that any crystalline, non-mobile regions can account for only a small (though unspecified) fraction of the fibre volume.

c.- The as-spun capture thread is laid down in a slack condition. Tautness is induced by water in the coating (Vollrath and Edmonds 1989). The glue has a low surface energy with respect to the fibre, but a high surface energy with respect to air. Therefore, it favours maximum contact with the fibre and minimum contact with air. A uniform thin coating of fluid glue on a straight fibre is not stable (Stewart and Golubitsky 1992), so the glue exists as a series of discrete droplets. When the thread is extended by the impact of prey, the glue is spread out over its surface; subsequently the droplets re-form, slack thread is coiled into the droplets, and coalescence of droplets restores tension in the fibre (Vollrath 1994).

d.- When the spider ingests the web to recycle the amino acid monomers of the silk, the glue provides a useful source of water.

10.2.5. Cobweb silk

Spiders such as the black widow (*Latrodectus*) produce three-dimensional, irregular meshes of silk (cobwebs) instead of two-dimensional, structured orb webs. Both cobwebs and orb webs serve to capture prey, but they achieve this in rather different ways. Orb webs are designed according to a "yield before break" criterion: the capture thread dissipates the kinetic energy of impacting prey by stretching and subsequent slow retraction. Because a cobweb is three-dimensional, individual fibres can be thinner than in an orb web; they dissipate energy by breaking, allowing the prey to fall deeper into the web while becoming increasingly tangled in the broken strands. The strength of *Latrodectus mactans* cobweb fibres can exceed that of *N. clavipes* MAS by a factor of 2 or more (Moore and Tran 1996; Holden 1997). Because the properties and mode of use of cobweb strands are different from those of other silks, one must expect the hierarchical microstructure to be different too. Initial studies using atomic force microscopy (Nguyen *et al.* 1994) indicate that the 660 nm diameter threads consist of parallel 80 nm diameter fibres, which in turn consist of 9-12 nm diameter parallel fibrils that are inclined at 20° to the long axis of the thread.

10.2.6. Comparison of silks and other high-performance fibres

The lack of standardisation of gauge length and strain rate among tensile tests of silks has already been commented on. Attempts to glean data about other high-performance fibres from the literature are also restricted by the difficulty of finding results that have been obtained under comparable conditions. Even the criteria for comparing performance are open to debate; for example, should parameters such as yield strength and initial stiffness be quoted at a standard temperature, or at a standard fraction of the glass transition temperature? While the latter basis of comparison could be helpful in the restricted context of polymers, it is useless if other material classes are to be included. Figure 10.1 presents breaking stress, initial modulus, and strain-to-failure data for MAS and selected metallic, polymeric and ceramic materials; it should be interpreted subject to the limitations already discussed. The combination of high stiffness, high strength and superlative strain to failure is responsible for the remarkable toughness exhibited by MAS.

10.3. HIERARCHICAL MICROSTRUCTURE OF SILK FIBRES

10.3.1. Molecules

From the small number of silks for which detailed sequence data are available, it is apparent that no two types of silk have identical amino acid sequences. A study of the major ampullate silk, capture thread and cocoon silk from *Araneus diadematus* (garden) spiders has shown that a gene family encodes gland-specific proteins with different proportions of glycine-rich, polyalanine and poly(glycine-alanine) repeat motifs (Guerette *et al.* 1996). This allows for a range of mechanical properties according to the crystal-forming potential of the exact primary structure of each silk. Which primary structures *are* necessarily crystalline is still the subject of some debate, though it is agreed that more than one type of ordered entity could be formed.

The simplicity of the *B. mori* silk microstructure is a direct consequence of the repetitive primary sequence of the constituent protein (Lucas *et al.* 1955; Strydom *et al.* 1977; Mita *et al.* 1988). The macromolecules feature a well-conserved sequence of $[\text{-Gly-Ala-Gly-Ala-Gly-Ser-}]_n$. It was, in fact, the simple chemistry of *B. mori* silk protein (with glycine, alanine, and serine in an approximately 3:2:1 ratio) that allowed

Pauling to deduce the first accurate description of ß-sheet crystals from XRD data (Marsh *et al.* 1955a). When these chains adopt an extended ß-strand conformation, the glycyl and non-glycyl side chains point in opposite directions, nominally perpendicular to the backbone (Figure 8.9 in Chapter 8). Folding such a chain into lamellae produces ß-sheets with chemically distinct faces: hydrogens on one side, and larger methyl and methanolic groups on the other. Hydrophobic packing of these sheets into three-dimensional structures results in crystals with a bimodal distribution of inter-sheet spacings: 3.5 Å for the glycyl-glycyl juxtaposed faces and 5.7 Å for the methyl-methyl juxtaposed faces. Amorphous regions occur where the molecules have an amino acid sequence that does not participate in ß-sheet formation. The simple chemistry of the constituent molecules thus produces a concomitantly simple composite microstructure of well-defined crystals distributed in an amorphous matrix — a model that has carried over into the literature of spider MAS (Gosline *et al.* 1986; Lewis 1992; Li *et al.* 1994; Mahoney *et al.* 1994).

The chemistry of the constituent proteins is also a useful starting point from which to approach an understanding of the supramolecular structure of spider MAS. The primary structures in MAS protein have been examined by partial sequencing of the corresponding cDNA (Xu and Lewis 1990; Hinman and Lewis 1992). There is some question as to whether these sequences pertain to distinct molecules, or to different segments of just one species of protein molecule (Lombardi and Kaplan 1990; Beckwitt and Arcidiacono 1994; Mello *et al.* 1994; Mello *et al.* 1995); the weight of evidence seems to favour the former interpretation. While this issue is peripheral to the description of microstructure, it is convenient to use Lewis' notation of Spidroin 1 and Spidroin 2 to distinguish between the sequenced portions, as they are dominated by different sets of residue repeat motifs.

Spidroin 1 is dominated by short runs (5-7 residues) of polyalanine separated by approximately five repeats of a loosely conserved -Gly-Gly-X- motif, where X is predominantly Gln, Tyr, and Leu (Xu and Lewis 1990). As will become apparent below, these sequences respectively are associated with the lower and upper limits of the range of inter-sheet spacings observed in the ordered regions of MAS. The most significant motifs in Spidroin 2 are slightly longer runs of polyalanine (6-10 residues), as well as several proline-containing pentapeptides, including -Gly-Tyr-Gly-Pro-Gly-, -Gly-Pro-Gly-Gly-Tyr- and -Gly-Pro-Gly-Gln-Gln- (Hinman and Lewis 1992). Spidroins 1 and 2 respectively are 719 and 628 residues long, each including a "tail" which is slightly more hydrophilic than the conserved regions. These C-termini contain approximately 60 residues that show no apparent repeat motif.

Whereas *B. mori* silk protein is dominated by a single repeating motif, the microstructure of MAS must accommodate several. This leads to the possibility of a significantly more complicated supramolecular microstructure for MAS. The extent to which the MAS microstructure is at all analogous to that of *B. mori* silk will depend on the ability of the various spidroin motifs to form ß-sheet crystals. Polyalanine may be regarded as an excellent candidate for assembly into ß-sheet crystals, given how it forms the crystalline phase in Tussah (*Antherea pernyi*) silk (Marsh *et al.* 1955b). The loosely conserved -Gly-Gly-X- motif in Spidroin 1 can also participate in ß-sheet formation (see below). In contrast, the proline-containing pentapeptides characteristic of Spidroin 2 are detrimental to extended ß-strand formation: the structure of each proline residue forces an abrupt permanent kink in the polymer backbone. Thus, if an attempt were made to construct ß-sheet crystals out of Spidroin 2 sequences, the frequently-occurring proline residues would severely disrupt their structural integrity, effectively terminating the crystals into disordered matrix.

10.3.2. Secondary structure

Perhaps the most striking feature of silk secondary structure is that silk does not in fact show a strong *intrinsic* propensity to form specific secondary structures! If secondary structure does form, it is influenced strongly by external factors. It has been demonstrated (Minor Jr and Kim 1994) that ß-sheet formation in polypeptides is significantly determined by tertiary context (initiated by shear in the case of silk), and not by intrinsic propensity to a ß-strand secondary structure.

10.3.2.1. Silk polymorphism. Silk proteins adopt random conformations with little or no discernable secondary structure when maintained in solution under equilibrium conditions in the gland (Asakura 1986; Zheng *et al.* 1989; Wellman *et al.* 1992; Asakura *et al.* 1994). However, the success of many silks as load-bearing materials is due to the fact that a *metastable* ß-strand conformation of individual strands can be induced by flow along a duct and through a spinneret. A greater-than-critical shear rate, the magnitude of which depends on the protein concentration, is needed to effect this conformational ordering (Iizuka 1966). The ß-strand conformation is stabilised by hydrogen bonds between the carbonyl oxygen and amide hydrogen on juxtaposed strands; hydrogen-bonded ß-strands form ß-sheets, which can stack into three-dimensional ß-sheet crystals (Figure 8.9 in Chapter 8). The separation of the sheets depends on the size of the side groups that must be accommodated between them. ß-sheet crystals in silk are often referred to as silk II, recognising that silk is polymorphic and forms crystalline phases that are affected by environment more than by intrinsic preference for particular schemes of ordering.

Assignment of a particular silk polymorph is made principally on the basis of XRD, taking into account only the *general* distribution and relative intensities of features in the diffraction patterns. The silk I polymorph is formed when silk undergoes bulk crystallisation from solutions that are quiescent (i.e. not undergoing flow or shear). It is also exhibited by some genetically engineered proteins which contain silk-like moieties — for example Silk-Like Polymer with Fibronectin cell attachment facility (SLPF; Figure 10.3), which combines the physical and chemical stability of silk and the cell attachment bioactivity of fibronectin (Anderson *et al.* 1994a; Anderson *et al.* 1994b). SLPF can be used to coat cell culture dishes to promote the adhesion and spreading of cells; the coating is resistant to autoclave treatment and harsh solvents. The silk-like segments in SLPF are based on the -Gly-Ala-Gly-Ala-Gly-Ser- repeat of *B. mori* fibroin. A number of different detailed models have been proposed for the silk I structure, and there is little agreement as to which is correct.

["Head"] — [**(Gly-Ala-Gly-Ala-Gly-Ser)$_9$** (Fibronectin segment)]$_{12}$ — ["Tail"]

The "head" contains a **(Gly-Ala-Gly-Ala-Gly-Ser)$_6$** sequence
The "tail" contains a **(Gly-Ala-Gly-Ala-Gly-Ser)$_2$** sequence

Fig. 10.3. SLPF (Silk-Like Polymer with Fibronectin cell attachment facility), showing the size and location of domains based on the principal crystallisable motif of *B. mori* silk.

While the argument about silk I structure is of limited relevance to fibrous silk, the fact that molecular modelling cannot yet produce a result in close agreement with experimental studies does emphasise that no single technique should be relied on to reveal all aspects of the hierarchical structure of complex molecules.

Yet another polymorph, silk III, is formed by crystallisation at an air-water interface, either in free-standing thin films of silk cast from dilute solution, or in films of silk produced by Langmuir-Blodgett methods (Valluzzi *et al.* 1996). If solubilised *B. mori* silk is used, the chains adopt a left-handed 3_2 helical conformation and become ordered into a hexagonally packed array.

10.3.2.2. Chou-Fasman predictions. Using the Chou-Fasman scheme for predicting secondary structure (Chou and Fasman 1978), probability ratings for helix ($\langle P_\alpha \rangle$) and ß-sheet ($\langle P_\beta \rangle$) formation in *N. clavipes* MAS can be assigned to the -Gly-Gly-Gln-Gly-Gly-Tyr- and polyalanine motifs (Thiel *et al.* 1997), the pentapeptides being disqualified from consideration on account of their proline content. The ratings are shown in Table 10.2, with -Gly-Ala-Gly-Ala-Gly-Ser- (*B. mori*) included for comparison. None of the motifs listed in Table 10.2 are intrinsically *strong* ß-sheet formers (Viney *et al.* 1992; Thiel *et al.* 1997). Both -Gly-Gly-Gln-Gly-Gly-Tyr- and polyalanine sequences are predicted to be *weak* ß-sheet formers with nearly identical scores. Polyalanine is also predicted to be a strong helix former while the -Gly-Gly-Gln-Gly-Gly-Tyr- motif is a mild helix breaker; acting together, these contrasting propensities for helix formation are consistent with the small (approximately 5% at most (Gillespie *et al.* 1994)) amount of helix actually found.

While the formation of ß-sheet crystals may represent a non-equilibrium conformation for the individual participating sequences, a shear-dependent mechanism of crystallisation has the advantage of not being directly driven by chemical equilibrium. Therefore, the nucleation and growth of the solid microstructure is not limited by reaction kinetics. Metastable ß-sheet conformations can persist indefinitely in the solid state, because there is no accessible mechanism to effect a change to a lower energy conformation.

Table 10.2. Chou-Fasman (1978) predictions for secondary structure formation by potentially crystallisable silk motifs.

	-Gly-Gly-Gln-Gly-Gly-Tyr-		Polyalanine		-Gly-Ala-Gly-Ala-Gly-Ser-	
	Score	*Rating*	*Score*	*Rating*	*Score*	*Rating*
$\langle P_\alpha \rangle$	0.65	b_α	1.45	H_α	0.88	i_α
$\langle P_\beta \rangle$	0.96	I_β	0.97	I_β	0.85	i_β

$b_\alpha \equiv$ helix breaker; $I_\beta \equiv$ weak ß-sheet former; $H_\alpha \equiv$ strong helix former; $i_{\alpha,\beta} \equiv$ indifferent to helix or ß-sheet participation.

10.3.2.3. Model peptides and biophysical measurements. Experimental support for the ability of -Gly-Gly-Gln-Gly-Gly-Tyr- and polyalanine to specifically form ß-sheet microstructures is provided by the behaviour of model polypeptides (Lewis 1992). Synthetic polypeptides based on the -Gly-Gly-X- and polyalanine motifs together, or the -Gly-Gly-X- motif on its own, were studied to determine conformations in a variety of chemical and thermal environments. It was concluded that these polypeptides are able to form a variety of secondary structures (including ß-sheet), depending on the experimental conditions. Also, the low level of bound water in MAS (less than 6 weight per cent) was shown to be appropriate to stabilising the polyalanine motif in a ß-sheet conformation. Given this *flexibility* of the dominant motifs to form ß-sheet structures, one can expect their incorporation into ß-sheet crystals to be promoted by an environment that favours extension and alignment of molecules.

10.3.2.4. NMR spectroscopy. NMR provides information about the *local* chemical environment of selected atomic species. Characterisation of *N. clavipes* MAS bundles by ^{13}C NMR has indicated that the polyalanine motif adopts a ß-strand conformation (Simmons *et al.* 1994). It was also concluded that there is no evidence of any α-helical secondary structure (although the experimental chemical shifts for glycine C_α and C=O were not explicitly compared with the shifts obtained from glycine in a known α-helical environment). Alanine was shown to be present in *two different motional environments*, suggesting its participation in regions that differ markedly in their degree of internal order (Simmons *et al.* 1996). This description is consistent with microstructural results obtained by transmission electron microscopy (TEM) (Thiel *et al.* 1994; Thiel and Viney 1995a; Thiel and Viney 1995b; Thiel *et al.* 1997; Thiel and Viney 1997), as will be discussed in sections 10.3.3.2 and 10.3.3.3 below.

The all-ß-sheet model for ordered regions in *N. clavipes* MAS is challenged by a study in which two-dimensional ^{13}C proton-driven polarisation-transfer data are compared with predictions from simple models (Kümmerlen *et al.* 1996). In that study, MAS bundles from *N. madagascariensis* were used, and it was argued that the alanine-rich segments form ordered ß-sheets while the glycine-rich segments adopt a 3_1-helical conformation. In the absence of relevant sequence information, it was assumed that *N. madagascariensis* MAS has the same sequence as *N. clavipes* MAS. Yet, strands of -Gly-Gly-Ala- in different conformations were used to model the NMR results for the glycine-rich segments, neglecting the significant fact that the -Gly-Gly-X- motif in *N. clavipes* MAS is predominantly substituted with X = Gln, Tyr and Leu, i.e. residues with large side chains. Also, the models assumed a greater degree of internal perfection for ordered regions than is consistent with the highly non-equilibrium conditions under which silk fibres are spun by the spider. No XRD or TEM evidence for any type of helical structures in MAS has been obtained – and it is within the capability of these techniques to detect such structures if they exist (Barghout *et al.* 1999).

10.3.2.5. Raman spectroscopy. Within the limits of experimental error (±5%), Raman spectroscopy of single fibres indicates anti-parallel ß-sheet as being the single most prevalent secondary structure (56%) in *N. clavipes* MAS (Gillespie *et al.* 1994). This quantity of ß-sheet can account for the volume fraction of crystalline material in MAS as determined by electron microscopy (Thiel *et al.* 1994), XRD (Guess 1995), or consideration of mechanical properties (Gosline *et al.* 1986), without recourse to additional ordered conformations.

The amount of ordered α-helix was found to be 5%, i.e. on the borderline of the resolution of the experiment, so there is no significant disparity with the NMR results described above. Any α-helices which are present also remain undetected by both x-ray and electron diffraction.

10.3.3. Crystallographic length scales

10.3.3.1. X-ray diffraction. Wide-angle XRD data from *N. clavipes* MAS have been interpreted (Work and Morosoff 1982; Becker *et al.* 1994) in terms of a simple composite microstructure: discrete polyalanine crystals dispersed throughout an amorphous (i.e., non-diffracting) protein matrix. This interpretation is rooted in several circumstantial pieces of evidence:

a.- The fibre XRD pattern of MAS qualitatively resembles patterns obtained from *B. mori* fibres (i.e., ß-sheet crystals, preferentially aligned with the fibre axis).
b.- XRD patterns from MAS are dominated by reflexions which are consistent with ß-sheets spaced at 5.3 Å, i.e. the spacing for polyalanine crystals in Tussah moth silk (Marsh *et al.* 1955b).
c.- The breadth of the XRD maxima indicates that these crystallites are on the order of 20-30 Å in size, which is consistent with polyalanine runs of six to eight residues.
d.- Amino acid analysis reveals a prevalence of alanine domains in *N. clavipes* MAS.

Although this microstructural description accounts for the gross features of fibre XRD patterns, it is not fully consistent with all available chemical, structural or mechanical data.

More recent work (Thiel *et al.* 1997), in which the diffraction data are processed to remove background scattering, reveals low intensity features corresponding to a range of lattice spacings that are much too large to be accounted for by polyalanine crystals. These features are attributed to the presence of additional crystalline structure, in which the inter-sheet spacings are *greater* than 5.3 Å. They had not been noted in previous XRD studies of MAS, and are only revealed by enhanced data collection equipment and digital image processing. The d-spacings are consistent with values determined by TEM. It is worth noting that a recent synchrotron x-ray study (Bram *et al.* 1997) also reveals diffuse peaks that are consistent with a range of larger inter-sheet spacings, even though, in that study, the indexing of intensities is confined to those which fit polyalanine ß-sheet crystals.

For all of the relative ease in data collection, and the scope for elegant interpretation, fibre XRD yields only a bulk average structure and provides little insight as to the specific nature of any one diffracting region. Even when a third-generation synchrotron radiation source is used to obtain diffraction from single fibres (Bram *et al.* 1997), the beam size is of the order of 10 μm (full width at half-maximum), i.e. two orders of magnitude greater than the largest ordered regions detected in MAS by TEM (Thiel *et al.* 1997).

10.3.3.2. Transmission electron microscopy. In contrast to x-ray methods, TEM can provide highly detailed information from very small regions of sample areas — individual crystals within a composite, for example. However, this detail is achieved at the expense of sensitivity to the bulk average microstructure. Additionally, sample preparation and electron radiation damage accumulated during examination may result in significant extrinsic artifacts. Radiation damage may be a problem in XRD too, if high incident fluxes generate heating that cannot be dissipated. In a synchrotron beam, the lifetime of MAS at room temperature is less than 30s (Bram *et al.* 1997); to obtain high resolution patterns, it is necessary to resort to cryogenic conditions, in which case lifetimes of a few minutes are possible.

TEM studies (Thiel *et al.* 1994; Thiel *et al.* 1997) have revealed relatively large diffracting (70 - 500 nm) regions in a non-diffracting matrix. The crystals exhibit diffraction behaviour which is consistent with ß-sheet crystals, but the intersheet spacings observed range from approximately 5.9 Å to approximately 7.0 Å. Individual crystals of polyalanine were not observed by TEM, nor were diffraction maxima with spacings characteristic of polyalanine. *Taken together*, TEM, XRD, and NMR structural characterisation results suggest that the MAS microstructure contains *two* types of crystalline (i.e. diffracting) region dispersed in a non-diffracting matrix. In addition to small polyalanine crystallites, there are much larger entities with a less perfect degree of internal positional and orientational molecular order. Various terms have been used to describe this second type of ordered region: Non-Periodic Lattice (NPL) crystals (Thiel and Viney 1995b; Thiel *et al.* 1997; Thiel and Viney 1997), protocrystals (Simmons *et al.* 1996) and oriented amorphous material (Grubb and Jelinski 1997).

The NPL crystallites in MAS are formed by forcing chemically inhomogeneous ß-strands of protein together in a ß-sheet crystal configuration. The backbones tend to pack on a three-dimensional lattice. However, this periodicity is frustrated by the imperfectly repeating sequence of amino acid side chains along each molecule and by the consequently necessary fluctuations of the inter-sheet spacings where the side chains are accommodated. The crystals are far too large to consist purely of just one type of crystallisable run, and so must contain both polyalanine and -Gly-Gly-X-sequences, i.e. the two potential ß-sheet formers in Spidroin 1. The effective crystallinity (characterised as the ability to diffract) varies from point to point within an NPL crystallite, depending on local composition.

Why are the polyalanine crystals, which are so prevalent in the wide-angle XRD patterns, not apparent in the electron microscope? The small size of the crystallites, approximately 20 Å, broadens the diffraction maxima approximately 50 times relative to those originating from the much larger NPL crystallites. Also, protein crystals diffract electrons weakly, even under the best conditions. The combination of intrinsically weak diffraction, spreading of diffraction maxima, and short specimen lifetime in the beam makes the crystallites difficult to detect by TEM. XRD experiments, which are exempt from the liability of radiation damage (if fluxes are low enough to avoid heat damage), can be configured to collect data over many hours if necessary, leading to satisfactory signal-to-noise ratios.

TEM studies support the existence of twisted crystalline structures in *A. diadematus* cocoon silk, in which the dominantly repeated crystallisable motifs (Guerette *et al.* 1996) are similar to those in *N. clavipes* MAS. It is possible, but remains to be proved, that these structures are NPL crystals, the twist being detectable in diffraction patterns for a restricted range of crystal sizes and orientations (Barghout *et al.* 1999). A twist parallel to the chain direction could explain the lower stiffness of the cocoon silk in comparison to MAS, where no twist of the ß-sheet crystals has been observed.

10.3.3.3. The case for NPL crystals. As outlined above, various structural characterisation techniques converge to a composite microstructure for MAS in which three phases are present: NPL crystals (from Spidroin 1), polyalanine crystals (with contributions possible from both Spidroin 1 and Spidroin 2) and amorphous matrix (From Spidroin 2). There is extensive interconnection of these phases, especially given the evidence (Lombardi and Kaplan 1990; Beckwitt and Arcidiacono 1994; Mello *et al.* 1994; Mello *et al.* 1995) in favour of the two Spidroins being different domains of a single species of molecule.

A microstructural model in which there are two types of reinforcing element is supported by observations of the stress-strain behaviour of MAS. The existence of a second yield point in MAS that can be extended sufficiently without breaking was noted in section 10.2.2.1. Yield occurs when microstructural resistance to deformation is overcome. The ability of crystalline domains to resist deformation depends on their size, orientation and internal perfection, so the reinforcing ability of polyalanine and NPL crystallites should be exceeded at different stages of the deformation process.

The concept of Non-Periodic Lattice crystals is an extension of the two-dimensional non-periodic *layer* (n.p.l.) crystals used to characterise ordered regions in the solid microstructures of many synthetic liquid crystalline random copolyesters (Windle *et al.* 1985; Viney and Windle 1987; Hanna and Windle 1988). The n.p.l. model describes an ordered molecular solid where structural stability is achieved (in the absence of long-range chemical periodicity) through local compatibility between residues on adjacent chains (Figure 10.4). A microstructure that incorporates *statistical* crystals of this kind offers a number of advantages in regard to properties, as is discussed further in Section 10.5. Given the relative novelty of NPL crystals as elements of microstructure, there is value in compiling a summary of the hard evidence for, and other observations consistent with, such crystals in MAS:

a.- Electron diffraction patterns can be indexed according to the orthogonal unit cell which is characteristic of ß-sheet crystals. The intrachain repeat expected for ß-strand backbones is used (20.88 Å for six residues, i.e. -Gly-Gly-Gln-Gly-Gly-Tyr), and the hydrogen-bonded inter-chain separation within sheets is fixed at 4.72 Å. The only variable is the inter-sheet spacing, which, for all patterns observed, lies in the range 5.9 Å to 7.0 Å (Thiel *et al.* 1997).

b.- These diffraction patterns are obtained from regions that are too large — and that have the wrong inter-sheet spacing — to consist solely of the available polyalanine runs. They are also an order of magnitude larger than the displacement lengths of the -Gly-Gly-X- based sequences. The diffracting regions must therefore be ß-sheet crystals made from *mixed* strands of polyalanine and -Gly-Gly-X-. The bulky residues in the -Gly-Gly-X- motifs necessarily dominate the inter-sheet spacing (but not the overall composition) of the mixed crystals in this model. Large diffracting structures, with at least one dimension exceeding 100 nm, can be inferred from *small* angle x-ray scattering (Yang *et al.* 1997).

c.- The scale of fine structure observed in (i) bright field (Thiel and Viney 1995b; Thiel and Viney 1995a) and (ii) dark field (Thiel *et al.* 1994) TEM images of regions associated with these diffraction patterns is consistent with the scale of internal compositional variation implied for an NPL crystal, i.e. the few-nanometer length scale of the two dominant repeat motifs.

d.- Within the TEM image of an NPL crystal, there can be some featureless areas that correspond to a region of crystal where positional correlations are insufficiently developed, or the layer spacings locally have the incorrect value, to give coherent scattering.

e.- The contrast of NPL crystallites relative to the amorphous matrix, and of coarse and fine structure within NPL crystals, can be enhanced by staining with tin. The tin is deposited preferentially in more disordered regions, making them more prone to scatter electrons (Thiel and Viney 1997).

f.- Molecular modelling demonstrates that the range of inter-sheet spacings needed to index TEM diffraction patterns on the unit cell of a ß-sheet crystal is consistent with a compositional range extending from pure polyalanine to pure -Gly-Gly-Gln-

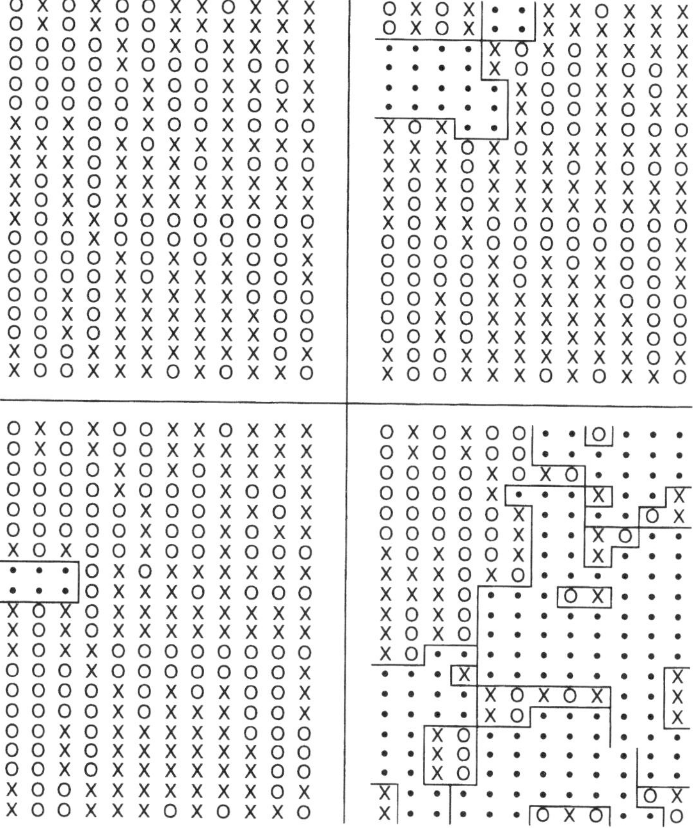

Fig. 10.4. Construction of NPL crystallites from aligned molecules containing two generic residue types O and X. The O and X residues are covalently bonded along the molecular axis (vertical), so only immediate left and right hand neighbours are important in determining local crystallinity of a region.

Top left: Twelve chains, each containing 20 residues, that form the microstructural features described in the remaining parts of this Figure.

Top right: Domains in which the composition is pure O. Residues that contribute to these domains are identified with filled circles. Locally, such compositionally pure domains will be highly crystalline. In silk, the corresponding microstructural features will involve silk ß-strands organised locally into uniformly spaced layers; the spacing would be unique to the local composition.

Bottom left: A domain in which the composition is pure X. Again, there will be a high degree of local crystallinity. In silk, the corresponding ß-sheet crystals would again have a uniform inter-sheet spacing, unique to the new local composition.

Bottom right: Domains of mixed composition. These are in general larger than the domains of pure O or pure X. Individual area or linear defects (seen in the largest domain) respectively correspond to bulk and planar defects in a three-dimensional microstructure. In silk, the corresponding NPL ß-sheet crystallites will have an inter-sheet spacing that varies with location within each crystallite.

Gly-Gly-Tyr-. Because the energy penalty for expanding the equilibrium inter-sheet spacing of polyalanine is small in comparison with the penalty for compressing -Gly-Gly-X- (Thiel 1995; Thiel *et al.* 1997), the local inter-sheet spacings in NPL crystals are most dependent on the specific local -Gly-Gly-X- sequences.

g.- Electron diffraction data obtained from the large ß-sheet crystals can be used to construct Patterson plots which are consistent with predicted scattering based on the NPL model of these crystals (Thiel *et al.* 1997).

h.- Formation of NPL crystals is achieved reliably over a range of silking rates. TEM characterisation of MAS spun at rates ranging from 0.5 to 10.0 cm.s^{-1} showed that NPL crystals which form at the fastest spinning rate are significantly smaller, and their collective volume fraction in the microstructure is reduced slightly, compared to those formed at the slowest rate (Thiel and Viney 1997). Molecular modelling confirms that the size and internal fine structure of NPL crystals is compatible with their originating from statistical rather than perfect matches between adjacent chains, which in turn is consistent with their ability to form under a range of highly non-equilibrium conditions. The NPL character of these crystals is also responsible for the greater sensitivity of microstructural *scale* to spinning rate (Hanna and Windle 1988): the lateral distances over which statistical correlations persist become smaller with increasing departure from equilibrium conditions of formation.

i.- A plausible relationship between thermal expansion coefficient and the rate at which MAS is reeled from spiders can be deduced with reference to NPL crystals. The magnitude of the expansion coefficient is an increasing function of the overall degree of molecular alignment in a fibre. In turn, the latter quantity increases with (i) the retained volume fraction of aligned material (greatest for *low* spinning rates, where molecules are better able to develop statistical matches with their neighbours), and (ii) the local order parameter for aligned material (greatest for *high* spinning rates, where extended conformations are afforded less opportunity to randomise before the fibre solidifies). A maximum in the overall degree of molecular alignment, detectable as a high value of expansion coefficient, is therefore to be expected at some intermediate spinning rate, in agreement with experimental observation. Because tensile modulus is also an increasing function of overall molecular alignment, the measurements of expansion coefficient provide compelling evidence that stiffness is maximised at the 1 cm.s^{-1} spinning rate typically used in web construction. By the same argument, the stiffness is significantly reduced at spinning rates used by spiders making a quick getaway by "abseiling" (Guess and Viney 1998).

j.- *A. diadematus* cocoon silk yields TEM diffraction patterns in which some crystalline reflexions are drawn out into streaks. The cocoon silk contains polyalanine and -Gly-Gly-X- runs that are similar to but shorter than those found in *N. clavipes* MAS, so it can be anticipated that NPL crystals in cocoon silk will be less blocky, i.e. a more continuous distribution of the intersheet spacing will be found within each NPL crystal. The diffraction pattern streaks can be interpreted in terms of the continuous rather than discrete variability of this lattice parameter (Barghout *et al.* 1999).

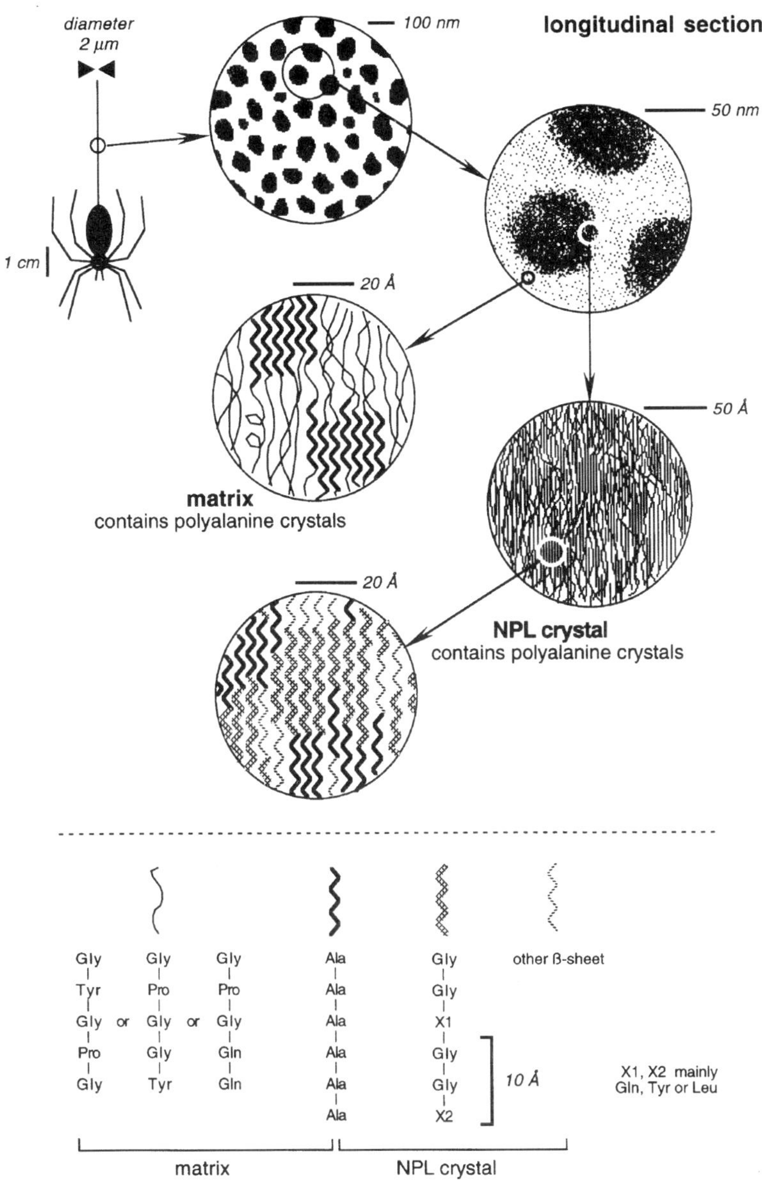

Fig. 10.5. Schematic representation of the hierarchical microstructure of spider MAS. All microstructural views are shown in longitudinal section. Only the most regular sequences are shown explicitly in the key. Short irregular sequences may occur as defects within the NPL crystals, and longer ones will be localised to the matrix.

10.3.4. Macroscopic length scales

A mechanical model, incorporating the time-dependent stress-strain characteristics of *A. diadematus* frame silk and capture thread, led to the discovery that aerodynamic damping is important in dissipating the kinetic energy of prey that impacts a web (Lin *et al.* 1995). The stretching and subsequent relaxation of threads (the mechanisms considered in Sections 10.2.2 and 10.2.4) cannot account for all the energy absorbed by a web. At the same time, aerodynamic drag increases the risk of the web being destroyed by wind, which may explain (Lin *et al.* 1995) why spiders favour the construction of webs that are not faced directly into the primary wind direction (Hieber 1984).

Tension in the radial threads of an orb web increases outwards from the centre of the web (Frank 1995). This fact, together with the finite strength of silk threads, must impose an upper limit on the size of orb webs. Spiders could attempt to overcome this problem by laying down additional radial threads; however this would increase the material and energy debits of web construction, and would increase the likelihood of wind damage. As a compromise, some large spiders add extra radials towards the periphery of the web (Vollrath 1995).

10.3.5. MAS and hierarchical microstructure

Figure 10.5 illustrates many of the features of MAS microstructure described in the preceding sections, covering five decades of length scale. It emphasises schematically the multi-phase nature of the microstructure, in which the amorphous matrix contains two types of region that have sufficient internal order to diffract x-rays or electrons. The two populations of diffracting regions differ in terms of (1) crystallite size, (2) the degree of order within crystallites, and (3) orientation distribution. While a high degree of orientational molecular order *within* individual NPL crystals is implied, this should not be interpreted as suggesting a high degree of orientational correlation across the *population* of NPL crystals.

10.4. SPINNING – THE ORIGINS OF SILK FIBRE MICROSTRUCTURE

10.4.1. Molecular and microstructural issues

10.4.1.1. Supramolecular liquid crystallinity. A shear-sensitive liquid crystalline phase occurs as a processable intermediate between the soluble form of silk (in the gland) and the insoluble form (in the fibre) (Kerkam *et al.* 1991b; Willcox *et al.* 1996; Viney 1997). Liquid crystallinity reduces the viscosity of the approximately 30 wt% protein solution (Iizuka 1985) to a level where spinning through a small aperture is possible. Both experimental and theoretical studies suggest that the liquid crystalline phase is *supramolecular* (Viney 1997); the rod-like structures responsible for orientational order are formed by the *non-covalent aggregation* of solubilised protein coils that have no significant secondary structure. The necessarily large axial (length-

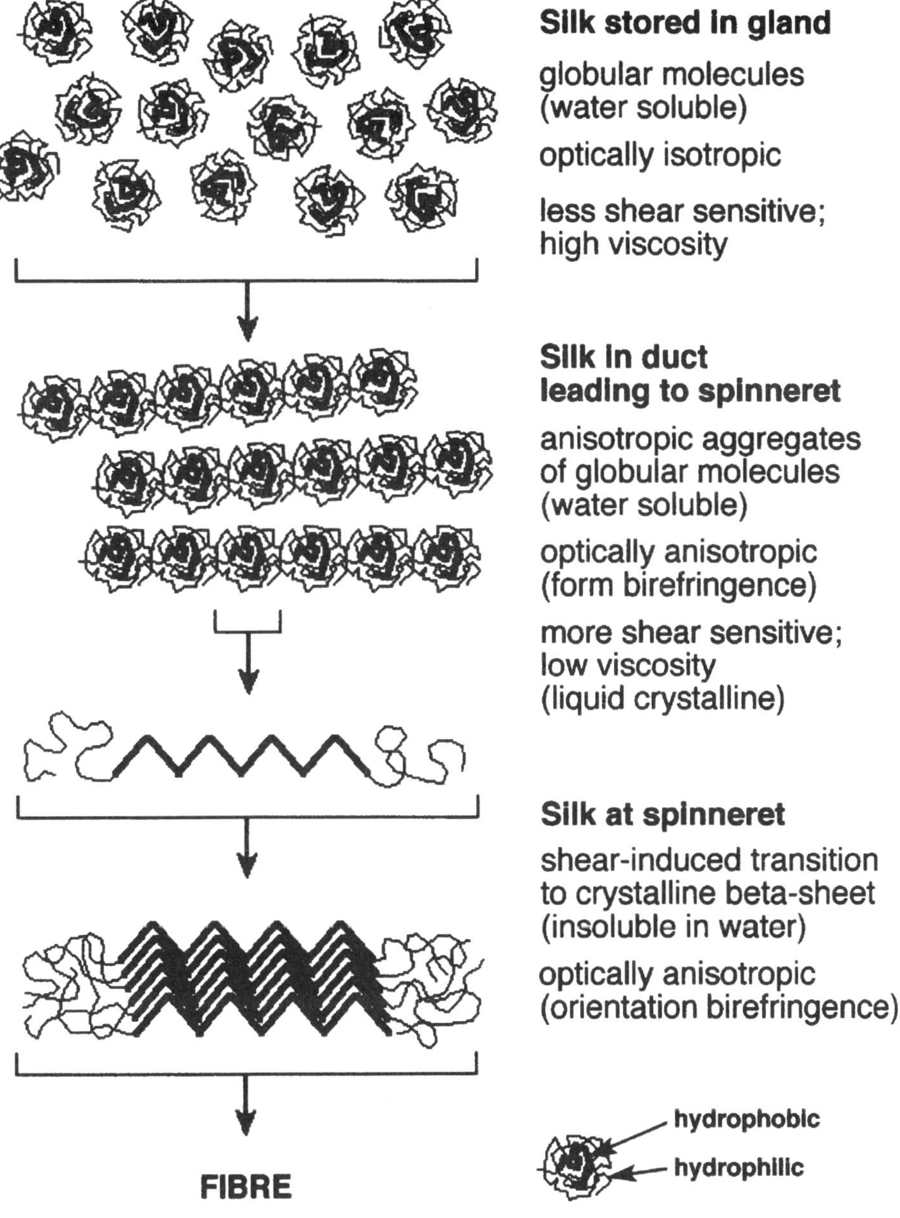

Fig. 10.6. Molecular order and properties of silk secretion at various stages in the spinning of water-insoluble fibre from fluid silk secretions in Nature. Thicker lines are used to denote more hydrophobic molecular sequences. The actual length-to-width ratio of the liquid crystalline aggregates is larger than shown.

to-width) ratio of rods that comprise the liquid crystalline fluid can only be accounted for if the individual globular molecules are allowed to form linear aggregates (Figure 10.6). Evidence for the supramolecular liquid crystallinity of *N. clavipes* MAS and *B. mori* cocoon silk secretions can be summarised as follows:

a.- The protein backbones are intrinsically flexible; their primary structure does not confer the rigid, rod-like characteristics necessary for liquid crystal phase formation by *individual* molecules (Hamodrakas and Kafatos 1984; Viney *et al.* 1992; Viney *et al.* 1994).

b.- Individual protein molecules exist as time-averaged random coils in aqueous solution, over a wide range of concentrations. Also, *in vivo* NMR characterisation of *B. mori* secretion points to a random coil conformation for the protein chains (Asakura *et al.* 1994). There is no significant stabilisation of rod-like secondary structures in solution (Zheng *et al.* 1989; Wellman *et al.* 1992), and nothing that can be aligned into a liquid crystalline phase exists at this scale.

c.- The liquid crystalline phase is exhibited by *quiescent* fluid. In other words, the anisotropy can develop *before* molecules are straightened and aligned by flow during spinning.

d.- The secretions are biphasic (i.e. consist of coexisting isotropic and liquid crystalline phases) over a narrow concentration range only (Viney 1992; Viney *et al.* 1993), which implies that they have the thermodynamic characteristics typical of an athermal liquid crystalline solution (Flory 1956; Flory and Ronca 1979; Flory 1984) (Figure 10.7). This in turn means that

(i) the rods (whatever their origin, and unlike the individual molecules in this system) are rigid (Papkov 1984);

(ii) the rods align primarily as a result of "hard" (excluded volume) interactions;

(iii) the rod axial ratio has an *upper* limit of around 30, since the biphasic regime requires a concentration greater than the approximate value of 30 weight % (Iizuka 1985) (equivalent to approximately 24 volume % if the relative density of dry silk is taken as 1.34 (Warner 1995)) that is typical of natural silk secretion prior to drying;

(iv) the rod axial ratio has a *lower* limit greater than the minimum value needed to sustain liquid crystallinity in an athermal solution (approximately 6.4, corresponding to neat polymer (Flory and Ronca 1979)).

e.- If Figure 10.6 shows an appropriate qualitative representation of molecular order in liquid crystalline silk secretion, the associated optical anisotropy is due to *form birefringence* only. This simple model accommodates the rod-like structures needed for liquid crystal formation, without recourse to anisotropy of individual molecules. The form birefringence can be modelled in terms of the refractive indices and relative amounts of water and isotropic fibroin (Viney 1997). A maximum value of 0.0097 is predicted for the birefringence of *B. mori* silk secretion, occurring at a polymer content close to 0.58 weight % (0.50 volume %, which is a plausible concentration for the partially dried secretion in which liquid

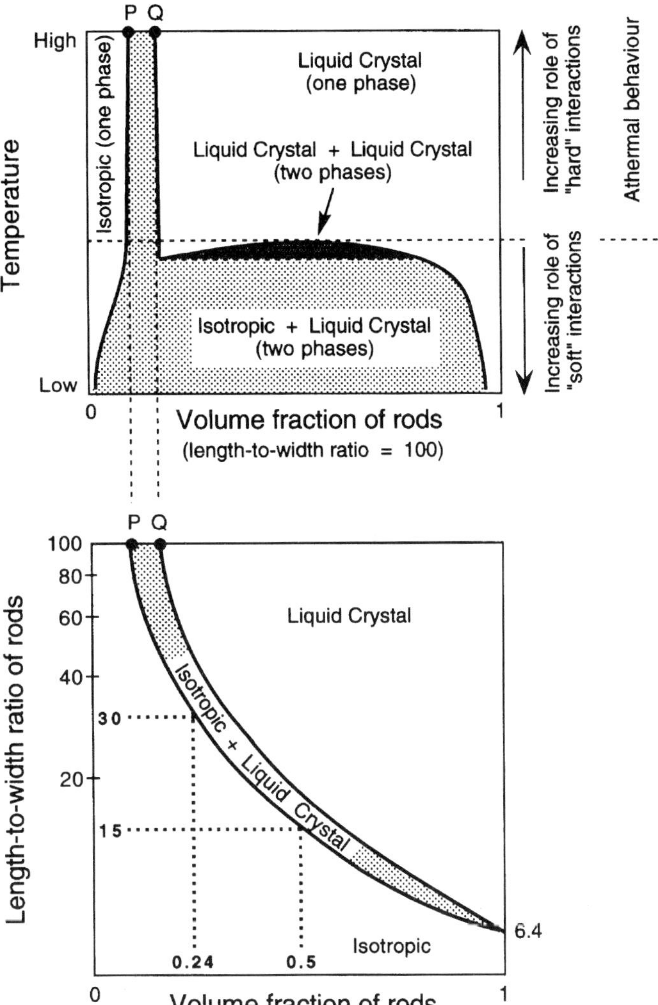

Fig. 10.7. *Top*: Solvent - rod phase diagram if the axial (length:diameter) ratio of the rods is 100; prediction of a simple lattice model (Flory 1956). The system exhibits athermal behaviour under conditions where the solvent - rod interactions are "hard", i.e. dominated by excluded volume effects rather than electrostatic attractions/repulsions. Athermal conditions cause the biphasic region on the phase diagram to form a "chimney" that encompasses a narrow range of concentrations.

Bottom: The concentration range covered by the "chimney" depends on the length:diameter ratio of the rods; prediction of a simple lattice model (Flory and Ronca 1979). The relationship to the phase diagram for rods having an axial ratio of 100 is emphasised by the vertical broken lines extending between the two parts of the diagram: concentrations P are identical in both parts, as are the concentrations Q. The significance of the highlighted concentrations, 24 vol% and 50 vol%, is explained in the text; they correspond to the likely upper and lower bounds of the rod axial ratio in liquid crystalline silk secretion.

crystalline order is observed). Experiments to determine the maximum birefringence of the liquid crystalline silk secretion recorded a value of 0.01, which corresponds closely to the predicted value. Using Figure 10.7, a refined estimate (approximately 15) can be obtained for the average rod axial ratio. In other words, if the rods are single-stranded, they consist on average of approximately 15 globular fibroin molecules.

Items (a, b) may be viewed as primarily molecular considerations, while items (c, d, e) are primarily microstructural.

While the conventional wisdom in polymer processing insists that interpenetrating coils are needed to maintain the cohesivity that ensures polymer spinnability, nature here demonstrates a successful alternative. This capacity of non-covalent associations to produce cohesive fibrous structures is not restricted to silk, and has no better illustration than the ability of muscle fibres (F-actin, composed of supramolecularly associated coils of G-actin) to generate the force needed to lift heavy weights (Stryer 1988).

Microscopically, MAS is spun by a "smart" process, i.e. the contents of the silk glands respond in a manner that facilitates the spinning. The processable liquid crystalline phase forms as concentration is increased by removal of water (Kerkam *et al.* 1991a; Kerkam *et al.* 1991b). Compared to independent molecules in the gland, aggregated fibroin coils in the duct leading to the spinneret will necessarily be more shear sensitive. The formation of water-insoluble fibre is initiated when the processable liquid crystalline fluid is denatured by shear, exposing hydrophobic molecular segments to the surrounding aqueous medium.

10.4.1.2. A role for ionic impurities. It has been proposed that small concentrations of physiological cations play a role in organising the secreted silk protein into the final fibre microstructure (Iizuka 1985). This view is supported by evidence that the critical shear rate needed to induce ß-sheet assembly in *B. mori* silk secretion is decreased by the presence of divalent cations such as Ca^{2+}. Also, it is well known that many proteins have binding sites for divalent cations such as calcium and zinc (Stryer 1988) – for example, many enzymes use this type of site to gain stability and/or functionality, using the metal as an electron reservoir. The distribution of such cationic species is therefore one aspect of control that a spider or silkworm might exert over the evolution of microstructure and properties in its silk during spinning. Similarly, if such ions are added to or removed from the secretion at a set rate during fibre spinning, their concentrations would be affected by varying the silking rate. It is of interest, therefore, to look for correlations between reeling rate and cation concentration (Figure 10.8).

Significant concentrations of the multivalent species Ca, Fe, Al and Zn are found in silk reeled at web-building rates, but not at faster rates. Only the levels of Na and K (monovalent cations which are highly mobile in physiological processes) do not drop very low for all reeling rates of 2 cm/sec and above. These observations suggest that the delivery mechanism for (especially multivalent) cations is a limiting factor in fibre spinning. Under natural conditions, spiders rarely need to produce even a few meters

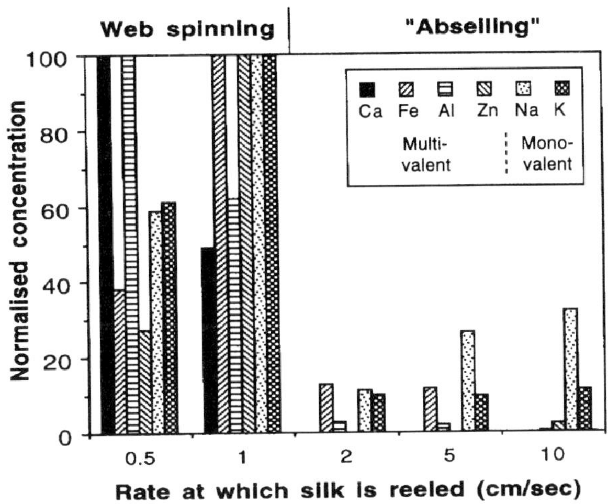

Fig. 10.8. Normalised analyte concentrations in *N. clavipes* MAS, determined by ICP-MS. An average concentration of each analyte was obtained from 5 measurements for each reeling rate. The plotted data for each analyte were normalised by setting the highest average concentration of the analyte to 100, and scaling its average concentration at the other four silking rates accordingly (Thiel and Viney 1997).

of silk at the highest rates covered by the data in Figure 10.8 — and then only when escaping from a predator. Spiders will often pause on a long descent, and one can speculate that this may afford an opportunity for the ion transport mechanisms to catch up with demand.

It is tempting to seek a microstructural consequence of the different cation contents as a function of production rate. However, fibre stiffness (as characterised via thermal expansion coefficient, on the microstructural basis discussed in section 10.3.3.3) passes through a maximum in the 0.5 to 10 cm/s range of reeling rates under discussion, while the relationship between multivalent ion concentration and reeling rate is better described by a step function. There is, therefore, no simple correlation between physical microstructure and multivalent cation content (chemical microstructure). However, there may be a more subtle interpretation of the dependence of multivalent cation concentration on reeling rate: the cation concentration affects the *process* of microstructural assembly rather than the final microstructure itself. The shear sensitivity of the liquid crystalline phase will be an increasing function of the number of molecules in each aggregate, since the co-operative response of the molecules to shear depends on their extent of interconnection. It is imperative that the transition from the water-soluble random coil conformation of silk protein to the water-insoluble, crystallisable conformation should not occur too soon, as this would block the duct and spinneret with insoluble material — indeed, this is why the silk is not stored as an aggregated, liquid crystalline phase in the gland (Viney *et al.* 1994)! To compensate for the higher shear rates associated with faster rates of silk spinning, the shear sensitivity of the silk secretion could be reduced by allowing a smaller degree of aggregation. Whether the spider does this actively, by controlling the supply of appropriate cations, or passively, due to the supply being intrinsically limited by the delivery mechanism, remains to be established.

10.4.2. Macro-scale issues

The silk spinning process in Nature may be macroscopically akin to extrusion, for example at the start of web frame construction (Foelix 1982) or during the production of strands on which spiders disperse by ballooning (Decae 1987). The process may be facilitated by various means. A spider may use a leg hooked around the dragline to pull it out of the spinneret during web building, or to act as a brake against the weight of the spider during a controlled descent. Air currents help to form the "parachute" as a spider prepares to balloon. Silkworms have to keep moving in order to pull their cocoon silk from the spinneret. In all these cases, silk-spinning organisms make do with a single processing step, because the conditions under which they have to produce fibre preclude post-spin drawing. Any drawing that does occur is achieved in *parallel* with, and as an integral part of, spinning (Figure 10.9a).

In contrast, processing of synthetic fibres, from both liquid crystalline and conventional polymers, depends on one or more *post-spin* drawing procedures for introducing most of the molecular alignment preserved in the product (Billmeyer 1984). Spinning and drawing therefore occur in *series* during the manufacture of synthetic fibres (Figure 10.9b), and it is apparent that the processing conditions used to optimise molecular order and mechanical properties in typical synthetic polymer fibres may not be similarly applicable in the context of silk-like polymers.

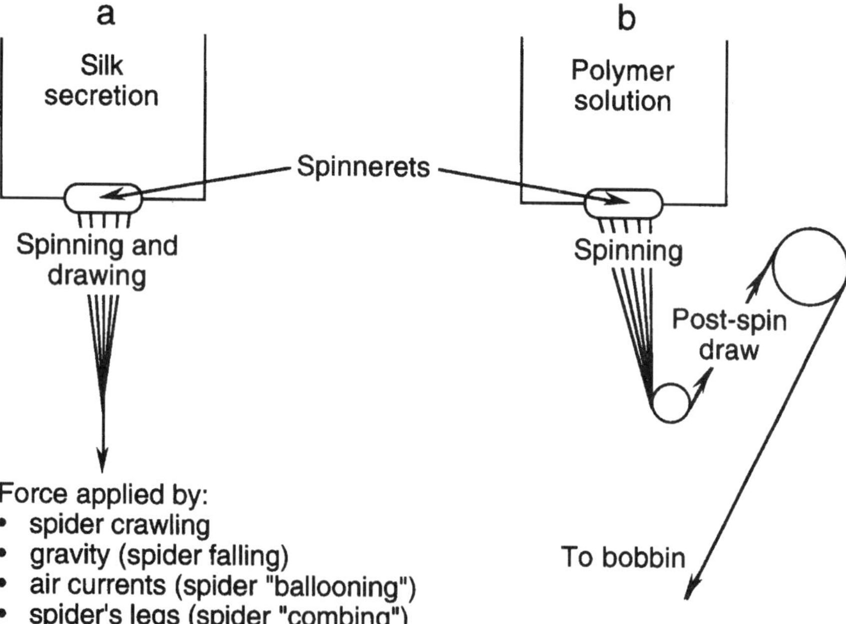

Fig. 10.9. Schematic illustration of a fundamental difference between the spinning of natural silk (a) and the spinning of synthetic fibres (b). In the latter case, spinning and drawing occur consecutively, while in the former case these two processes occur simultaneously.

Optical birefringence measurements have been used to characterise how the molecular order of *N. clavipes* MAS depends on the rate at which MAS is reeled from the spider, the extent to which the fibre is *subsequently* drawn, the rate at which drawing is performed, and the opportunity for relaxation (Carmichael and Viney 1999). Results were consistent with a microstructural model in which birefringence depends on both the overall degree of molecular orientation and the extent to which crystalline reinforcement is present. On drawing, two types of microstructural change occur:

a.- Ordered regions — in particular NPL crystals, but also polyalanine crystallites — are degraded, so that birefringence increases.
In ß-sheet crystals, there is transverse interchain bonding as well as longitudinal intrachain bonding; the *difference* between the longitudinal and transverse polarisabilities will therefore be increased if the interchain bonding is disrupted (Figure 10.10).
The chains in the remaining crystalline regions, as well as the chains that previously belonged to crystalline material, become more highly aligned, which also increases birefringence. These increases in birefringence are permanent when the fibre is allowed to relax: crystals do not reassemble in the solid state, and molecules constrained by the immediately adjacent presence of remaining crystal do not easily reorient.

b.- Amorphous material aligns, again increasing birefringence. This component of birefringence increase is temporary and recoverable.

A quantitative basis for this microstructural interpretation, confirming that *both* of the above factors must contribute to the experimentally characterised birefringence changes, has been developed through birefringence modelling (Carmichael *et al.* 1999).

The two types of microstructural change discussed above have opposite consequences for fibre stiffness. Increased orientational order will enhance the tensile modulus, while the concomitant lower volume fraction of ordered regions will diminish it. The two effects can mutually cancel: an experimental demonstration of this is obtained in the case of *B. mori* silk, where increased extents of post-spin drawing leaves the elastic stiffness unchanged (Pérez-Rigueiro *et al.* 1998).

These considerations are significant from the standpoint of processing. Post-spin plastic strain enhances microstructural and therefore optical anisotropy, some of which is preserved. However, the increased anisotropy does not necessarily herald an increase in tensile modulus. In fact, if the permanent component of birefringence increase is principally due to degradation of ordered regions, there may even be a concomitant *decrease* in stiffness, which would become more evident with the relaxation of strain-induced molecular alignment. In contrast to the methods conventionally employed to

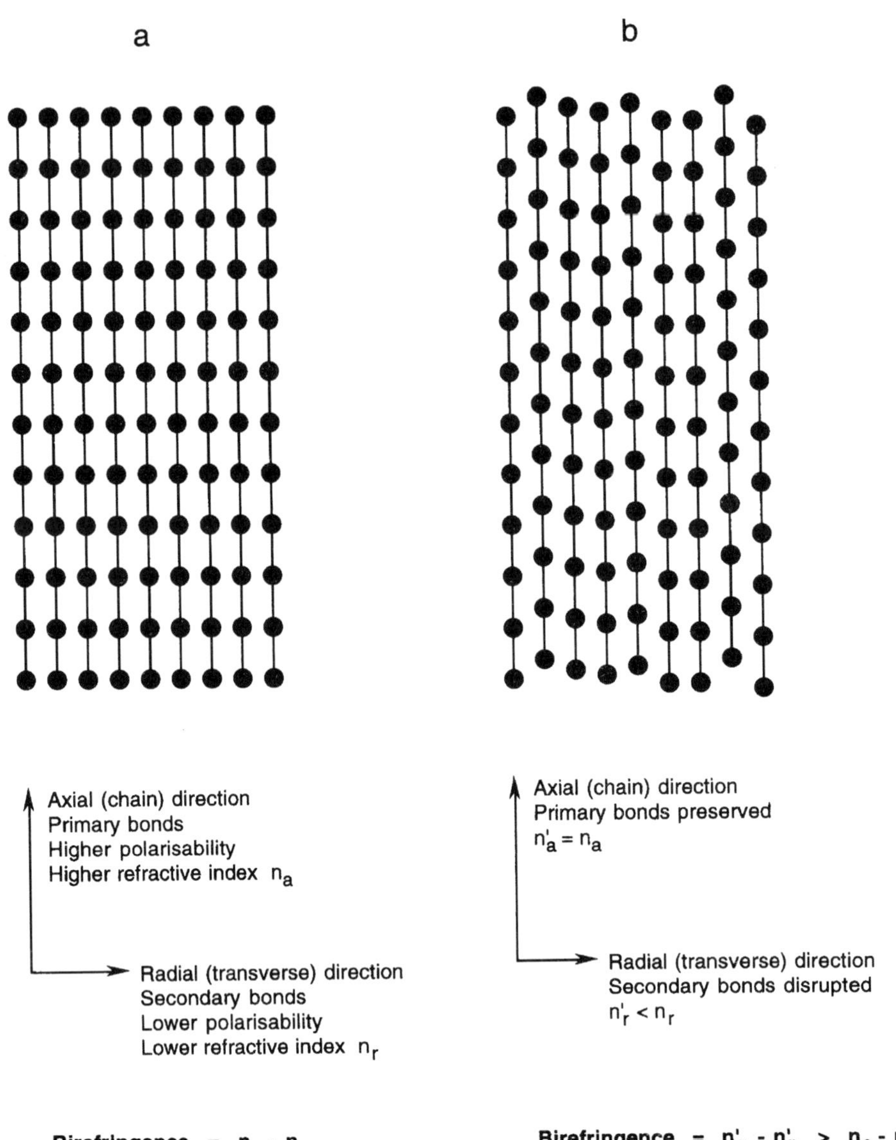

Fig. 10.10. The value of birefringence exibited by the aligned chains in (a) is increased if the molecules undergo random longitudinal displacements which disrupt the interchain or secondary bonding (b).

maximise stiffness in synthetic polymers, it appears that silk analogues should *not* be post-spin drawn. The maximum stiffness will be obtained by selecting a spinning rate that establishes an optimum balance between overall molecular alignment and internally ordered reinforcing entities in the microstructure. As discussed in section 10.3.3.3, measurement of thermal expansion indicates that this optimum is achieved at spinning rates close to 1 $cm.s^{-1}$ (Guess and Viney 1998). It is unlikely, though, that centimetre-per second rates can form the basis of an economically viable production process. Recent work (Trabbic and Yager 1998) has shown that *B. mori* silk can be solubilised, spun into fibre, immersed in a swelling agent, and then hand-drawn to generate molecular order resembling that found in naturally spun material. However, this process is limited by the lengthy immersion period and, again, by slow production rates.

The challenge, then, is to find a processing route that yields an aligned microstructure with the optimum level of crystalline reinforcement at high spinning rates. One approach might be to try and separate the steps of making the fibre and evolving the microstructure. A water-soluble crystallisation inhibitor (another of Nature's lessons – see section 10.2.4) could be incorporated in protein solution that is spun at satisfactory industrial rates into a coagulating medium. Subsequent exposure to a water bath could leech out the inhibitor, and the plasticised fibre could be drawn between rapidly rotating spools whose *difference* in rotation speeds corresponds to the speed of spinning/drawing used in natural silk production.

10.5. LESSONS FOR THE MOLECULAR AND MICROSTRUCTURAL DESIGN OF ENGINEERING POLYMERS

10.5.1 Types of lesson

Nature's successes with silk offer lessons in each of the four principal interacting areas that typically concern the materials technologist: *synthesis, processing, hierarchical microstructure* and *optimised properties*. These lessons will be consolidated in the sections that follow.

The sequence of consideration is important, because ingredients limit the possibilities for processing, while ingredients and processing act together to determine microstructure; in turn, all three of these factors directly affect properties (Figure 10.11). Some of the lessons merely reinforce what materials technology has already discovered (offering reassurance that "science has got it right"), while other lessons offer new perspectives on what might be achieved in the future.

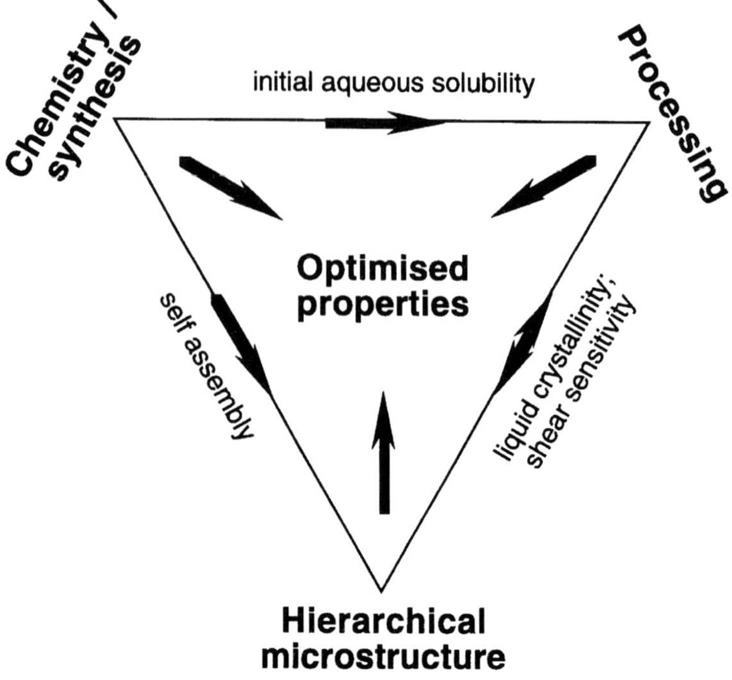

Fig. 10.11. The interrelationship between molecular synthesis, processing, hierarchical microstructure and material properties, with reference to silk.

10.5.2 Synthesis — materials chemistry

There are several advantages to assembling the fibre from a single macromolecular species. As optimised in *N. clavipes* MAS, the primary structure is complex and imperfectly repeating; it contains two different types of crystallisable sequence, both of which are more hydrophobic than the non-crystallising segments. The length and relative amounts of the different intramolecular repeat motifs are subject to genetic control. In viscid silk, there is additionally a water-soluble component that inhibits crystallisation, affording further control of microstructure.

The macromolecules do not intrinsically favour particular local conformations or secondary structures. Therefore, they fold according to the dictates of their environment. In solution, the molecules can fold to form coils in which their solvent-avoiding sequences are screened by solvent-seeking domains. Metastable, crystallisable ß-sheet conformations can be induced by shear during spinning. The molecules become insoluble as a result of a rapid physical (as opposed to conventional, slow chemical) phase transformation.

Solid microstructures can form quickly, without reliance on chemical reaction or long range diffusion of the initially solvated molecules. It is not possible for large, internally uniform crystalline regions to develop. Each polymer molecule participates in a number of different microstructural features, that vary in regard to their local composition and degree of crystallinity. The solid fibre is effectively a nanocomposite, with limited scope for coarsening or phase separation.

The interconnectivity of regions having various degrees of internal perfection precludes the existence of discrete interfaces that could weaken the material or provide easy crack paths. For the same reason, the fibre is resistant to buckling in compression.

10.5.3 Processing

Nature demonstrates that a fibre-forming, supramolecular liquid crystalline phase can be assembled from globular molecules. In the case of silk, this provides a processable intermediate between water-soluble polymer and insoluble fibre. Prior to aggregation, the globular molecules act independently; the solution can be stored, transported and even sheared without the risk of precipitating insoluble material. Aggregation is effected by a combination of concentration increase (the liquid crystalline phase forms on partial drying *in vitro*, in the absence of any other compositional change) and possible binding by ionic species. After aggregation, the supramolecular liquid crystalline phase promotes *co-operative* extension and alignment of molecules under the action of shear at or near the spinneret. This fibre processing route accommodates constraints on material, time and energy that favour (i) a high initial solution concentration, (ii) a low solution viscosity during processing, and (iii) avoidance of extensive modification to the polymer or the solution chemistry during processing.

10.5.4 Hierarchical microstructure

Both the reinforcement and the matrix are elements in a complex hierarchical microstructure that extends over length scales ranging from molecular to macroscopic. Collectively, this is responsible for the unique combination of mechanical properties exhibited by MAS. The fibre delivers a useful, optimised response to a variety of loading conditions.

Incorporation of NPL crystals in the fibre microstructure has many desirable consequences. Because these crystals evolve through the chance association of compatible sequences on adjacent chains, they do not rely on near-equilibrium conditions to form. NPL crystal formation is relatively insensitive to processing kinetics (spinning rates, and, by inference, drying rates as dictated by ambient temperature and humidity). As a result, there is no "skin-core" structure, so the entire fibre cross-section can contribute uniformly and reliably to the desired mechanical properties. Reinforcement can extend continuously, though not necessarily directly, over relatively large distances to confer strength and especially stiffness. Yet, there are included disordered regions that are capable of significant extension once the yield stress is exceeded; these regions confer toughness despite the absence of discrete "weak" interfaces. The NPL microstructure is not susceptible to phase separation / coarsening with time.

REFERENCES

American Ceramic Society (Eds.) (1990) *Ceramic Source* Vol. 6, (American Ceramic Society, Columbus, OH) p. 380.

Anderson, J.P., Cappello, J. and Martin, D.C. (1994a) *Biopolymers* **34**, 1049.

Anderson, J.P., Stephen-Hassard, M. and Martin, D.C. (1994b) in *Silk Polymers: Materials Science and Biotechnology,* ed. Kaplan, D., Adams, W.W., Farmer, B. and Viney, C. (American Chemical Society, Washington, DC) p. 137.

Asakura, T. (1986) *Makromoleculare Chemie, Rapid Communications* **7**, 755.

Asakura, T., Demura, M., Uyama, A., Ogawa, K., Komatsu, K., Nicholson, L.K. and Cross, T.A. (1994) in *Silk Polymers: Materials Science and Biotechnology,* ed. Kaplan, D., Adams, W.W., Farmer, B. and Viney, C. (American Chemical Society, Washington, DC) p. 148.

Barghout, J.Y.J., Thiel, B.L. and Viney, C. (1999) *International Journal of Biological Macromolecules* **24**, 211.

Becker, M.A., Mahoney, D.V., Lenhert, P.G., Eby, R.K., Kaplan, D. and Adams, W.W. (1994) in *Silk Polymers: Materials Science and Biotechnology,* ed. Kaplan, D., Adams, W.W., Farmer, B. and Viney, C. (American Chemical Society, Washington, DC) p. 185.

Beckwitt, R. and Arcidiacono, S. (1994) *Journal of Biological Chemistry* **269**, 6661.

Billmeyer, F.W. (1984) *Textbook of Polymer Science*, John Wiley and Sons, New York.

Bonthrone, K.M., Vollrath, F., Hunter, B.K. and Sanders, J.K.M. (1992) *Proceedings of the Royal Society of London* **B248**, 141.

Bram, A., Bränden, C.I., Craig, C., Snigireva, I. and Riekel, C. (1997) *Journal of Applied Crystallography* **30**, 390.

Buerger, M.J. (1959) *Vector Space and its Application in Crystal-Structure Investigations*; Wiley, New York.

Carmichael, S., Barghout, J.Y.J. and Viney, C. (1999) *International Journal of Biological Macromolecules* **24**, 219.

Carmichael, S. and Viney, C. (1997) Unpublished observation, Department of Materials, University of Oxford.

Carmichael, S. and Viney, C. (1999) *Journal of Applied Polymer Science* **72**, 895.

Case, S.T., Powers, J., Hamilton, R. and Burton, M.J. (1994) in *Silk Polymers: Materials Science and Biotechnology,* ed. Kaplan, D., Adams, W.W., Farmer, B. and Viney, C. (American Chemical Society, Washington, DC) p. 80.

Chou, P.Y. and Fasman, G.D. (1978) *Annual Reviews in Biochemistry* **47**, 251.

Craig, C.L. (1997) *Annual Reviews of Entomology* **42**, 231.

Cunniff, P.M., Fossey, S.A., Auerbach, M.A. and Song, J.W. (1994) in *Silk Polymers: Materials Science and Biotechnology,* ed. Kaplan, D., Adams, W.W., Farmer, B. and Viney, C. (American Chemical Society, Washington, DC) p. 234.

Decae, A.E. (1987) in *Ecophysiology of Spiders,* ed. Nentwig, W. (Springer-Verlag, Berlin) p. 348.

Dunaway, D.L. (1994) MSE Thesis, University of Washington, Seattle, WA.

Dunaway, D.L., Thiel, B.L., Srinivasan, S.G. and Viney, C. (1995a) *Journal of Materials Science* **30**, 4161.

Dunaway, D.L., Thiel, B.L. and Viney, C. (1995b) *Journal of Applied Polymer Science* **58**, 675.

Edmonds, D.T. and Vollrath, F. (1992) *Proceedings of the Royal Society of London* **B248**, 145.

Flory, P.J. (1956) *Proceedings of the Royal Society of London* **A234**, 73.

Flory, P.J. (1984) *Advances in Polymer Science* **59**, 1.

Flory, P.J. and Ronca, G. (1979) *Molecular Crystals and Liquid Crystals* **54**, 289.

Foelix, R.F. (1982) *Biology of Spiders*, Harvard University Press, Cambridge, MA.

Fornes, R.E., Work, R.W. and Morosoff, N. (1983) *Journal of Polymer Science: Polymer Physics Edition* **21**, 1163.

Fouda, I.M. and El-Tonsy, M.M. (1990) *Journal of Materials Science* **25**, 4752.

Frank, F.C. (1995) *Science and Public Affairs* **10** (Spring), 61.

Gillespie, D.B., Viney, C. and Yager, P. (1994) in *Silk Polymers: Materials Science and Biotechnology,* ed. Kaplan, D., Adams, W.W., Farmer, B. and Viney, C. (American Chemical Society, Washington, DC) p. 155.

Gosline, J., Guerette, P. and Ortlepp, C. (1996) in *Smart Structures and Materials 1996: Smart Materials Technologies and Biomimetics,* ed. Crowson, A. (SPIE, Bellingham, WA) p. 296.

Gosline, J., Nichols, C., Guerette, P., Cheng, A. and Katz, S. (1995) in *Biomimetics: Design and Processing of Materials,* ed. Sarikaya, M. and Aksay, I.A. (American Institute of Physics, Woodbury, NY) p. 237.

Gosline, J.M., DeMont, M.E. and Denny, M.W. (1986) *Endeavour* **10**(1), 37.

Gosline, J.M., Denny, M.W. and DeMont, M.E. (1984) *Nature* **309**, 551.

Grubb, D.T. and Jelinski, L.W. (1997) *Macromolecules* **30**, 2860.

Guerette, P.A., Ginzinger, D.G., Weber, B.H.F. and Gosline, J.M. (1996) *Science* **272**, 112.

Guess, K.B. (1995) MSE Thesis, University of Washington, Seattle, WA.

Guess, K.B. and Viney, C. (1998) *Thermochimica Acta* **315**, 61.

Hamodrakas, S.J. and Kafatos, F.C. (1984) *Journal of Molecular Evolution* **20**, 296.

Hanna, S. and Windle, A.H. (1988) *Polymer* **29**, 207.

Hayashi, C.Y. and Lewis, R.V. (1998) *Journal of Molecular Biology* **275**, 773.

Hieber, C.S. (1984) *Zeitschrift für Tierpsychologie - Ethology* **65**(3), 250.

Hillyard, P. (1994) *The Book of the Spider*, Hutchinson, London.

Hinman, M.B. and Lewis, R.V. (1992) *Journal of Biological Chemistry* **267**, 19320.

Holden, C. (1997) *Science* **275**, 163.

Hyde, N. (1984) *National Geographic* **165**(1), 3.

Iizuka, E. (1966) *Biorheology* **3**, 141.

Iizuka, E. (1985) *Journal of Applied Polymer Science: Applied Polymer Symposia* **41**, 173.

Kaplan, D.L., Adams, W.W., Farmer, B.L. and Viney, C., Eds. (1994) *Silk Polymers: Materials Science and Biotechnology*, American Chemical Society, Washington, DC.

Kaplan, D.L., Lombardi, S.J., Muller, W.S. and Fossey, S.A. (1991) in *Biomaterials: Novel Materials from Biological Sources,* ed. Byrom, D. (Stockton Press, New York) p. 1.

Kaplan, D.L., Mello, C.M., Arcidiacono, S., Fossey, S., Senecal, K. and Muller, W. (1997) in *Protein-Based Materials,* ed. McGrath, K. and Kaplan, D. (Birkhäuser, Boston, MA) p. 103.

Kerkam, K., Kaplan, D.L., Lombardi, S.J. and Viney, C. (1991a) in *Materials Synthesis Based on Biological Processes,* ed. Alper, M., Calvert, P.D., Frankel, R., Rieke, P.C. and Tirrell, D.A. (Materials Research Society, Pittsburgh, PA) p. 239.

Kerkam, K., Viney, C., Kaplan, D.L. and Lombardi, S.J. (1991b) *Nature* **349**, 596.

Kümmerlen, J., van Beek, J.D., Vollrath, F. and Meier, B.H. (1996) *Macromolecules* **29**, 2920.

Lewis, R.V. (1992) *Accounts of Chemical Research* **25**, 392.

Li, S.F.Y., McGhie, A.J. and Tang, S.L. (1994) *Biophysical Journal* **66** (April), 1209.

Lin, L.H., Edmonds, D.T. and Vollrath, F. (1995) *Nature* **373**, 146.

Lombardi, S.J. and Kaplan, D.L. (1990) *Journal of Arachnology* **18**, 297.

Lucas, F. and Rudall, K.M. (1968) in *Comprehensive Biochemistry: Extracellular and Supporting Structures,* ed. Florkin, M. and Stotz, E.H., Vol. 26B (Elsevier, Amsterdam) p. 475.

Lucas, F., Shaw, J.T.B. and Smith, S.G. (1955) *Journal of the Textile Institute* **46**, T440.

Mahoney, D.V., Vezie, D.L., Eby, R.K., Adams, W.W. and Kaplan, D.L. (1994) in *Silk Polymers: Materials Science and Biotechnology,* ed. Kaplan, D., Adams, W.W., Farmer, B. and Viney, C. (American Chemical Society, Washington, DC) p. 196.

Marsh, R.E., Corey, R.B. and Pauling, L. (1955a) *Biochimica et Biophysica Acta* **16**, 1.

Marsh, R.E., Corey, R.B. and Pauling, L. (1955b) *Acta Crystallographica* **8**, 710.

Mello, C.M., Arcidiacono, S., Senecal, K. and Kaplan, D.L. (1995) in *Industrial Biotechnological Polymers,* ed. Gebelein, C.G. and Carraher Jr., C.E. (Technomic, Lancaster, PA) p. 213.

Mello, C.M., Senecal, K., Yeung, B., Vouros, P. and Kaplan, D. (1994) in *Silk Polymers: Materials Science and Biotechnology,* ed. Kaplan, D., Adams, W.W., Farmer, B. and Viney, C. (American Chemical Society, Washington, DC) p. 67.

Minor Jr, D.L. and Kim, P.S. (1994) *Nature* **371**, 264.

Mita, K., Ichimura, S., Zama, M. and James, T.C. (1988) *Journal of Molecular Biology* **203**, 917.

Moore, A.M.F. and Tran, K. (1996) *American Zoologist* **36**, 54A.

Nguyen, A.N., Moore, A.M.F. and Gould, S.A.C. (1994). in *52nd Annual Meeting of the Microscopy Society of America / 29th Annual Meeting of the Microbeam Analysis Society,* ed. Bailey, G.W. and Garrattreed, A.J. (San Francisco Press, San Francisco, CA) p. 1056.

Papkov, S.P. (1984) *Advances in Polymer Science* **59**, 75.

Parkhe, A.D., Seeley, S.K., Gardner, K., Thompson, L. and Lewis, R.V. (1997) *Journal of Molecular Recognition* **10**, 1.

Pérez-Rigueiro, J., Viney, C., Llorca, J. and Elices, M. (1998) *Journal of Applied Polymer Science* **70**, 2439.

Prevorsek, D.C. (1995) *Trends in Polymer Science* **3**(1), 4.

Simmons, A., Ray, E. and Jelinski, L.W. (1994) *Macromolecules* **27**, 5235.

Simmons, A.H., Michal, C.A. and Jelinski, L.W. (1996) *Science* **271**, 84.

Stauffer, S.L., Coguill, S.L. and Lewis, R.V. (1994) *Journal of Arachnology* **22**, 5.

Stewart, I. and Golubitsky, M. (1992) *Fearful symmetry*, Blackwell, Oxford, UK.

Strydom, D.J., Haylett, T. and Stead, R.H. (1977) *Biochemical and Biophysical Research Communications* **79**, 932.

Stryer, L. (1988) *Biochemistry*, W.H. Freeman and Company, New York.

Termonia, Y. (1996) *Macromolecular Symposia* **102**, 159.

Thiel, B.L. (1995) PhD Dissertation, University of Washington, Seattle, WA.

Thiel, B.L., Guess, K.B. and Viney, C. (1997) *Biopolymers* **41**, 703.

Thiel, B.L., Kunkel, D.D. and Viney, C. (1994) *Biopolymers* **34**, 1089.

Thiel, B.L. and Viney, C. (1995a) in *Industrial Biotechnological Polymers,* ed. Gebelein, C.G. and Carraher Jr., C.E. (Technomic, Lancaster, PA) p. 221.

Thiel, B.L. and Viney, C. (1995b) *MRS Bulletin* **20**(9), 52.

Thiel, B.L. and Viney, C. (1997) *Journal of Microscopy* **185**(2), 179.

Tillinghast, E.K. and Townley, M. (1987) in *Ecophysiology of Spiders,* ed. Nentwig, W. (Spinger-Verlag, Berlin) p. 203.

Tillinghast, E.K. and Townley, M.A. (1994) in *Silk Polymers: Materials Science and Biotechnology,* ed. Kaplan, D., Adams, W.W., Farmer, B. and Viney, C. (American Chemical Society, Washington, DC) p. 29.

Trabbic, K.A. and Yager, P. (1998) *Macromolecules* **31**, 462.
Valluzzi, R., Gido, S.P., Zhang, W.P., Muller, W.S. and Kaplan, D.L. (1996) *Macromolecules* **29**, 8606.
Vincent, J.F.V. (1993) in *Biomolecular Materials,* ed. Viney, C., Case, S.T. and Waite, J.H. (Materials Research Society, Pittsburgh, PA) p. 35.
Viney, C. (1992) *ACS Polymer Preprints* **33**(1), 757.
Viney, C. (1997) *Supramolecular Science* **4**, 75.
Viney, C., Huber, A. and Verdugo, P. (1993) in *Biodegradable Polymers and Packaging,* ed. Ching, C., Kaplan, D.L. and Thomas, E.L. (Technomic, Lancaster, PA) p. 209.
Viney, C., Huber, A.E., Dunaway, D.L., Kerkam, K. and Case, S.T. (1994) in *Silk Polymers: Materials Science and Biotechnology,* ed. Kaplan, D., Adams, W.W., Farmer, B. and Viney, C. (American Chemical Society, Washington, DC) p. 120.
Viney, C., Kerkam, K., Gilliland, L.K., Kaplan, D.L. and Fossey, S. (1992) in *Complex Fluids,* ed. Sirota, E.B., Weitz, D., Witten, T. and Israelachvili, J. (Materials Research Society, Pittsburgh, PA) p. 89.
Viney, C. and Windle, A.H. (1987) *Molecular Crystals and Liquid Crystals* **148**, 145.
Vollrath, F. (1994) in *Silk Polymers: Materials Science and Biotechnology,* ed. Kaplan, D., Adams, W.W., Farmer, B. and Viney, C. (American Chemical Society, Washington, DC) p. 17.
Vollrath, F. (1995) *Science and Public Affairs* **10** (Spring), 61.
Vollrath, F. and Edmonds, D.T. (1989) *Nature* **340**, 305.
Vollrath, F., Holtet, T., Thøgersen, H.C. and Frische, S. (1996) *Proceedings of the Royal Society of London* **B263**, 147.
Warner, S.B. (1995) *Fiber Science*, Prentice Hall, Englewood Cliffs, NJ.
Wellman, S.E., Hamodrakas, S.J., Kamitsos, E.I. and Case, S.T. (1992) *Biochimica et Biophysica Acta* **1121**, 279.
Willcox, P.J., Gido, S.P., Muller, W. and Kaplan, D.L. (1996) *Macromolecules* **29**, 5106.
Wilson, R.S. (1962a) *Quarterly Journal of Microscopic Science* **104**(4), 557.
Wilson, R.S. (1962b) *Quarterly Journal of Microscopic Science* **103**(4), 549.
Windle, A.H., Viney, C., Golombok, R., Donald, A.M. and Mitchell, G.R. (1985) *Faraday Discussions of the Chemical Society* **79**, 55.
Work, R.W. (1976) *Textile Research Journal* **46**(July), 485.
Work, R.W. (1977) *Textile Research Journal* **47**(October), 650.
Work, R.W. (1981) *Journal of Arachnology* **9**, 299.
Work, R.W. (1985) *Journal of Experimental Biology* **118**, 379.
Work, R.W. and Morosoff, N. (1982) *Textile Research Journal* **52**(May), 349.
Xu, M. and Lewis, R.V. (1990) *Proceedings of the National Academy of Sciences, USA* **87**, 7120.
Yang, Z., Grubb, D.T. and Jelinski, L.W. (1997) *Macromolecules* **30**, 8254.
Zemlin, J.C. (1968) A study of the mechanical behavior of spider silks. Report no. 69-29-CM (AD 684333), U.S. Army Natick Laboratories, Natick, MA.
Zheng, S., Li, G., Yao, W. and Yu, T. (1989) *Applied Spectroscopy* **43**(7), 1269.

Chapter 11

Molecular Modeling of the Stress/Strain Behavior of Spider Dragline

Chapter 11

Molecular Modeling of the Stress/Strain Behavior of Spider Dragline

YVES TERMONIA

11.1. INTRODUCTION

Spider dragline represents one of the strongest materials available to date. The fiber is stronger than steel and has a tensile strength approaching that of Kevlar® (see Table 11.1). In contrast to the latter, however, the dragline is also characterized by a very high strain at break of the order of 20-30%. That unusual combination of high strength and elasticity leads to toughness values never achieved in synthetic high performance polymeric fibers. In man-made fibers, indeed, any improvement in tensile strength is always associated with a decrease in the strain at break and vice-versa. As a result, the exceptional toughness properties of spider dragline remain a mystery.

Other attractive feature of the dragline include its excellent compressive strength, ease of dyeability and foremost, its ability to dissolve in an aqueous environment. This is in contrast to high performance synthetic fibers, like Kevlar®, which require processing in very caustic and aggressive solvents such as highly concentrated solutions of sulfuric acid.

Spider dragline is a protein polymer in which the repetition unit consists of various amino acids [CO-CHR-NH] which differ in their side group R. The exact amino acid sequence has been determined see Xu and Lewis (1990). Their study indicates a

Table 11.1. Comparison of the tenacity and strain at break for different materials (10 g/d ≈ 1 Gpa)

	Tenacity (g/d)	*Strain (%)*
Steel	6	2
Nylon	9	20
Kevlar®	22	3
Spider dragline	20	30

preponderance of the two smallest amino-acids: glycine (R≡H) and alanine (R≡CH_3). The next largest fraction is made of glutamine, leucine and proline, which are characterized by very bulky side groups (D.L. Kaplan, C.M. Mello, S. Arcidiacono, S. Fossey, K. Senecal and W. Muller 1997). The identification of the amino acid sequence for the dragline has led recently to a series of experimental ventures aimed at synthesizing analogs of spider silk using recombinant DNA techniques (Tirrell, Fournier and Mason 1991). In that approach, one starts by solid-state synthesizing DNA strands which code for a short string of amino acids, which appears to be representative of the whole sequence. These strands are ligated into multimers and fractionated. They are then inserted into a plasmid and introduced into a strain of *Escherichia coli* for expression. Although the process should produce chains having the same length and amino-acid sequence, it frequently leads to very broad molecular weight distributions because of occasional random deletions and post-translational chain cleavage (O'Brien 1993). Thus, although freshly spun fibers from Major Ampullate have a very narrow molecular weight distribution immediately after spinning (M_w/M_n = 1.05), that distribution considerably widens after aging for 6 months (M_w/M_n = 2.42) (O'Brien, Fahnestock, Termonia and Gardner 1998).

From a theoretical standpoint, there is at present no basic understanding of the molecular origin of the unusual mechanical properties of spider dragline. Issues such as the importance of its narrow molecular weight distribution and small crystal size remain obscure. It is the purpose of the present work to address these problems using the molecular modeling techniques described in Chapter 9. Preliminary reports on our study can be found in (Termonia 1994).

11.2. MODEL

Spider dragline has been clearly identified as a semi-crystalline material made of amorphous flexible chains reinforced by crystallites. The latter are believed to be made of hydrophobic polyalanine sequences arranged into beta-pleated sheets. The amorphous part, on the other hand, can be attributed to oligopeptide chains rich in glycine. In sharp contrast to the case of polyethylene, extensively studied in Chapter 9, the chains in spider dragline are strongly hydrogen-bonded which hinders drawability. Figure 11.1 shows previous model results (Termonia 1996) for the dependence of the drawability of polymeric materials on the ratio between the elastic modulus of the attractive bonds (E_h) between chains and that originating from the entropic restoring force of the chains (E_a). In the case of polyethylene, which was extensively studied in Chapter 9, the attractive bonds between chains consist of weak van der Waals forces and the ratio E_h/E_a is small. As a result, the maximum draw ratio is essentially controlled by the density of entanglements along the chains and its value is high (9-10). In hydrogen-bonded polymers on the other hand, such as spider dragline, the ratio E_h/E_a is high and drawability is restricted. For a given E_h/E_a, the maximum attainable draw ratio is also a strong function of the crystalline volume fraction (see Fig.11.2), as crystals do not deform during drawing (for more details, the reader is referred to Termonia, 1996).

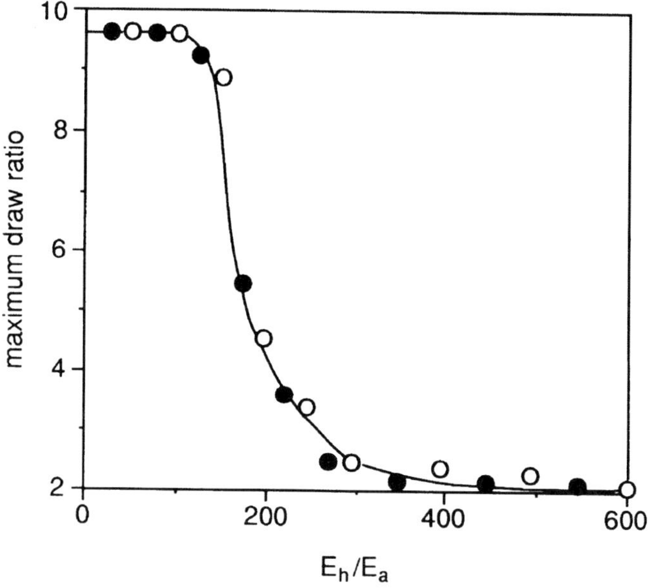

Fig. 11.1. Dependence of the maximum draw ratio of semi-crystalline polymers on E_h/E_a for two different values of the modulus E_a of the amorphous chain network. Symbols are as follows: (○): E_a=1 MPa; (●): E_a=3MPa. The figure is for a crystalline volume fraction V_c=0. For details, see (Termonia 1996).

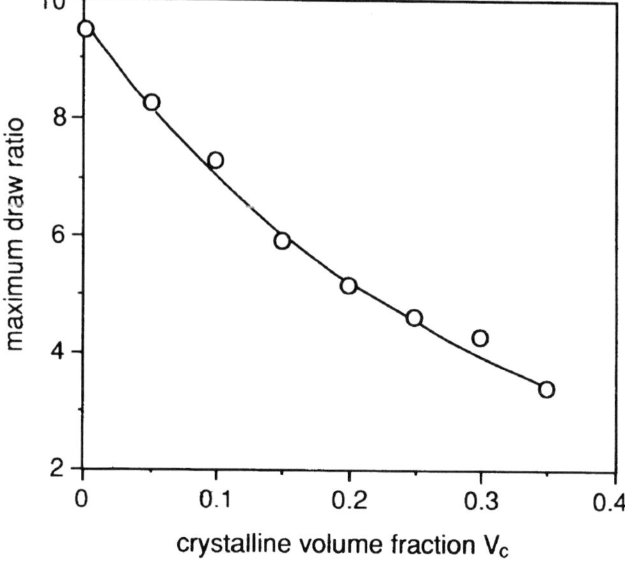

Fig. 11.2. Dependence of the maximum draw ratio on crystalline volume fraction V_c. The figure is for E_h/E_a=71. For details, see (Termonia 1996).

The above considerations require that our original model of Chapter 9 be refined in order to explicitly account for the volume fraction, initial size and shape of the crystallites in spider silk. Our model for the dragline is depicted in Fig.11.3a and it can be further simplified as in Fig.11.3b (for more details see Termonia (1994). In view of their very small size (6x2x21 nm for *Bombyx mori* cocoon silk) (Fraser and MacRae 1973), the crystallites can be viewed as multifunctional crosslinks which create inside the amorphous region a thin layer with a modulus of elasticity (E_{layer}) higher than that (E_a) in the bulk. Chains within that layer indeed retain some of the orientation present in the crystallites. This is clearly exemplified in Fig.11.4, which shows the decrease in the order parameter of the chains with an increase in distance (in nm) from the crystallite surface. For more details, the reader is referred to (Termonia 1995). The figure clearly reveals that the effective thickness of the ordered layer is of the order of 5-10 nm, which also corresponds to the end-to-end vector length of the trapped chains (Flory 1983). It should also be noted that the presence of such an interfacial region has been clearly identified in polyethylene samples using NMR (Kitamaru, Nakaoki, Alamo and Mandelkern 1996; Eckman, Henrichs and Peacock 1997) and Raman spectroscopy (Strobl and Hagedorn 1978), as well as small angle X-ray scattering (Stribeck, Alamo, Mandelkern and Zachmann 1995). Arguments based on the number of chains exiting the crystal surface (Termonia 1994) lead for that layer to a modulus value $E_{layer} = 6E_a$. The presence of that rubbery region of higher modulus has been schematically represented in Fig. 11.3b through the use of a three-line vector length for the chain strands. More information about the structure of spider silk can be learned from the effect of water on its components. Water is well known to have a plasticizing effect on the amorphous phase by preventing the formation of hydrogen bonds between chains. That plasticizing effect is responsible for the 50% shrinkage of the dragline when exposed to water (Gosline, Denny and DeMont 1984). The potential for supercontraction in the dry dragline can be easily implemented in our model of Fig.11.3. We start with the "wet" structure in which hydrogen bonds are absent and the amorphous chains assume a random coil configuration. That structure is stretched on the computer to a draw ratio $\lambda \approx 2$ and the orientation induced in the amorphous chains is then frozen-in through the imposition of hydrogen bonds between nodes (dotted lines in Fig.11.3b).

To summarize: We start with the model of Fig.11.3b in which the chains in the amorphous phase are not in a purely random coil configuration because of their pre-stretching to a draw ratio $\lambda \approx 2$. The semi-crystalline network is then deformed in a succession of very small increments δL. As in our original model described previously, after each increment, our model allows for four processes to occur:

(i) Breaking of the hydrogen bonds both in the amorphous and in the crystalline regions.

That process is assumed to be thermally activated and is performed according to Eqs.9.1-9.3 of Chapter 9 with appropriate values of the activation energies and volumes. For hydrogen bonds, we use U=35Kcal/mol (Termonia and Smith 1986) which ensures breaking, in the absence of stress, at temperatures above 250°C, which

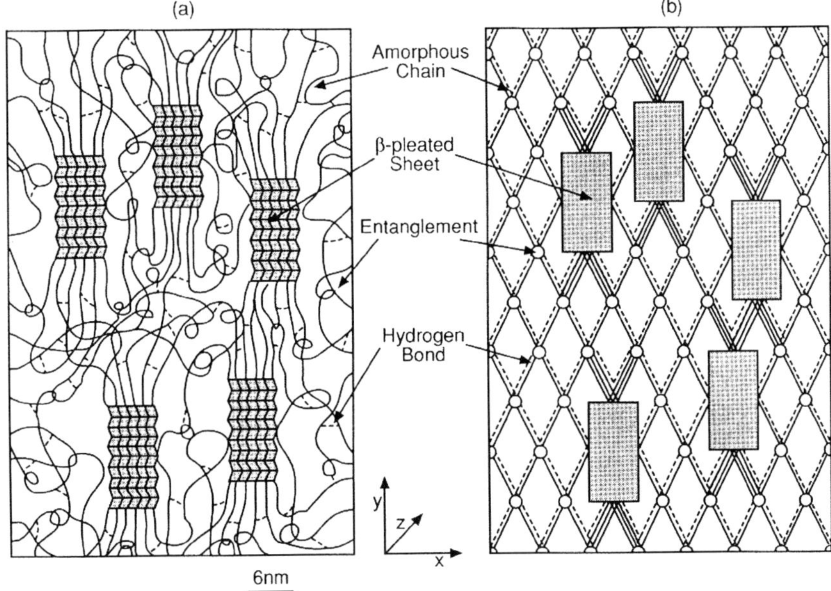

Fig. 11.3. Molecular model for spider dragline. (a) System of amorphous and crystalline chains. For the purpose of easy representation, the figure is for a 15% volume fraction of β-pleated sheets. (b) More schematic representation in which the details of the amorphous chains have been omitted and only end-to-end vectors are shown. Individual hydrogen bonds have been replaced by "overall" bonds (dotted lines) connecting every entanglement to its neighbors. The 3-lines vectors indicate the high modulus layer in the amorphous phase.

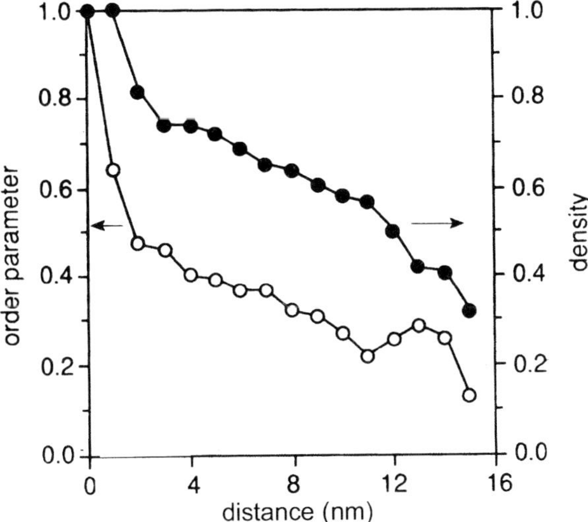

Fig. 11.4. Variation of the order parameter of chains exiting a crystallite with the distance in nm from the crystal surface. For details, see (Termonia 1995).

is in the range of the melting temperature of the dragline (Cunniff, Fossey, Auerbach and Song 1994) and other flexible hydrogen-bonded polymers. For the activation volume, we take $\beta = (4.74Å)^3$, which leads to breaking near the experimental yield point at 2% strain.

(ii) Stretching of the chains in the amorphous regions
Upon breaking of the hydrogen bonds acting along a particular chain strand, the latter is allowed to stretch and its stress is calculated using the classical theory of rubber elasticity, see Chapter 9. Thus, the stress on an amorphous chain *i* with local draw ratio λ_i is obtained from

$$\sigma_i = E_a n_e^{1/2} (1/3) \mathcal{L}^{-1} (\lambda_i / n_e^{1/2}) - \sigma_o \tag{11.1}$$

in which n_e denotes the number of statistical segments between entanglements and σ_o represents the stress in the absence of strain $(\lambda_i = 1)$. We choose $n_e = 14$, thereby assuming that the elastic properties of the chains can be approximated by those of synthetic polyethylene (see Chapter 9). For simplicity, we do not consider the possibility of chain slippage.

(iii) Breaking of the chain strands in the amorphous regions
The latter occurs when the local draw ratio exceeds its maximum value $\lambda = n^{1/2}$ in which n denotes the number of statistical segments for the strand.

(iv) Network relaxation
All the lattice nodes are relaxed towards mechanical equilibrium using the same techniques as those described in Chapter 9.

11.3. RESULTS AND DISCUSSION

11.3.1 Stress-draw ratio curves

Figure 11.5 shows our calculated stress-strain curve for a dragline first immersed in water and then strained at a rate $\lambda = 1.42$/min. To recall, our model assumes that the only effect of water on the fiber is to prevent the formation of hydrogen bonds between chains in the amorphous phase. As anticipated, the effect of water is to contract the structure by as much as 50%, thereby releasing the residual stress locked-in in the amorphous region (see model description in Section 11.2). Upon subsequent stretching of the network, now free of hydrogen bonds in the amorphous phase, the stress-strain curve exhibits a purely rubber-like behavior with a marked upturn near the breaking point. Also represented in the Figure is a typical experimental curve for a wet dragline, as obtained from (Work 1977). A good agreement between theory and experiment is found, which leads to confidence in the validity of our model.

Our model predictions for a dry dragline are given in Fig.11.6. At small strains (<2%), the curve is linear with modulus E=10GPa, in perfect agreement with

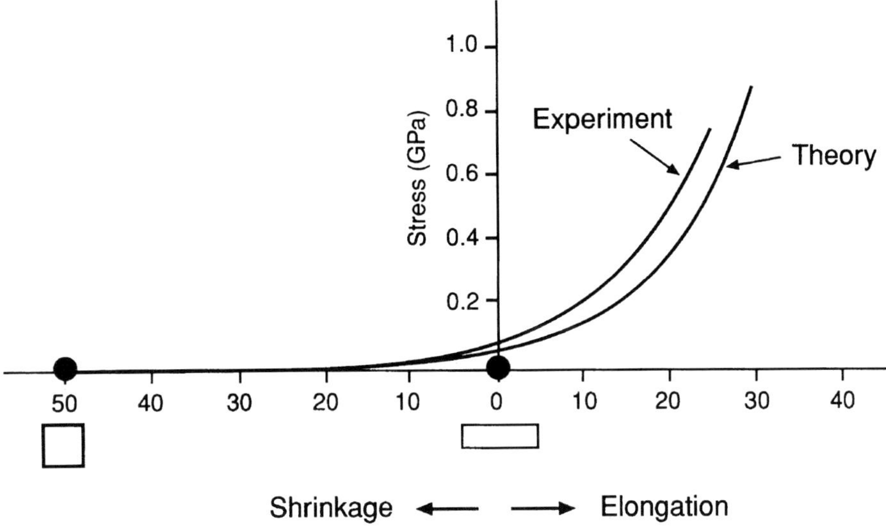

Fig 11.5. Calculated and experimental stress-strain curves for a dragline first immersed in water and then strained at a rate $\lambda = 1.42$/min. The experimental curve is taken from (Work 1977).

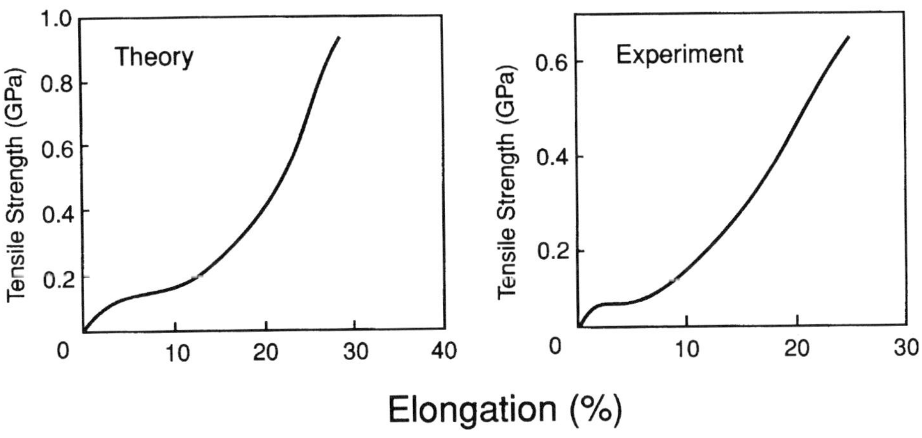

Fig. 11.6. Calculated and experimental stress-strain curves for a dry dragline. The experimental curve is taken from (Work 1977).

experimental observation (Gosline, DeMont and Denny (1986). At ~2% strain, the hydrogen bonds between chains in the amorphous regions start to break, leading to the formation of a yield point at which the stress-strain curve reaches a plateau. At 10% strain and higher, the hydrogen bond breaking process is almost complete and the stress resumes its increase with draw ratio. Our model results in Figure 11.6 also predict a draw ratio at break λ=1.3 and a tensile strength approaching 1GPa. All of the above model predictions are in excellent agreement with a typical experimental stress-strain curve reproduced from (Work 1977).

We now turn to a possible explanation for the unusual toughness properties obtained from our model results of Fig.11.6. As clearly explained in Section 11.2, our approach explicitly takes into account the role of an interfacial layer of higher modulus in the amorphous region. In an attempt to investigate the importance of that layer, we have also looked at our model results in the absence of that layer thus, taking $E_{layer}=E_a$. Our predictions are presented in Fig.11.7 and compared to those previously reported for the full model. The figure clearly indicates a substantial decrease in modulus and tensile strength in a fiber with $E_{layer} = E_a$, which reveals the crucial role played by that interfacial layer.

11.3.2. Effect of Crystal Size

Obviously, the reinforcing role of the high modulus layer will be strongly dependent on its volume fraction, hence on the crystallite size, as the layer has a constant thickness value around 5-10nm. This is clearly indicated by the schematic representation in Figure 11.8a, which illustrates the increase in volume fraction of the high modulus region (shaded region) with a decrease in crystallite size. Figure 11.8b

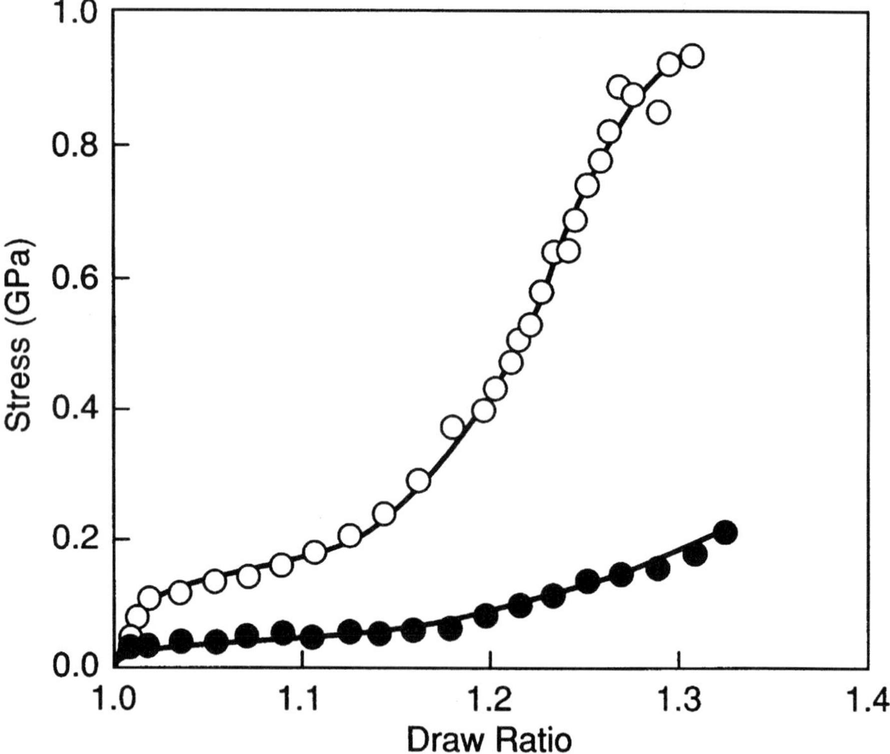

Fig. 11.7. Calculated stress-strain curves for a dry dragline in the presence (symbol ○) and absence (symbol ●) of an interfacial layer of higher modulus in the amorphous region.

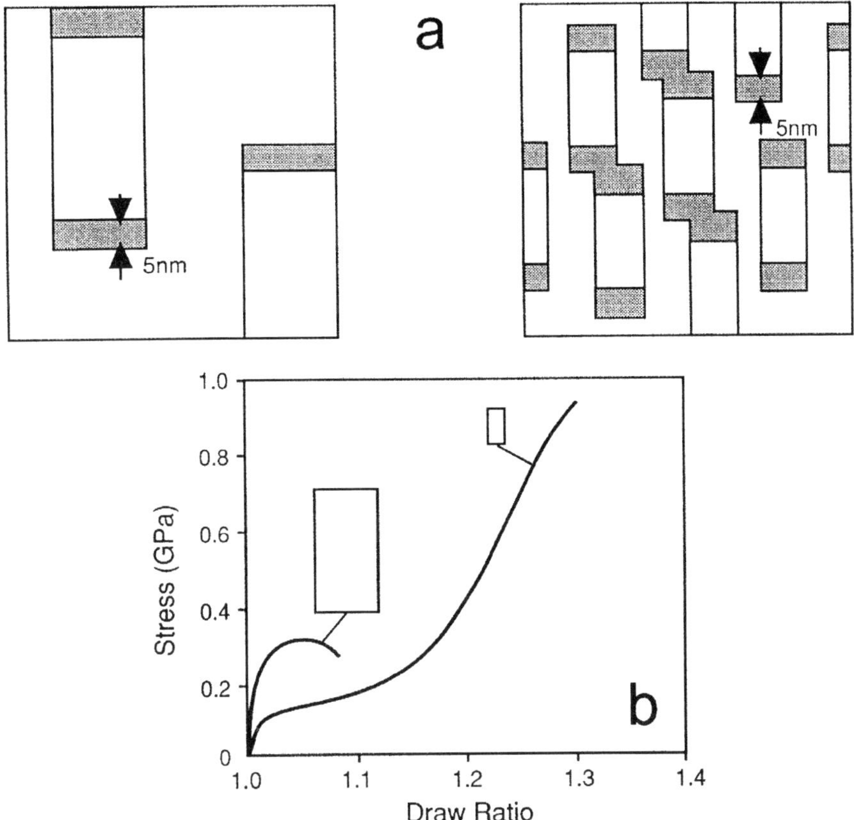

Fig. 11.8. (a) Schematic illustration of the increase in volume fraction of the high modulus layer (shaded region) with a decrease in crystallite size. (b) Nominal stress-draw ratio curves for the typical dragline with its small crystal size and for a fiber with crystallites nine times as large.

compares our calculated stress-strain curve for the typical dragline with small crystal size to that obtained with the model for a fiber with crystallites nine times as large. Large crystals are seen to lead to very high initial modulus values. However, they also act as network defects creating high local stress concentrations. As a result, premature failure of the samples occurs near 10% strain, leading to low toughness and tenacity values.

From the model results of Figures 11.7 and 11.8, it appears that the beta-crystallites in the dragline have an optimum size. On one hand, the crystals are small enough to ensure a high volume fraction of the thin reinforcing layer whereas, on the other, they are also large enough to guarantee a high modulus for that layer ($E_{layer} = 6E_a$). The molecular origin of the small crystal size in dragline silk has been discussed in a recent paper by Simmons, Michal and Jelinski (1996). Looking at the sequence of amino-acid for dragline silk (Xu and Lewis 1990), these authors

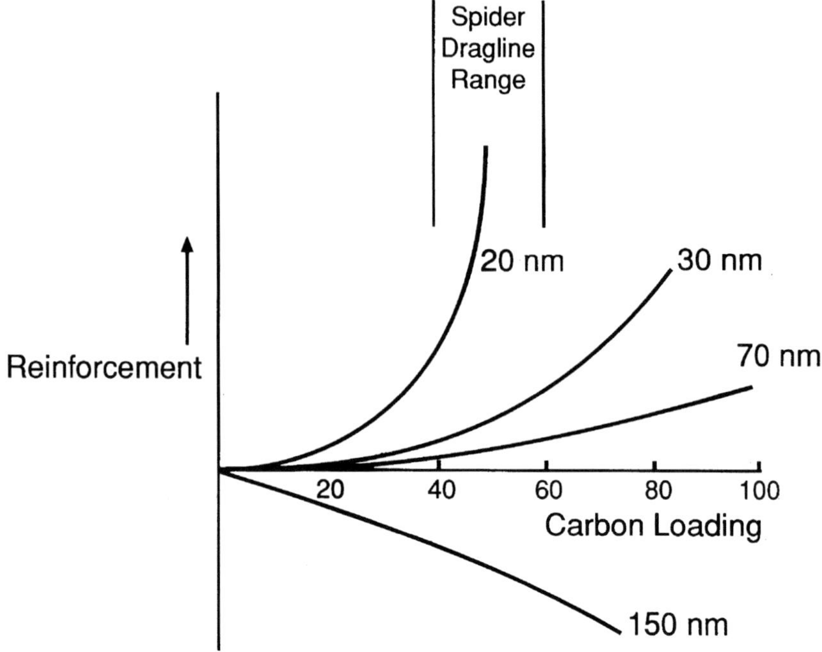

Fig. 11.9. Effect of carbon particle size on their reinforcement efficiency in elastomeric materials. The data are taken from (Donnet and Vidal 1986).

conjecture that a molecular chain reverses at the points in the sequence where a glycine is followed by a serine or an asparagine residue. This produces a secondary structure with small clusters of alanine-rich regions. Another possible explanation for the small size of the β-crystallites comes from the observation that the alanine sequences are usually flanked on each side by glutamine residues. These amino-acids are characterized by very bulky side groups, which, because of steric hindrance, may prevent the lateral growth of the β-crystallites.

There is a surprising similarity between the reinforcing effect of the crystallites in spider dragline and that of carbon particles in synthetic rubbers (Donnet and Vidal 1986). Figure 11.9 shows the effect of carbon particle size on their reinforcement efficiency in elastomeric materials. The data are reproduced from (Donnet and Vidal 1986). For large particle diameters of the order of 100nm and higher, the data clearly indicate a negative reinforcement efficiency (compare with our model results for large β-crystallites in Fig. 11.8). For smaller diameters, a true reinforcement is found which also increases with carbon loading. Note the large effect of small carbon black particles with their diameters of 20-30nm, which lie within the range of the size of the crystallites in spider dragline. As for the dragline, carbon black particles typically lead to the formation of a thin interphase, 3nm thick, within which the mobility of the chains is very constrained.

11.3.3 Effect of molecular weight and its distribution

Another peculiar feature of spider dragline resides in its molecular weight distribution which is very close to being monodisperse with M_w/M_n = 1.02 and M_w = 725,000 (O'Brien, Fahnestock, Termonia and Gardner 1998). Such monodisperse distributions are never attained in synthetic man-made fibers, which typically have M_w/M_n values in the range 2-5. As alluded to in the introduction, although we have succeeded in spinning dragline fibers with M_w/M_n = 1.05 (O'Brien, Fahnestock, Termonia and Gardner 1998), that value increases considerably after aging for only a few months because of chain scission effects related to proteolysis.

In order to shed some light on the mystery residing around the presence of a true monodisperse molecular weight distribution in spider dragline, we wish to return to some of our model predictions for synthetic polyethylene presented in Chapter 9. To recall our results of Section 9.3.3 of that Chapter, we found that a monodisperse molecular weight distribution substantially increases the drawability of the polymer chains. Our calculated data for the dependence of the maximum achievable draw ratio on drawing rate are summarized in Fig. 11.10 for two monodisperse polyethylenes with M_w = 143,000 and M_w = 6,800 (for more details, see Termonia, Allen and Smith (1988). We start by studying our results for M_w = 143,000. At high rates of deformation (>10^{-1} min^{-1}), our results indicate that all samples break near their "natural" draw ratio value around 5-10. As the rate decreases, calculated data indicate

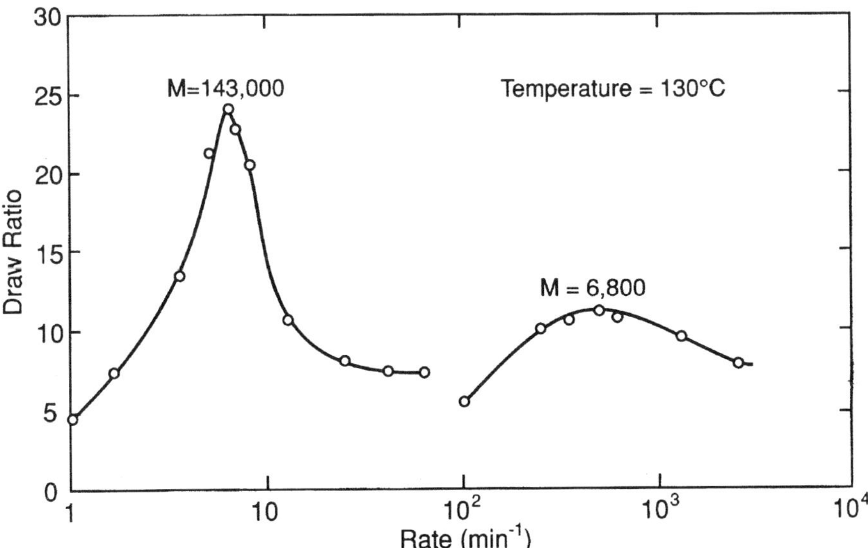

Fig. 11.10. Calculated dependence of the maximum achievable draw ratio on rate of drawing for (close to) monodisperse synthetic polyethylenes with M_W=143,000 and M_W=6,800. The temperature of drawing is kept constant.

that chains start to slip through entanglements and drawability increases up to maximum value $\lambda_{max} = 30$, reached at a rate 8 min^{-1}. At still lower rates, drawability is lower because the rate of slippage now becomes higher than that at which the sample is being drawn. Our results therefore point to an optimum drawing rate around 8 min^{-1}. Turning to the second curve for M_w = 6,800, we find -again- a bell shape curve with a well-defined maximum. A most important observation, however, is that the optimum rate of deformation is two orders of magnitude higher than that for M_w = 143,000. In other words, every molecular weight value has its own optimum drawing rate which is itself controlled by the rate of slippage through entanglements. From our model results, it therefore transpires that polydisperse systems will never exhibit the behavior described in Fig. 11.10 as every single molecular weight value will have its own optimum rate different from the others (see also Fig. 9.15 in Chapter 9).

Turning to application to spider dragline, it is now well accepted that the rate of deformation is easily controlled by a fine tuning of the valves at the exit of the spinnerette. Recent experimental observations (Guess and Viney 1988) indicate that the spinning rates can be varied by an order of magnitude, leading to draglines with different modulus values. In view of our model results of Fig. 11.10, the possibility of fine tuning the spinning rate of a polymer with a true monodisperse polymer allows for high draw ratios but also for a very uniform and affine stretching. The latter, in conjunction with small crystal size, leads to a very homogeneous deformation and to exceptional toughness properties never achieved in synthetic man-made fibers.

11.4. CONCLUSIONS

Spider dragline is a strongly hydrogen-bonded polymer in which the crystallite size and molecular weight distribution play a crucial role. Our model has been quite successful in reproducing the complex stress strain curves found experimentally for the dragline in both the wet and the dry states. More importantly, our approach provides the first comprehensive analysis of the factors controlling spider silk elasticity. In that connection, our model clearly reveals the importance of the small crystalline β-sheets which create inside the amorphous phase a thin layer with modulus higher than in the bulk. Our approach also provides the first plausible explanation for the presence of a monodisperse molecular weight distribution.

We are perfectly aware that our dragline model may be too simplistic to describe all the aspects of spider silk elasticity. The approach, however, brings out very clearly essential points like the effect of water and the role of the crystalline and amorphous phases. It is our hope that such a simplified approach will foster further theoretical and experimental research aimed at designing synthetic materials which would either mimic or improve on spider silk properties.

REFERENCES

Cunniff P.M., Fossey S.A., Auerbach M.A. and Song J.W.(1994) *ACS Symp. Ser.* **544**, 234.
Donnet J.B. and Vidal A. (1986) in *Pharmacy, Thermomechanics, Elastomers, Telechelics,* ed. Dusek, K. (Springer-Verlag. Berlin) p. 104.
Eckman R.R., Henrichs P.M. and Peacock A.J. (1997) *Macromolecules* , **30**, 2474.
Flory P.J. (1983) *Principles of Polymer Chemistry*, Cornell University Press, Ithaca NY.
Fraser R.D.B. and MacRae T.P. (1973) *Conformation in Fibrous Proteins*, Academic Press. New York.
Gosline J.M., Denny M.W. and DeMont M.E. (1984) *Nature* , **309**, 551.
Gosline J.M., DeMont M.E. and Denny M.W. (1986) *Endeavor* , **10**, 37.
Guess K.B. and C. Viney (1998) *Thermochimica Acta,* **315**, 61.
Kaplan D.L., Mello C.M., Arcidiacono S., Fossey S., Senecal K. and Muller W. (1997) in *Protein-Based Materials* ed. McGrath, K. and Kaplan, D. (Birkhauser. Boston) p. 103.
Kitamaru R., Nakaoki T., Alamo R.G. and Mandelkern L. (1996) *Macromolecules,* **29**, 6847.
O'Brien J.P. (1993) *TRIP*, **1**, 228.
O'Brien J.P., Fahnestock S.R., Termonia Y. and K.H. Gardner (1998) *Adv. Mater.,* **10**, 1185.
Simmons A.H., Michal C.A. and Jelinski L.W. (1996)*Science* , **271**, 84.
Stribeck N., Alamo R.J., Mandelkern L. and Zachmann H.G. (1995) *Macromolecules,* **28**, 5029.
Strobl G.R. and Hagedorn W. (1978) *J. Polym. Sci.: Polym. Phys.Ed.* , **16**, 1181.
Termonia Y. and Smith P. (1986) *Polymer* , **27**, 1845.
Termonia Y., Allen S.R. and Smith P. (1988) *Macromolecules,* **21**, 3485.
Termonia Y. (1994) *Macromolecules* , **27**, 7378.
Termonia Y. (1995) *Macromolecules*, **28**, 7667.
Termonia Y. (1996) *Macromolecules,* **29**, 4891.
Tirrell J.G., Fournier M.J., Mason T.L. and Tirrell D.A. (1994) Biomolecular Materials, *C&EN,* December 19, p. 40.
Work R.W. (1977) *Textile Res. J.*, **47**, 650.
Xu M. and Lewis R.V. (1990) *Proc. Natl. Acad. Sci.* **87**, 7120.

Glossary

Actuators: Transducers of electrical energy to mechanical energy by changes of volume proportional to an electrical magnitude.

Allograft: See **implants**.

Amino acid: The monomeric building blocks of a protein. See Figures 8.1 and 8.2 and associated text in Chapter 8.

Amorphous: This term refers to regions of material where the local secondary structure (e.g. β-strand; see "conformation" below) of the protein possesses insufficient long range order in three dimensions to produce detectable diffraction of x-rays or electrons. 2. State of a polymer in which the chains are in a coiled conformation.

Arthroscopy: A local surgical procedure by which the internal structures of the joint may be examined and repaired without opening up the joint.

Articular cartilage: The soft bearing material covering the bone ends in a synovial joint. It can be considered to be a biological composite composed of collagen fibres reinforcing a proteoglycan gel.

Artificial muscle: Actuator able to transduce electrical charge to mechanical energy by electrochemical stimulation of conformational changes along polymeric chains, interchanging ions and water molecules with the surroundings.

Autograft: See **implants**.

Bioartificial or **tissue engineered implants**: Implants composed of living cells (autologous, allogeneic or xenogeneic) within a synthetic or semi-synthetic substrate. This gives rise to terms such as bioartificial "tissues", "grafts" or "materials", depending on complexity and maturity of the construct. These have never previously been an intact living tissue but are designed to become fully integrated with surrounding biological structures. Hence terms such as tissue (dermal or more layers; skin) substitute or replacements.

Bio-impersonation: is a term coined to describe the use of artificial or semi-artificial materials, bio-control processes, diffusible regulators of cell function etc., to simulate aspects of the normal bio-environment required. Thus, cellular functions are preserved within limits, compatible with acceptable normal function, but outside a natural in vivo tissue environment. That is critical environmental cues are mimicked, not reproduced perfectly.

Biological polymer: This term refers to any polymer made by a living organism. The organism is one that is found in Nature. A polymer that has been produced by a genetically modified host is referred to as a *genetically engineered* polymer - whether or not that polymer is also produced in Nature. Some authors use the term *biopolymer* as a synonym for biological polymer, but others use *biopolymer* to denote a polymer (of whatever origin) that is used in medical implants; we therefore avoid this term in order to minimise possible ambiguity.

Biomaterial: A material intended to interface with biological systems to evaluate, treat, augment or replace any tissue, organ or function of the body.

Bio-prostheses: are non-living implants prepared from biological materials which do not normally become integrated with surrounding biological tissues.

Birefringence: In fibrous material, and other materials in which the microstructure is cylindrically symmetric, birefringence is the difference between the refractive indices measured along and transverse to the cylinder axis.

Buckling: Mode of deformation in which an instability occurs in a structural member, usually under compressive loads, resulting in a twisting or bending out of shape. Generally leads to plastic deformations and eventual collapse.

Cancellous bone: Porous bone tissue which consists in a network of septa or **trabeculae** intercommunicated and occupied by bone marrow. It is also called **spongy bone** and **trabecular bone**.

Cellular engineering: These are used in many cases synonymously to mean "the use of engineering principles and design practices, with biology, *to fabricate implantable tissues*". This is best reserved for the term **tissue engineering** (TE). Cellular engineering is regarded by some to be the small subsection of TE where isolated cells are implanted into a defect without a supporting matrix, i.e. in cell suspension (e.g. some forms of cartilage resurfacing treatment). A broader definition is used in Europe where cellular engineering (CE) is regarded as a distinct and larger discipline, in which "engineering principles are used in the control or measurement of cellular function". This definition makes CE a large umbrella term including elements of biomedical sensors and diagnostic devices (cyto-monitoring) as well as the field of tissue engineering.

Collagen: A structural protein which is present in fibrous form in soft tissues.

Compact bone: Dense bone tissue with a continuous solid mass aspect in which the only empty spaces are meant for blood vessels and bone cells or **osteocytes**. Usually it is also called **cortical bone**.

Compliance: The easy with which a body can be deformed elastically or viscoelastically. It is measured in units of deflection/force. Formally, it is the reciprocal of **stiffness**.

Conducting polymers: Monodimensional electronic conductors at molecular level formed by a cross-linked network of polyconjugated chains. They can be oxidized and reduced as inorganic metals. During oxidation their properties change as a function of the composition.

Configuration: This is a synonym for the chemical or *primary* structure of a molecule. It refers to the composition and connectivity of the molecule: what atoms are used, which ones are linked, and what is the stereochemistry of linking? To change the configuration of a polymer, it is necessary to break covalent bonds. Unfortunately, many older texts use the term configuration to denote what a modern text would call **conformation**.

Conformation: This is a synonym for the physical structure (shape) of a molecule, and encompasses secondary and tertiary structure. Conformation is determined by bond rotations; it is not associated with altering the scheme of covalent bonds. *Secondary* structure refers to the local shape of molecular segments, while *tertiary* structure refers to the shape of entire molecules. For example, some segments of the molecule might have an α-helical secondary structure, while the molecule as a whole is globular.

Conformational movements: Change of chain conformation, electrochemically induced by extraction or injection of electrons.

Cortical bone: See **compact bone**.

Counterions: Compensating charges interchanged between the conducting polymer and the solution during oxidation, or reduction, processes in order to keep the electroneutrality inside the material.

Creep: The increase of deformation of materials with time under constant stress (see **stress relaxation**).

Crystalline: A term that describes regions of materials where the local secondary structure (e.g. β-strand; see **conformation** above) of the protein possesses sufficient long range order in three dimensions to produce detectable diffraction of x-rays or electrons. 2. State of a polymer in which the chains are in an extended and well ordered conformation.

Chaotropic: A chaotropic agent helps to break up any structure which is imposed on a solvent by interactions between the solvent and a polymeric solute. In other words, the chaotropic agent favours disorder in the solvent, increasing the solubility of the polymer.

Chiral: A molecule that cannot be superimposed on its mirror image is said to be chiral.

Chondrocytes: A mature cartilage cell embedded in a small cavity of lacuna, in the cartilage matrix. It is responsible for the synthesis and maintenance of the extracellular matrix of cartilage.

Damage ratio: The ratio of a specific mechanical parameter, prior to and following a period of mechanical damage, such as is associated with fatigue.

Diaphysis: Cylinder of **compact bone**, the internal surface of which closes the medullar cavity.

Dragline: High strength silk fiber used by the spider to lower itself from the web.

Draw ratio: Unit of deformation defined as $\lambda = 1 + \varepsilon$ $(\varepsilon = \delta L/L_0)$.

Dynamic modulus: A complex modulus, which describes the behaviour of viscoelastic materials. It is made up of a real elastic component and an imaginary viscous component.

Electrochromic property: Change of color in films of conducting polymers as a function of the oxidation depth. Color can be changed in a continuous, infinitesimal and reverse way, as the oxidation depth.

Electron-ion transducer: Material able to translate an electronic pulse to a pulse of ions. Conducting polymers store ions which can be liberated by electric pulses, acting as electron-ion transducers.

Entanglement: Inter- or intra-chain knot along a chain contour.

Ephiphysis: Extreme parts of a long bone, which are mainly formed by **trabecular bone** covered by a thin layer of **compact bone**.

Fatigue resistance: The ability of a material to resist failure when it is subjected to a series of repetitive load cycles.

Fibroblasts: Cells found in a range of soft tissues, such as tendon, ligament and skin, which are responsible for the production of an aligned collagenous matrix.

Form birefringence: The particular type of birefringence that occurs when elongated, optically isotropic particles or microstructural features are at least partially aligned in a matrix that is also optically isotropic. The elongate particles and the matrix have different refractive indices and the scale of the microstructure is smaller than the wavelength of light.

Fracture toughness: A measure of the capacity of a cracked material to withstand loads. Under elastic behaviour, the critical value of the stress intensity factor K is used to predict the fracture toughness.

Glycosaminoglycans (GAG): A series of molecules, such as chondroitin sulphate and keratan sulphate, containing disaccharide units, which are negatively charged. One exception is hyaluronan, which is an uncharged glycosaminoglycan present in articular cartilage and synovial fluid.

Graft: See **implants**.

Haversian system: see **osteon**.

Haversian tissue: In **cortical bone**, **secondary osteons** can be distributed either highly dispersed or tightly packed. In this later case successive generations of **secondary osteons** may substitute one another. Each one of these generations is called, 1st, 2nd, 3rd, ... generation and constitute **Haversian tissue**.

Hydrogen bonds: Strong attractive bonds between polymer chains.

Hydroxyapatite: The main mineral component of mature bone, with stoichiometric formula $Ca_{10}(PO_4)_6(OH)_2$. Hydroxyapatite in bone is calcium deficient with a deficiency ranging between 5 and 10%.

Hysterisis: The energy lost within a material when it is subjected to a load/unload cycle.

Implants: Implants come with a baffling array of descriptions depending on whether they are moved within the same organism (auto-), between individuals of the same species (allo-) or between species (xeno-). **Grafts** can be any of these three, whilst the term transplant is not normally used for autologous movements. Both **grafts** and **transplants** are living tissues. Non-living implants would be termed **prostheses** whilst **implants** covers all eventualities.

Integration: refers to the process by which biological tissues grow together, such that any interfaces present in the first place are obliterated and indistinguishable. This can be used to refer to sites of repair integration, where wound site margins naturally become obscured. It can also refer to the process by which an independently functioning implanted structure eventually takes on a role within the whole biological tissue or structure. Hence an *integrated* implant becomes part of the functional whole tissue/organ.

Interfacial region: Thin layer of semi-ordered polymeric materials in-between the crystalline and amorphous phases.

Lacunae: Array of ellipsoidally shaped cavities contained in the interfaces between the **lamellae**, which contain bone cells or **osteocytes**.

Lamellae: In mature bone, the collagen fibres run parallel to each other to form laminae, called lamellae. The lamellae can be arranged in concentric cylindrical layers, in osteons, or parallel.

Liquid crystal: The liquid crystalline state combines characteristics of an ordinary fluid with others that would usually be associated with crystalline solids. For example, the low viscosity of many liquid crystals permits them to flow easily, so they adopt the shape of their container. Meanwhile, transmitted polarised light microscopy performed on thin undisturbed specimens of the same fluid materials may reveal a high degree of local structural anisotropy. Such hybrid properties must imply an underlying scheme of molecular order which is intermediate between the conventional fluid and crystalline state. X-ray diffraction reveals that it is specifically long-range molecular *orientation* that is preserved in a liquid crystal; while long range positional order may also be present, it is not fully developed in three dimensions.

Lyotropic: A liquid crystalline phase (Section 8.3) is lyotropic if its formation depends on the presence of a greater-than critical concentration of orientable moieties.

MAS: Major Ampullate Silk (see p. 302).

Mechanotransduction: The ability of a cell to sense and respond to a mechanical environment. The associated pathways in articular cartilage may be resolved into extracellular components followed by intracellular signaling events.

Metaphysis: Bone region of transition between the **epiphysis** and the **diaphysis**. The ossification of the epiphysary plate determines the fusion of the epiphysis and the diaphysis meaning the end of the period of active growth of bone.

Microstructure: *Microstructure* is a generic term relating to one or more aspects of the order within a material. The description may or may not be confined to one length scale, and it may be based on a single characterisation technique or on several techniques. Traditionally, the term refers to structure at greater-than-micrometer scales, i.e. features that are resolvable with a conventional light microscope. It is now used colloquially to encompass structure down to atomic length scales, i.e. it includes what is technically called *nanostructure*.

Modulus: Slope of stress-strain curve (same units as stress).

Monte-Carlo process: Process commonly used in modeling in which thermodynamic equilibrium of a system is reached using a series of elementary moves controlled by a random lottery.

Nervous interface: Array of electron-ion transducers being biocompatibles with dendrites or axons termianls suitable to transform electronic pulses into ionic pulses, which can be understood by neurons.

NPL: Non-Periodic Lattice crystals (see p. 312 and 314).

n.p.l.: Non-periodic layer crystals (see p. 314).

Organic battery: Battery formed by a reduced conducting polymer (able to store cations), a thin film of a polymeric electrolyte having a high ionic conductivity, and an oxidized polymer blend of a conducting polymer and a polyelectrolyte. Reverse movement of cations from a conducting polymer to the other occurs during discharge or charge.

Osmotic swelling pressure: The pressure exerted by a hydrated polymer gel which, in articular cartilage, is associated with the proteoglycan component.

Osteoarthritis: Degenerative joint condition which is characterised by the loss of articular cartilage and the exposure of underlying bone.

Osteocyte: Bone living cells physiologically active which are mutually connected through cytoplasmatic prolongations inside very thin channels called canaliculi.

Osteon: Vascular channel surrounded by concentric lamellar bone. If bone is of centripetal deposition and without previous resorbtion at the periphery of the channel a **primary osteon** is formed. Structures originated from a process of erosion initiated from the vascular channel towards the periphery, and followed by a later centripetal deposition of concentric lamellar bone are **secondary osteons** or **Haversian systems**.

Oxidation depth: Is the percentage of oxidized polymer, considering 0% the polymeric chains without positive charges and 100% of the polymeric chain bearing the maximum density of charges. It can be controlled through the oxidation charge or by the oxidation potential.

Patterson plot (function): The autocorrelation function (self-convolution) of electron density, often projected onto a specified direction or plane (Buerger 1959; Marsh *et al.* 1955b). The distances of peaks from the origin correspond to interatomic vectors; the height of a peak is an increasing function of the product of the atomic numbers of the corresponding atoms, and to the number of times that the interatomic distance occurs in the crystallographic unit cell.

Polyethylene: Polymer made of hydrocarbon chains CH_3-$(CH_2)_n$-CH_3.

Primary osteon: See **osteon**.

Primary structure: The composition and connectivity of a molecule, i.e. a description of what atom types are used, which ones are linked, and the stereochemistry of linking. If this word is used in the context of a protein polymer, the primary structure is adequately described by the sequence of amino acid residues. See **configuration**.

Prostheses: See **implants**.

Proteoglycans: High molecular weight macromolecules of connective tissues composed of a protein core to which glycosaminoglycans are covalently attached. In articular cartilage, proteoglycans are generally present in aggregate form.

Reeling: In the context of spider silk, this term refers to the controlled collection of fibre (e.g. on a motorised spindle) from a live restrained spider. The spider may or may not be anaesthetised during this process. In the context of silkworm silk, reeling refers to the unraveling of a degummed cocoon to yield a single long thread.

Relaxation: Return of system to equilibrium after sudden disturbance. When the return is exponential, the time constant of exponential function is the *relaxation time*.

Representative volume element (RVE): The smallest volume over which the average of mechanical or physical properties, such as Young's modulus or coefficient of thermal expansion, for example, are representative of the whole (see p. 5).

Secondary osteon: See **osteon**.

Secondary structure: See **conformation.**

Spongy bone: See **cancellous bone.**

Statistical segment: Unit length of polymer chain beyond which the chain can be viewed as flexible (l = 14 nm for polyethylene).

Stiffness: The ability of a material to resist elastic or viscoelastic deformation. It is measured in units of force/deflection. Formally, it is the reciprocal of **compliance.**

Strain: Unit of deformation defined as $\varepsilon = \delta L/L_0$, in which δL is the deformation and L_0 is the initial length.

Strength: Maximum stress reached at the breaking point.

Stress: Force per unit area; represented by symbol σ and often expressed in GPa units (1GPa = 10^9 Pascals; 1 Pascal = $1N/m^2$).

Stress Relaxation: The decrease of stress of materials with time under constant strain. See **creep.**

Tangent modulus: A measure of material stiffness, estimated from the gradient of a stress-strain curve at a particular point. The gradient is commonly taken within the linear section of the curve for soft tissues.

Tendon: A fibrous structure of connective tissue by which a muscle is attached to bone.

Tertiary structure: See **conformation.**

Tissue engineered implants: See **Bioartificial.**

Tissue engineering: The application of engineering principles and the life sciences towards the development of biological substitutes that restore, maintain or improve tissue function. See also **cellular engineering.**

Toughness: Area under a stress-strain curve. See **fracture toughness.**

Trabeculae: See **cancellous bone.**

Trabecular bone: See **cancellous bone.**

Translation: In the context of protein synthesis, this term refers to the process of protein synthesis as mediated by messenger-RNA in a living cell. In other words, translation is the process by which information coded in the "alphabet" of nucleic acids is converted to information expressed in the "alphabet" of amino acid sequence in a protein.

Tritiated thymidene: A radioactive marker for cell proliferation.

Tropocollagen: The molecular unit of collagen fibrils. It is composed of three polypeptide chains, made up of approximately 1000 amino acid units, arranged in a helical structure.

Van der Waals (vdW) bonds: Weak attractive bonds between polymer chains.

Viscoelastic tissue: A material description of all soft tissues, whose properties are partly those of a viscous fluid and partly those of an elastic solid.

Xenograft: See **implants.**

Subject Index

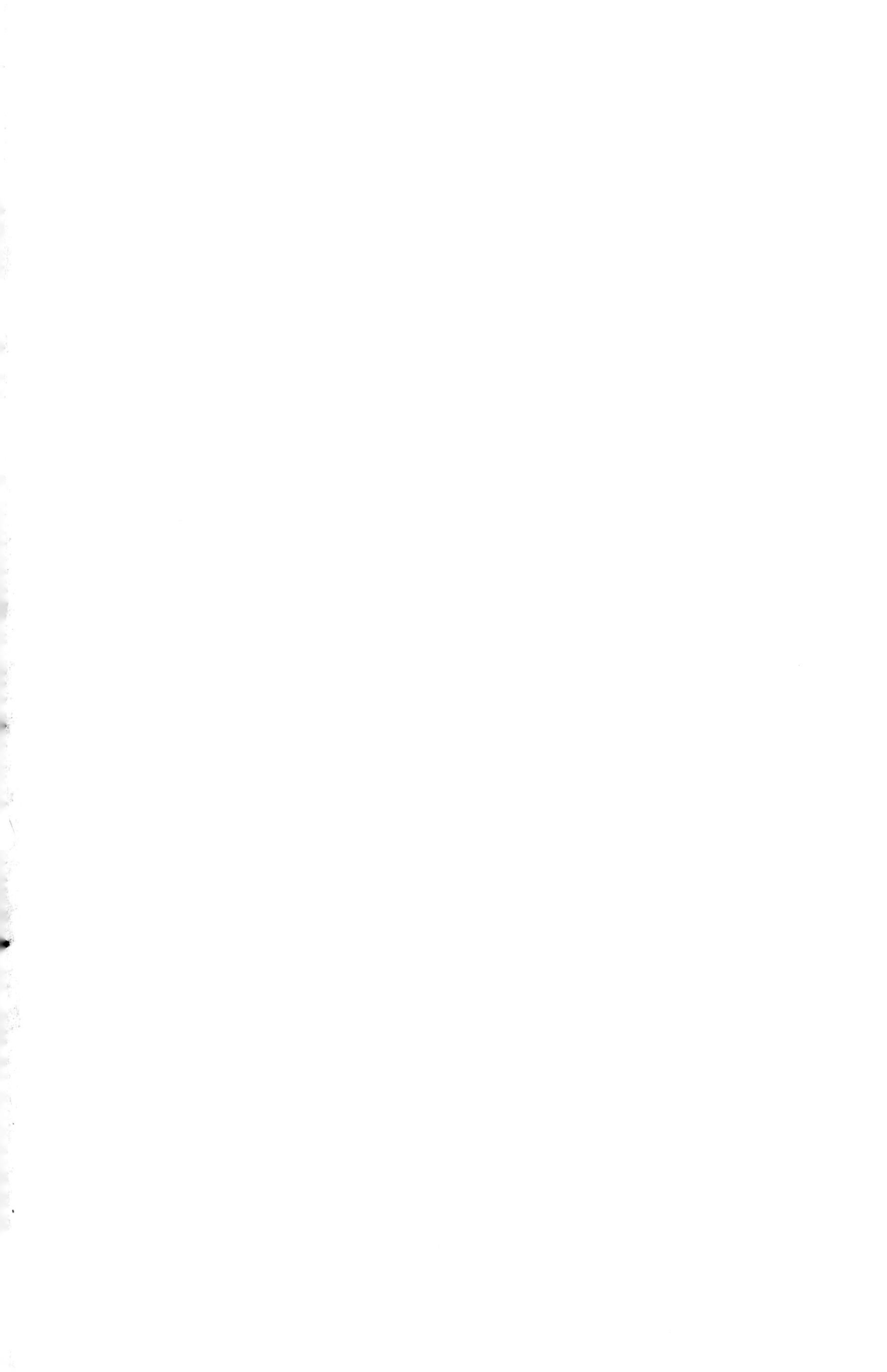